SEROTO-NATION

A DRIVER OF THE STATUS QUO

I0841009

BY

ADONIS SFERA, MD

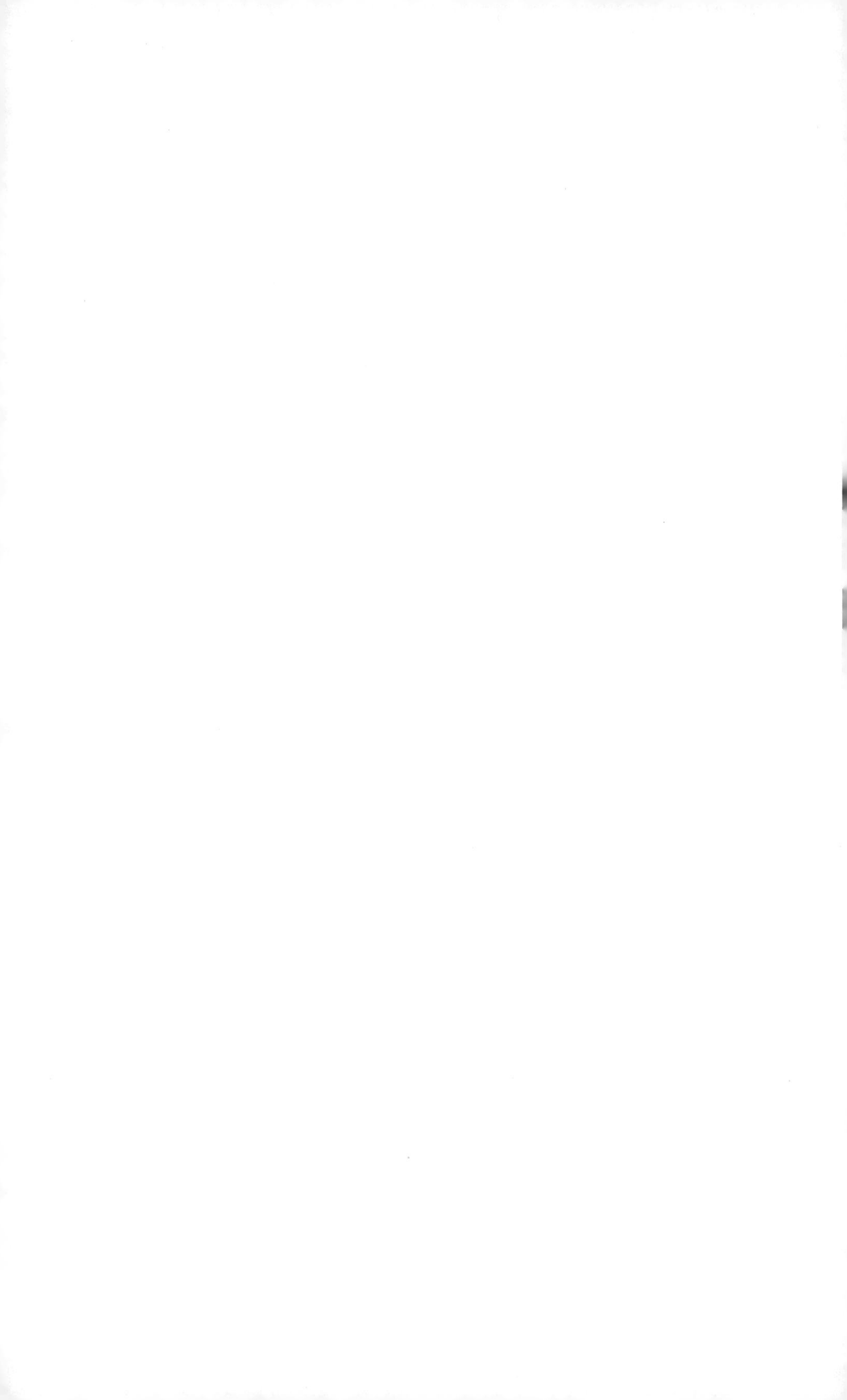

Copyright © 2024 by
Adonis Sfera

ALL RIGHTS RESERVED. No part of this book may be reproduced or transmitted by any means, electronic or mechanical, including photocopying and recording, or by any information storage and retrieval system, except as may be expressly permitted in writing from the author.

Printed in the United States of America

To my patients and staff at Patton State Hospital.

To Maggie, my Brown Lab, who spent many nights
with me while writing this book.

A Glance at the Book

For over six decades, the psychiatric treatment of depression and psychosis has been guided by the serotonin and dopamine hypotheses, respectively. Yet, despite the advent of numerous antipsychotic and antidepressant drugs, the prevalence of both conditions has increased dramatically since the 1980s. For example, depression is the most significant cause of disability worldwide, while State hospitals are still standing as proof of concept that sustained recovery in schizophrenia (measured by return to the premorbid level of functioning without relapses) is dismal. Indeed, after the first psychotic episode, less than 15% of patients can hold a job, and 26% are homeless at 5 years follow up..

As brain dopamine opposes gray matter depletion, long-term treatment with dopamine blockers may contribute to cortical thinning and decreased mitochondrial abundance. This may induce iatrogenic cognitive deficit, negative symptoms, and depression, suggesting that chronic psychotic disorders may need to be managed without lowering brain dopamine.

In patients with severe mental illness, loss of gray matter volume, associated with aggressive behavior, can be a consequence of both neuropathology and dopamine-blocking therapeutics. This prompts the question of whether schizophrenia maintenance treatment may enhance aggression or negative symptoms, hindering sustained recovery.

Aryl hydrocarbon receptor (AhR), best known as a dioxin sensor, has numerous other ligands, including dopamine, serotonin, melatonin, vitamin D, environmental pollutants, phenothiazines, and clozapine.

Located at the gut barrier and blood-brain barrier, AhR senses luminal microbes, metabolites, and xenobiotics. Moreover, AhR regulates gastrointestinal permeability and cellular senescence by its action on tight junction (TJ) molecules, tryptophan catabolism, and IL-22, the "guardian" of the gut barrier. For example, AhR binds indoleamine 2,3-dioxygenase, shifting tryptophan catabolism from the serotonin/melatonin branch to kynurenine and the downstream quinolinic acid, a toxin previously implicated in schizophrenia, PTSD, autism spectrum disorders, and suicide.

The AhR model can explain several characteristics of schizophrenia that are difficult to reconcile with the dopamine hypothesis, including increased prevalence at higher latitudes, association with pollutants or plasticizers, and comorbidity with inflammatory bowel disease.

This model can yield several novel antipsychotic and antidepressant strategies, including AhR antagonists, recombinant IL-22, mitochondrial transplantation, membrane lipid replacement, and plasmalogen replacement therapy, as well as biophysical approaches such as gamma band entrainment, phototherapy, or transcranial magnetic stimulation.

The larger picture: a unifying hypothesis of schizophrenia

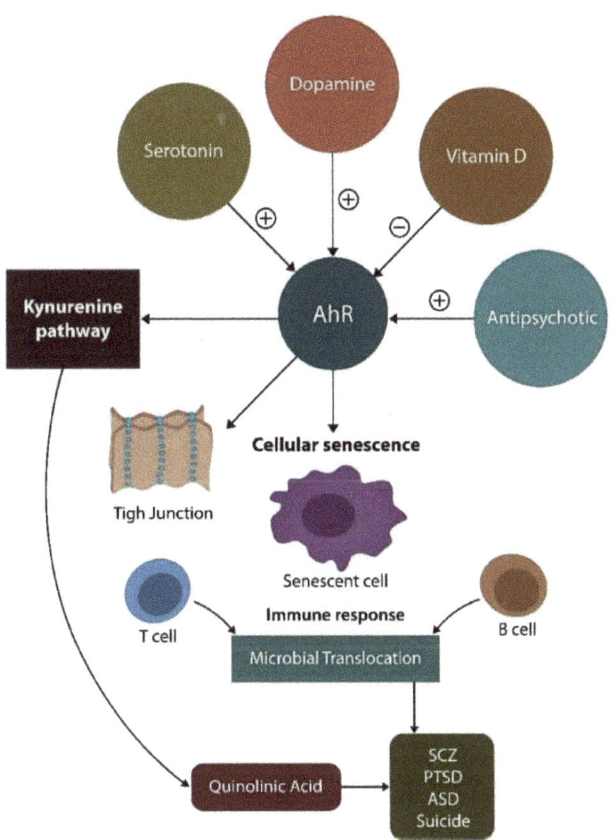

Aryl hydrocarbon receptor (AhR) is a transcription factor downstream from dopamine and serotonin. Under normal circumstances, AhR regulates tight junctions (TJs), cellular senescence, and tryptophan catabolism. Several antipsychotics and vitamin D are AhR ligands. Dysfunctional AhR disrupts TJs and induces cellular senescence in the cells of the intestinal barrier, enabling microbial translocation from the gut into host circulation. The immune system's response to "trespassing" bacteria consists of inflammation and immunogenicity, predisposing to neuropsychiatric syndromes. Quinolinic acid, derived from tryptophan, is a toxin that contributes further to the development of schizophrenia, posttraumatic stress disorder, autism spectrum disorder, and suicide.

Table of Contents

About the Author

Dr. Sfera graduated from medical school in 1980 and has been practicing medicine for over forty years. From 1984 to 1989, Dr. Sfera worked in analytical psychotherapy research at the Carl Gustav Jung Institute of Los Angeles, where he participated in the production of a documentary entitled "A Matter of Heart" on the life and work of Swiss psychiatrist C.G. Jung.

In 1998, Dr. Sfera completed a psychiatry residency and a consultation and liaison psychiatry fellowship at the University of Southern California in Los Angeles. Dr. Sfera worked at USC as a principal investigator in schizophrenia research.

In 1999, Dr. Sfera started a schizophrenia research company named South Coast Clinical Trials in Anaheim, California. During this time, he wrote over 100 articles and book chapters on biological psychiatry, herbal medicine, and lifestyle medicine. Since 2006, Dr. Sfera has been working for the California Department of State Hospitals at Patton as the chief of professional education.

Preface

In 1994, Elizabeth Wurtzel, an American writer, journalist, and lawyer, published her first book, "Prozac Nation," an autobiographical account in which she described her experience with the "night of the soul," depressive episodes, thoughts of suicide, cocaine use, aggression, etc. The selective serotonin reuptake inhibitor (SSRI), Prozac (fluoxetine), the drug she was taking at that time, came on the market in 1988 and was believed to be a psychopharmacological breakthrough compared to the older tricyclic antidepressants.

The timing of "Prozac Nation" coincided with the emergence of confessional literature, a genre promoting socially acceptable approaches to mental illness and suicide. "If Prozac Nation has any particular purpose," Wurtzel wrote, "it would be to come out and say that clinical depression is a real problem, that it ruins lives, that it ends lives, that it very nearly ended my life, that it afflicts many, many people, many very bright and worthy and thoughtful and caring people, people who could probably save the world or at the very least do it some real good." This stigma-averting approach was started by other poets and writers, including Sylvia Plath, whose tragic death by suicide on February 11, 1963, led to the acceptance of her confessional, "The Bell Jar," but only three decades later, when suicide gained more public understanding.

The epidemic of depression of the 80s and early 90s prompted others, including Kay Redfield Jamison with "An

Unquiet Mind," Susanna Kaysen's "Girl Interrupted," and William Styron with "Darkness Visible," to join the suicide advocacy forum and defeat stigma. By the 1990s, talk about depression became almost fashionable, and SSRI treatment became a sort of "cosmetic psychopharmacology" aimed at making one feel better instead of just good. This may have represented a countercurrent to Elisabeth Kübler-Ross, who 1969 published "On Death and Dying", bringing these topics into the forefront of societal discourse.

During three decades of research and clinical practice, including at Patton State Hospital, the largest forensic institution in the country, I have witnessed a continuous surge in mental illness compared to the previous years, despite the advent of novel psychopharmacological treatments. For example, between 1988 and 1994, only 3 percent of older adults were taking antidepressant drugs, while from 2015 to 2018, 19% were treated with these agents. Among college students, the use of SSRIs and stimulants, such as Adderall, went up 25%, likely a direct result of DTCPA (Direct-to-Consumer Pharmaceutical Advertising) passed in 1981. However, despite the newer and perhaps better drugs, sustained recovery (return to the premorbid level of functioning) is low in severe mental illness (SMI) and rarely discussed. Why is the pharmaceutical industry ignoring the neuropsychiatric disease outcome?

For the past six decades, we have been told that increasing serotonin (5-HT) and lowering dopamine (DA) in the synaptic cleft is the reason SSRIs and antipsychotic drugs ease the symptoms of depression and alleviate acute psychosis, respectively. During all this time, we have been ignoring the measurable indicators of severe mental illness (SMI) such as gray matter volume (GMV) reduction, loss of rapid gamma band (30-100 Hz) on electroencephalogram (EEG), mitochondrial depletion, and the presence of microbial molecules and bacterial translocation markers in the peripheral circulation. Moreover, since antipsychotic drugs also contribute to GMV loss, what is the evidence (other than industry-sponsored research) that psychotropic medications should be taken for long periods, if not for the entire life? (1).

Although symptomatic relief can be attained in SMI, sustained recovery is rare, and disability rates remain unchanged compared to the pre-psychopharmacological era. In other words, despite newer and more expensive drugs, the prevalence of depression has increased globally by 49.8% between 1990 and 2017, while schizophrenia (SCZ) by 62.74% during the same interval (2) (3).

At present, thirty years after the "Prozac Nation," it may be the right time to take a closer look at contemporary and future psychiatric treatments, focusing on the outcomes.

How do we see today the serotonin and dopamine hypotheses of depression and psychosis? Most importantly, are we as a Nation less "chemically imbalanced" in 2024 compared to the pre-psychotropic era?

Putting it all together, several questions beg for answers:

1. What are the consequences of the "serotonization" of America?

2. How is serotonin-induced indifference impacting the population? (4)

3. Does serotonin alter the human moral judgment?

A recent study found that serotonin made people more likely to judge harmful actions as forbidden, but only when the harm was emotionally relevant (5). In other words, serotonin makes us see the world through emotional glasses. Since emotion can be manipulated by input from society or mass media, SSRIs likely increase suggestibility and passivity of the populace. Furthermore, is "mass serotonization" akin to water fluoridation and perhaps with a similar impact on the brain? Indeed, SSRIs contain halogen-binding sites that attach to fluoride, altering the properties of serotonin transporters (SERTs), the molecules inhibited by SSRIs (6). Along this line, a preclinical study found upregulated serum 5-HT in fluoride-treated mice, indicating a direct link (7).

Another question: does serotonin affect human cholesterol metabolism? For example, lowering brain cholesterol lowers serotonin levels, predisposing to depression, anxiety, and aggressive behavior (8). Interestingly, statins, which came on the market in the late 1980s, may have contributed to the massive uptick in depression in the 1980s and 1990s. Indeed, between 1987 and 1997, the proportion of the U.S. population receiving antidepressants increased by 300 percent, probably implicating statins (9).

The arrival of the COVID-19 pandemic and the mRNA "vaccine" has revealed common mechanisms driving viral infections, cancer, and SMI. These include the Endocytic

Pathway (EP), cell membrane lipids, and human endogenous retroviruses (HERVs).

This book tackles these and many other questions to encourage patients and the public to research rather than rely on the opinion of "authorities," many of whom may have ulterior motifs or narratives on their agenda.

Preface References:

1. Sfera A. Targeted intermittent treatment in chronic schizophrenia. Front Psychiatry. 2013 Mar 14;4:13. doi: 10.3389/fpsyt.2013.00013. PMID: 23505392; PMCID: PMC3596804.

2. Liu Q, He H, Yang J, Feng X, Zhao F, Liu J. Changes in the global burden of depression from 1990 to 2017: Findings from the Global Burden of Disease study. J Psychiatr Res. 2020 Jul;126:134-140. doi: 10.1016/j.jpsychires.2019.08.002

3. Solmi, M., Seitidis, G., Mavridis, D. et al. Incidence, prevalence, and global burden of schizophrenia - data, with critical appraisal, from the Global Burden of Disease (GBD) 2019. Mol Psychiatry 28, 5319–5327 (2023). https://doi.org/10.1038/s41380-023-02138-4

4. Sansone RA, Sansone LA. SSRI-Induced Indifference. Psychiatry (Edgmont). 2010 Oct;7(10):14-8. PMID: 21103140; PMCID: PMC2989833.

5. Siegel JZ, Crockett MJ. How serotonin shapes moral judgment and behavior. Ann N Y Acad Sci. 2013 Sep;1299(1):42-51. doi: 10.1111/nyas.12229. PMID: 25627116; PMCID: PMC3817523.

6. Zhou Z, Zhen J, Karpowich NK, Law CJ, Reith ME, Wang DN. Antidepressant specificity of serotonin transporter suggested by three LeuT-SSRI structures. Nat Struct Mol Biol. 2009 Jun;16(6):652-7. doi: 10.1038/nsmb.1602.

7. Lu F, Zhang Y, Trivedi A, Jiang X, Chandra D, Zheng J, Nakano Y, Abduweli Uyghurturk D, Jalai R, Onur SG, Mentes A, DenBesten PK. Fluoride-related changes in behavioral outcomes may be related to increased serotonin.

Physiol Behav. 2019 Jul 1;206:76-83. Doi
10.1016/j.physbeh.2019.02.017.

8. Thomas, Jaya Mary; Varkey, Joyamma; Augustine, Bibin
    Baby. Association between serum cholesterol, brain
    serotonin, and anxiety: A study in simvastatin administered
    experimental animals. International Journal of Nutrition,
    Pharmacology, Neurological Diseases 4(1):p 69-73, Jan–Mar
    2014. | DOI: 10.4103/2231-0738.124617

9. Olfson M, Marcus SC, Druss B, Elinson L, Tanielian T,
    Pincus HA. National Trends in the Outpatient Treatment of
    Depression. Journal of the American Medical Association.
    2002; 287:203–9

Chapter 1
What is Decentralized Cognition?

Cognition and memory are precious human assets as they make each one of us unique and distinct from the Animal Kingdom. For this reason, cognitive functions are distributed throughout the body, lowering of losses due to injuries or pathology. They are probably encoded in the molecular networks of every cell. For example, the cellular cytoskeleton communicates with the proteins of the extracellular matrix via integrins and lipid rafts (membrane windows that unite intra- and extracellular molecular networks).

Proteins are part of a molecular network and are believed to encode memory in a quantum manner via conformational dynamics (folding). They have unique properties that facilitate information storage. Proteins fold along specific lines, like in origami art, connect instantly with each other in a Lego-like fashion, and, like Transformers, build new structures from the existing components. Moreover, proteins can exist as two-state systems, engendering logic gates, the building blocks of quantum circuits.

The molecular network-mediated memory allows information to be stored not only in neurons but also in most body cells, generating a decentralized "blockchain" cognition. Indeed, phantom limb, pseudocyesis (false pregnancy), psychogenic blindness, or cardiac transplant recipients adopting donor personality traits show that cells and molecules can harbor memories and behavioral patterns.

In severe mental illness (SMI), cells throughout the body undergo premature cellular senescence triggered by dysfunctional TJs.

Senescent cells spread senescence to neighboring healthy cells and may increase gut and blood-brain barrier (BBB) permeability, enabling microbial migration into the host circulation, eventually reaching the brain. Senescent glial cells and pluripotent stem cells stop replicating or replicating sporadically, promoting organismal aging; the opposite occurs in cancer, where there is uncontrolled replication.

Ancient viruses inherited from our predecessors, human endogenous retroviruses (HERVs), dwell in our DNA, comprising approximately 8% of the human genome. HERVs are activated by different pathologies, including cancer, schizophrenia (SCZ), or contemporary viruses, including SARS-CoV-2, the etiologic agent of the COVID-19 pandemic. Some HERVs have become "domesticated" and "work" for us. For example, HERV-W ENV. Encodes for a placental protein that, under pathological circumstances, may cause infertility. Another example is the Activity-regulated cytoskeleton-associated (Arc) gene, an ancestral virus expressed primarily in the brain, which promotes synaptic plasticity, facilitating learning and long-term potentiation (LTP).

A patient with cysticercosis, whom I saw years ago, comes to mind. He behaved, walked, and talked adequately. The only complaint he had was some forgetfulness and word-finding difficulties. The resident physician did a dementia work-up, including an MRI of the brain. We were surprised when the results arrived and wondered how this patient could live. He had very little brain tissue left. Numerous large cysts were seen throughout the parenchyma, yet the patient seemed minimally affected. This individual and others like him are proof that information and memories are stored not only in the brain but also in cells throughout the body. This may explain the patient's normal functioning despite extensive loss of cerebral mass.

Indeed, consider the amount of information in the DNA, which is present in every single cell in the body, ensuring that the genetic information is not lost. Furthermore, our muscles and tendons "remember" old postures we have long abandoned. Immune cells recall previous infections, while 36.2% of patients with heart transplants inherit bits and pieces of the donor's personality.

Experiments in the 1960s showed that unicellular organisms can learn without a central nervous system (CNS), suggesting that rudimentary information processing can occur within a single cell. In the chapter on facial recognition, the reader can follow this train of thought and see that single neurons can "recall" a familiar face and distinguish it in a crowd.

A growing body of evidence has implicated the cellular cytoskeleton (tubules and filaments that maintain cell shape) in recall and information processing. For example, in eukaryotic organisms (such as humans and animals), cells communicate with each other by exchanging molecules directly through the cell membrane or indirectly via extracellular vesicles (EVs) or tunneling nanotubules (TNTs).

Indeed, SMI is not something "in your head" only but in every cell in the body. For example, patients with SCZ exhibit cellular senescence, affecting the neurons and most cells at the body's periphery. Since senescence is an anticancer defense, this may explain why SCZ patients are more refractory to cancer compared to the general population.

What is cellular senescence?

In 1961, Leonard Hayflick found that human somatic cells do not replicate indefinitely but exit the cell cycle after 40-60 divisions

(Hayflick's limit). These cells enter a state of replicative senescence marked by proliferative arrest. They remain alive, have an active metabolism, and release toxic molecules, known as the senescence-associated secretory phenotype (SASP).

A few decades later, it was discovered that aside from replicative senescence, human cells can activate the senescence program in response to various insults, including damaged plasma membrane or damaged DNA, suggesting that senescence is a default state in charge of averting neuronal loss.

Over the past few years, it became clear that SMI also triggers cellular, including neuronal and endothelial senescence, which disrupts the BBB, a characteristic of many neuropsychiatric disorders.

At present, the exact mechanism of how mental illness triggers senescence is unclear. However, it may involve viruses as virus-induced lipid peroxidation may activate the senescent phenotype. For example, under normal circumstances, cholesterol synthesis regulates cellular senescence, while oxidized cholesterol likely disrupts this process, leading to premature senescence, as observed in SMI (1).

Contrasting SMI to cancer: in neuropsychiatric illness, cells become senescent before reaching the Hayflick limit, while cancer cells do not undergo senescence and continue to replicate indefinitely (2). An anticancer strategy involves inducing malignant cell senescence by viral infection to stop replication (4). Furthermore, the replicative capacity of human hippocampal progenitor neurons is low in patients with SMI, probably reflecting the cognitive deficit associated with these pathologies (3). In contrast, cancer or HeLa cells proliferate excessively and may never stop replicating.

Cellular Immortality vs. Human mortality

In contrast to SMI, cancer cells replicate and increase for many decades, as seen in HeLa cells, suggesting that these conditions and cell cycle disorders may be related.

The name HeLa comes from Henrietta Lacks, an African American woman from Baltimore who had cervical cancer and died in the early 1950s at the age of 31. Cells taken from her body (without her knowledge or consent) comprise the HeLa cell line, which has been used for research ever since, contributing to several innovations, including the human papillomavirus (HPV) vaccine, HIV medications, and recently, COVID-19 vaccines. The HeLa case has sparked legal and ethical debates, some of which are still ongoing, over the rights of an individual to their genetic material and tissues.

HeLa cell line has been kept alive for over 70 years, highlighting that cancer cells are immortal and not subject to Hayflick limit.

There were exciting developments and anecdotes regarding HeLa cells during the Cold War. For example, in the 1960s, scientists in the Soviet Union became interested in HeLa cells as they intended to study cancer behavior at zero gravity. For this reason, HeLa cells, obtained from John Hopkins University, were sent on the first orbit flight around the earth in 1961 with Yuri Gagarin, the first Soviet astronaut. HeLa cells were sent again in other Soviet missions, including Vostok 4 in 1962, Vostok 5 and 6 in 1963, Voskhod 1 in 1964, and Zond 5 in 1968 (5) (6). The outcome of these space experiments was that, compared to normal cells, which generally grew normally in orbit, HeLa cells became more aggressive, dividing faster with each trip, suggesting that zero or low gravity accelerates cancer growth.

In 1971 Richard Nixon signed the National Cancer Act, called the "War on Cancer." As part of this act, the US and the USSR began cooperating in cancer research. However, due to bilateral mistrust, the HeLa cells they exchanged were contaminated, which sabotaged many research projects by infecting other cell cultures in both countries, ultimately exacerbating the Cold War tensions (7).

Taken together, both cancer and mental illness ignore the Hayflick limit, the former by driving uncontrolled proliferation and immortality, while the latter by deficient proliferation and premature mortality.

Do viruses induce cellular senescence in severe mental illness?

Why discuss viruses in a book on mental illness?

Several reasons:

1. Viral illness during pregnancy or shortly after birth has been associated with SMI later in life.

2. Several viruses implicated in SCZ are also known to thrive for a long time in viral reservoirs, such as macrophages and microglia.

3. Several exogenous viruses can activate Human Endogenous Retroviruses (HERVs) that were previously implicated in SCZ,

4. Viruses are a part of the microbiome, known as the virome.

5. A brain virome was recently documented in the general population (8).

SMI has been associated with premature cellular/neuronal senescence, a direct driver of organismal aging. Indeed, patients with SCZ live on average 15-20 years shorter than the general population and develop late-life disorders at an earlier age. In senescence, individual neurons may attempt to reenter the cell cycle; however, as they lack the molecular machinery to complete replication, they may undergo apoptosis or remain fused indefinitely. Some viral infections, including SARS-CoV-2, fuse host cells to each other to induce senescence, a phenotype rich in iron and calcium that is ideal for viral replication (9) (10) (11) (12). Interestingly, some of these fused and senescent cells may comprise viral reservoirs.

Viral reservoirs are cell types in which viruses can accumulate, replicate, and thrive after the acute phase of illness. For example, microglia are well-known reservoirs for the human immunodeficiency virus (HIV), as the pathogen can thrive in a latent state, averting exposure to highly active antiretroviral therapy (HAART) (9).

Other known viruses that can maintain latency in humans are herpes simplex virus (HSV), varicella-zoster virus (VZV), and Epstein–Barr virus (EBV), pathogens that were associated with SMI (13) (14)

The SARS-CoV-2 virus promotes premature cellular senescence in many cell types, including macrophages and microglia. It thrives in a latent state in these cells, maintaining low-grade inflammation.

COVID-19 can induce premature cellular senescence in host cells by generating syncytial structures (fused cells), also called multinucleated giant cells. Fused cells are resistant to cell death and challenging to eliminate. For example, cancer induces multinucleated malignant cells resistant to radiation therapy (15) (16). The SARS-CoV-2 spike (S) protein contains arginine-rich peptides that drive cell-cell fusion by perforating cell membranes (17) (18) (19).

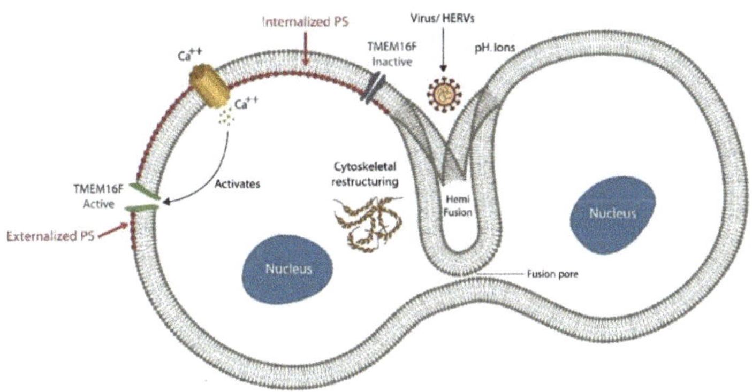

Fig. 1.1 Exogenous viruses and HERVs hijack human physiological fusogenic molecules, fusing host cells. The fusion process is comprised of 3 steps: (1) cytosolic Ca2+ upregulation (via extracellular uptake or endoplasmic reticulum release), (2) TMEM16F activation, and (3) phosphatidylserine (PS) externalization (ePS). Cells undergo fusion or apoptosis (death), depending on the extracellular pH. Viruses benefit from ePS and elevated cytosolic Ca2+ as the former induces immunosuppression and the latter cellular senescence.

Arc, a virus to remember

Arc protein is a remnant of an ancient retrovirus expressed by the neurons and plays a critical role in learning and memory. Like HERV-W ENV, this viral fossil has been domesticated and participates in human cognition (20).

Multinucleated giant cells (syncytia) were found not only in SARS-CoV-2 infected individuals but also after vaccination with messenger RNA (mRNA) therapeutics (21) (22) (23). For example, giant cell myocarditis was documented after COVID-19 vaccine (24).

Exogenous viruses, including SARS-CoV-2, have been demonstrated to activate HERVs, a pathology documented in myalgic encephalomyelitis/chronic fatigue syndrome (ME/CFS) and long COVID (25) (26) (27) (28).

Taken together, the SARS-CoV-2 virus induces premature cellular senescence and usurps the elimination of senescent and virus-infected cells. This triggers inflammation and disruption of the gut barrier and BBB, allowing gut microbes to migrate into host tissues and organs, including the brain.

Chapter 1 References:

10. Ziegler, D.V., Czarnecka-Herok, J., Vernier, M. et al. The cholesterol biosynthetic pathway induces cellular senescence through ERRα. npj Aging 10, 5 (2024). https://doi.org/10.1038/s41514-023-00128-y

11. Mahadik SP, Mukherjee S, Laev H, Reddy R, Schnur DB. Abnormal growth of skin fibroblasts from schizophrenic patients. Psychiatry Res. 1991 Jun;37(3):309-20. doi: 10.1016/0165-1781(91)90066-x. PMID: 1891511.

12. Palmos, A.B., Duarte, R.R.R., Smeeth, D.M. et al. Telomere length and human hippocampal neurogenesis. Neuropsychopharmacol. 45, 2239–2247 (2020). https://doi.org/10.1038/s41386-020-00863-w

13. Seoane R, Vidal S, Bouzaher YH, El Motiam A, Rivas C. The Interaction of Viruses with the Cellular Senescence Response. Biology (Basel). 2020 Dec 9;9(12):455. doi: 10.3390/biology9120455.

14. Beskow LM. Lessons from HeLa Cells: The Ethics and Policy of Biospecimens. Annu Rev Genomics Hum Genet. 2016 Aug 31;17:395-417. doi: 10.1146/annurev-genom-083115-022536. Epub 2016 Mar 3. PMID: 26979405; PMCID: PMC5072843.

15. Skloot R. The Immortal Life of Henrietta Lacks. New York: Crown; 2010.

16. Michael Gold. A Conspiracy of Cells; One Woman's Immortal Legacy and the Medical Scandal it Caused—State University of New York Press (1986). ISBN:9780887060991, 0887060994

17. Masaldan, S.; Clatworthy, S. A. S.; et al. Iron Accumulation in Senescent Cells Is Coupled with Impaired Ferritinophagy and

Inhibition of Ferroptosis. Redox Biol 2018,14, 100–115.
https://doi.org/10.1016/j.redox.2017.08.015

18. Sato, T.; Shapiro, J. S.; et al. Aging Is Associated with Increased Brain Iron through Cortex-Derived Hepcidin Expression. Elife 2022, 11. https://doi.org/10.7554/eLife.73456.

19. Di Micco, R.; Krizhanovsky, V.; et al. Cellular Senescence in Ageing: From Mechanisms to Therapeutic Opportunities. Nat Rev Mol Cell Biol 2021, 22 (2), 75–95.https://doi.org/10.1038/s41580-020-00314-w.

20. Dang X, Hanson BA, Orban ZS, Jimenez M, Suchy S, Koralnik IJ. Characterization of the brain virome in human immunodeficiency virus infection and substance use disorder. PLoS One. 2024 Apr 17;19(4):e0299891. doi: 10.1371/journal.pone.0299891. PMID: 38630782; PMCID: PMC11023569.

21. Masaldan, S.; Clatworthy, S. A. S.; et al. Iron Accumulation in Senescent Cells Is Coupled with Impaired Ferritinophagy and Inhibition of Ferroptosis. Redox Biol 2018,14, 100–115.
https://doi.org/10.1016/j.redox.2017.08.015

22. Sato, T.; Shapiro, J. S.; et al. Aging Is Associated with Increased Brain Iron through Cortex-Derived Hepcidin Expression. Elife 2022, 11. https://doi.org/10.7554/eLife.73456.

23. Di Micco, R.; Krizhanovsky, V.; et al. Cellular Senescence in Ageing: From Mechanisms to Therapeutic Opportunities. Nat Rev Mol Cell Biol 2021, 22 (2), 75–95.https://doi.org/10.1038/s41580-020-00314-w.

24. Martin, N.; Bernard, D. Calcium Signaling and Cellular Senescence. Cell Calcium 2018,70, 16–23.
https://doi.org/10.1016/j.ceca.2017.04.001

25. 13. Wallet, C.; De Rovere, M.; et al. Microglial Cells: The Main HIV-1 Reservoir in the Brain. Front Cell Infect Microbiol 2019, 9. https://doi.org/10.3389/fcimb.2019.00362.

26. Kavanagh, E. Long Covid Brain Fog: A Neuroinflammation Phenomenon? Oxf Open Immunol 2022, 3 (1). https://doi.org/10.1093/oxfimm/iqac007.

27. Mirzayans, R.; Andrais, B.; et al. Multinucleated Giant Cancer Cells Produced in Response to Ionizing Radiation Retain Viability and Replicate Their Genome. Int J Mol Sci 2017, 18 (2), 360. https://doi.org/10.3390/ijms18020360.

28. Martin-Rodriguez, O.; Gauthier, T.; et al. Pro-Resolving Factors Released by Macrophages After Efferocytosis Promote Mucosal Wound Healing in Inflammatory Bowel Disease. Front Immunol 2021, 12. https://doi.org/10.3389/fimmu.2021.754475.

29. Gal, H.; Krizhanovsky, V. Cell Fusion Induced Senescence. Aging 2014, 6 (5), 353–354.https://doi.org/10.18632/aging.100670.

30. Chuprin, A.; Gal, H.; et al. Cell Fusion Induced by ERVWE1 or Measles Virus Causes Cellular Senescence. Genes Dev 2013, 27 (21), 2356–2366. https://doi.org/10.1101/gad.227512.113.

31. Burton, D. G. A.; Krizhanovsky, V. Physiological and Pathological Consequences of Cellular Senescence. Cellular and Molecular Life Sciences 2014, 71 (22), 4373–4386. https://doi.org/10.1007/s00018-014-1691-3.

32. Pastuzyn ED, Day CE, Kearns RB, Kyrke-Smith M, Taibi AV, McCormick J, Yoder N, Belnap DM, Erlendsson S, Morado DR, Briggs JAG, Feschotte C, Shepherd JD. The Neuronal Gene Arc Encodes a Repurposed Retrotransposon Gag Protein that Mediates

Intercellular RNA Transfer. Cell. 2018 Jan 11;172(1-2):275-288.e18. doi: 10.1016/j.cell.2017.12.024.

33. Zhao, W.; Huang, Y.; et al. Dopamine Receptors Modulate Cytotoxicity of Natural Killer Cells via CAMP-PKA-CREB Signaling Pathway. PLoS One 2013, 8 (6), e65860. https://doi.org/10.1371/journal.pone.0065860.

34. Stadlmann, S.; Hein-Kuhnt, R.; et al. Viropathic Multinuclear Syncytial Giant Cells in Bronchial Fluid from a Patient with COVID-19. J Clin Pathol 2020, 73 (9), 607–608. https://doi.org/10.1136/jclinpath-2020-206657.

35. Buchrieser, J.; Dufloo, J.; et al. Syncytia Formation by SARS-CoV-2-infected Cells. EMBO J 2020, 39 (23). https://doi.org/10.15252/embj.2020106267

36. Sung, K.; McCain, J.; et al. Biopsy-Proven Giant Cell Myocarditis Following the COVID-19 Vaccine. Circ Heart Fail 2022, 15 (4). https://doi.org/10.1161/CIRCHEARTFAILURE.121.009321.

37. Giménez-Orenga, K.; Pierquin, J.; et al. HERV-W ENV Antigenemia and Correlation of Increased Anti-SARS-CoV-2 Immunoglobulin Levels with Post-COVID-19 Symptoms. Front Immunol 2022, 13. https://doi.org/10.3389/fimmu.2022.1020064.

38. Rodrigues, L. S.; da Silva Nali, L. H.; et al. HERV-K and HERV-W Transcriptional Activity in Myalgic Encephalomyelitis/Chronic Fatigue Syndrome. Autoimmunity Highlights 2019, 10 (1), 12. https://doi.org/10.1186/s13317-019-0122-8.

39. Zhang, M.; Liang, J. Q.; et al. Expressional Activation and Functional Roles of Human Endogenous Retroviruses in Cancers. Rev Med Virol 2019, 29 (2). https://doi.org/10.1002/rmv.2025.

40. Qie, S.; Ran, Y.; et al. Candesartan Modulates Microglia Activation and Polarization via NF-KB Signaling Pathway. Int J Immunopathol Pharmacol 2020, 34, 205873842097490. https://doi.org/10.1177/2058738420974900

Chapter 2
The Bugs or the Synapses

This chapter discusses the background of synaptic serotonin (5HT) and dopamine (DA) hypotheses of depression and SCZ respectively and contrasts this model with the non-synaptic, Aryl hydrocarbon/microbial translocation hypothesis. Although not mutually exclusive because aryl hydrocarbon receptor is located downstream from dopamine and serotonin, the translocation paradigm can explain several characteristics of SCZ that are difficult to account for by DA hypothesis. These include autoantibodies, higher prevalence in cold climate, and association with pollutants or plasticizers as well as with inflammatory bowel disease (IBD).

In depression, it has been highlighted that although about 50% of depressed patients respond to SSRIs, there is no data to demonstrate that serotonin levels are decreased in individuals with this condition. As a rule of thumb, depressed people likely lose a disproportionate number of mitochondria, accounting for low energy, psychomotor retardation, attention, and concentration difficulties. SSRIs facilitate mitochondrial import from astrocytes into neurons, likely correcting the energy deficit. This non-synaptic mechanism of action could explain the efficacy of SSRIs.

For over six decades, dysfunctional 5-HT and DA signaling in the synaptic cleft have been hypothesized to cause depression and psychosis, respectively. Antidepressant and antipsychotic drugs are believed to normalize neurotransmission at the synapse, restoring the premorbid affective and cognitive homeostasis. However, this is rarely the case in clinical practice, suggesting that other mechanisms may be at work. Lately, non-synaptic action of antidepressant and antipsychotic agents have been discovered, as well as non-synaptic communication pathways among brain cells. In addition, as more 5-HT and DA are generated in the GI tract than in the brain, the GI tract may be the primary cause of SMI.

Despite the belief that psychotropics "work" at the synapse, these agents' beneficial effects may occur at the intestinal level and consist of decreasing permeability and lowering microbial migration outside the gut. For example, SSRIs drive mitochondrial transfer from astrocytes to neurons via tunneling nanotubules (TNTs) or extracellular vesicles (EVs), placing these energy-producing organelles at the epicenter of SMI pathogenesis. This raises the question: Is it possible that a decreased abundance of mitochondria causes depression? And the next question is, can SSRIs "work" by facilitating mitochondrial transfer to neurons?

Neurons are postmitotic cells that live almost as long as we do and work very hard, spending over 20% of the body's energy to support brain work. For this reason, mitochondria undergo rapid wear and tear, leading to their early demise. Depletion of neuronal mitochondria likely manifests clinically as depressed mood, low energy, mental fatigue, loss of interest in activities previously enjoyed, psychomotor retardation, poor concentration, and attention.

Regarding DA, the brain tracts producing this neurotransmitter are certainly affected by antipsychotic drugs. However, these agents may also work at the gut level, optimizing permeability by repairing plasma and mitochondrial membranes. Many antipsychotics enter the lipid bilayer of cell and mitochondrial membranes and (due to their antioxidant properties) rescue lipids from peroxidation, averting cell death by ferroptosis. In addition, as antipsychotics and antidepressants exhibit antibacterial and antiviral properties, these drugs may simply "kill" the translocated microbes, preventing them from causing further damage.

The sustained recovery from severe mental illness has been low for two reasons:

Focusing on the synapse - we are treating the symptoms and not the etiopathogenetic cause of these conditions, the gut.

Maintenance treatment with antipsychotic drugs induces gray matter loss, making it difficult for the brain to revert to the premorbid level of function.

How do serotonin and dopamine work?

After decades of treating psychiatric patients, I can say that, in general, about 50% of individuals with clinical depression feel better upon treatment with SSRIs. The same is true of patients with acute psychosis treated with antipsychotic medication. Acute psychosis may sometimes clear in a matter of hours or days. However, despite the amelioration of symptoms, long-term outcomes do not improve much, and many patients with MDD and SCZ progress in time to cognitive impairment, negative symptoms, and overall disability. Indeed, despite novel antidepressant strategies, MDD remains the leading cause of disability worldwide (1).

It appears that despite medications, SMI pathology continues to run unabated in the background and, from time to time, manifests as relapses.

The question begs for an answer: Why does an improved clinical picture not translate into better outcomes?

To answer this question, first, let us examine the serotonergic and dopaminergic hypotheses of MDD and SCZ, respectively, as well as sustained recovery and employment data during the 20th century.

Serotonergic and dopaminergic hypotheses

In a nutshell, these models propose that:

1. Since increasing 5-HT lowers the symptoms of depression, depressed individuals must be low in 5-HT. Therefore, treatment with 5-HT-increasing drugs would make them well.

2. Since lowering DA in psychotic disorders clears the psychotic symptoms, patients with psychosis must have too much brain DA. Therefore, treatment with DA-blocking drugs would be beneficial.

I propose that increasing 5-HT and lowering brain DA may be of limited relevance for the overall treatment of depression and psychosis. Antidepressant and antipsychotic drugs likely work at the gut level, reducing intestinal permeability by upregulating TJs and the regulatory T cells (T regs). Decreasing gut barrier permeability limits the abundance of microbial translocation from the lumen into the host tissues and organs, including the brain.

Tregs are lymphocytes that maintain immunological tolerance to food proteins and gut microbiota, lower inflammation, and the permeability of the gut barrier.

This hypothesis is based on the following data:

1. Patients with MDD and those with SCZ exhibit low levels of Tregs (2) (3).

2. Under physiological circumstances, Tregs decrease intestinal permeability and microbial translocation outside the GI tract (4).

Conversely, decreased Tregs facilitate microbial translocation from the GI tract into the host tissues and organs, including the brain.

3. Patients with MDD and SCZ exhibit "leaky gut" (increased gut barrier permeability) and increased comorbidity with IBD (5) (6).

4. Patients with MDD and SCZ have elevated levels of bacterial translocation markers, including sCD14, lipopolysaccharide-binding protein (LBP), and cf-mDNA (7) (8)

5. Antipsychotic and antidepressant medications increase Treg levels, lowering microbial translocation (9) (10).

6. Gut microbiota components and antibodies against these molecules were detected in patients with MDD and SCZ, emphasizing translocation (11) (12).

Taken together, the efficacy of antidepressant and antipsychotic drugs is better accounted for by their action at the gut level than the synaptic cleft. Decreasing gut barrier permeability and microbial translocation averts aberrant AhR activation, inflammation, and immunogenicity directed at the microbes and their components, In addition, several antipsychotic drugs can over-activate AhR, leading to gray matter volume (GMV) reduction. GMV reduction is not only a hallmark of aggressive behavior but also of negative and cognitive pathology.

Therefore, since SCZ-related GMV depletion is augmented by chronic use of antipsychotics, it is suggested that chronic SMI patients should not be maintained on DA blockers and may need replacement therapy with DA agonists. This is substantiated further by the fact that DA prevents gray matter loss. In contrast, depleting the brain of DA is a significant obstacle to post-psychotic recovery as negative and cognitive symptoms hinder this process.

Background of serotonergic and dopaminergic hypotheses

The serotonin hypothesis of depression originated in the 1960s and was based on the observation that lowering monoamines with reserpine generates a syndrome resembling MDD. Conversely, upregulating monoamines via tricyclic antidepressants or monoamine oxidase inhibitors elevates the mood and increases 5-HT. Therefore, blocking dopamine D2 receptor (D2R) and upregulating 5-HT transmission is believed to ease the psychotic and depressive symptoms, respectively.

Recently, a new study has found that although many depressed patients experience symptomatic relief with SSRIs, there is no evidence that low 5-HT levels result in depression (13). This study suggests that 5-HT may work at non-synaptic sites to produce antidepressant effects. Indeed, it is not counterintuitive to link the low-energy symptoms of MDD to mitochondrial depletion.

GMV reduction is known to occur in both non-medicated and medicated SCZ patients. In this regard, a new study has shown that GMV loss is directly correlated to the levels of gut microbes translocated from the GI tract into the brain (14). It is also well-established that DA prevents GMV loss, indicating that chronic treatment with DA-blockers may lead to iatrogenic cortical thinning and cognitive deficit.

Why do nonmedicated patients with SCZ present with GMV reduction? This raises another question: does DA depletion rather than excess cause SCZ? This question was raised previously by Davis KL et al al. and is in line with psychosis occurring in untreated Parkinson's disease (PD) patients.

Neuropsychiatric illnesses are systemic conditions that likely originate in the gut. Therefore, to improve SMI outcome, the treatment should focus on correcting the intestinal barrier, lowering GMV loss, adding dopaminergic agonists to antipsychotics, or maintaining patients on non-DA-depleting agents, such as recombinant human IL-22 or AhR antagonists.

Sustained recovery in schizophrenia

SCZ is a multifactorial disorder marked by remission and exacerbation of positive and negative symptoms. The outcome of SCZ is variable and difficult to measure as the concept of recovery may mean different things to different people. For example, patients often envision recovery as being able to work or go to school, live independently, and raise a family. On the other hand, clinicians may think of recovery as remission of positive and negative symptoms, while patients' families may want a better quality of life for their loved ones (3). In general, sustained recovery, measured by return to the premorbid level of functioning without relapse, is rare in SCZ. For example, novel studies have shown that 33% of SCZ patients relapse during the first 12 months after an initial psychotic episode, 26% remain homeless at two years follow-up, while five years after the first psychotic outbreak, only 10% are employed (15) (16) (17). Recovery at 15 and 25 years of follow-up is somewhat better at 16%. However, sustained recovery in chronic SCZ is an exception rather than the rule (18). Indeed, only 13.5% of patients meet recovery criteria at any time after the first psychotic episode (19).

A large meta-analysis of 114 follow-up studies by Warner R. looked at the entire 20th century (from 1900 to 1996) and found that the overall SCZ recovery rate during the 20th century (from 1900 to 1996) was no different in the early years compared to the late 1990s:

1. 1901–1920, complete recovery 20%, employed 4.7;

2. 1921–1940, complete recovery 12%, employed 11.9%;

3. 1941–1955, complete recovery 23%, employed 4.1%;

4. 1956–1975, complete recovery 20%, employed 5.1%;

5. 1976–1995, complete recovery 20%, employed 6.9%.

Surprisingly, sustained recovery after the introduction of antipsychotic drugs was not higher compared to that of the pre-antipsychotic era. In addition, the employment rate of patients with SCZ stayed below 12% throughout the 20th century (20). This suggests that the psychotropic drugs do not suppress the neuropathology despite the attenuation of symptoms.

This data is consistent with SCZ neuroimaging studies, which show progressive and lifelong GMV reduction, starting in the temporoparietal region and spreading slowly in all directions (21) (22). Moreover, the existence of long-term public institutions for the treatment of chronic mental illness, such as State hospitals, is proof of concept that outcomes in neuropsychiatry are dismal. In contrast, public hospitals for tuberculosis and leprosy were closed more than half a century ago as antibiotics rendered these institutions obsolete. Furthermore, upregulating DA in the CNS would likely cause euphoria, increased motivation, and alertness rather than hallucinations or delusions, and negative symptoms, suggesting that altered dopaminergic transmission may be a secondary event in this disorder.

Since DA and 5-HT are AhR ligands, this transcription factor may play a key role in MDD and SCZ. AhR is found in the BBB and gut barrier and regulates the migration of microbes and their components into the host tissues and organs, including the brain. As pollutants and vitamin D3 are AhR ligands, this receptor may explain the link between toxicants and SCZ and the higher prevalence of this disorder at higher latitudes.

It is worth mentioning that numerous neuroimaging studies over the past three decades have shown that not only first but also second-generation antipsychotic drugs deplete the GMV, suggesting that long-term administration of these drugs may likely induce iatrogenic brain atrophy (23) (24). This likely emphasizes that chronic psychosis may require different treatment strategies than the acute phase of illness.

Taken together, although there is no doubt that antipsychotic drugs are highly effective for the treatment of acute psychosis, chronic SCZ may be the result of GMV reduction. A different treatment approach may be required to avert iatrogenic loss of brain parenchyma.

Non-synaptic antidepressant/antipsychotic mechanisms

5-HT and DA are likely implicated in MDD and SCZ, respectively. However, these neurotransmitters may not be the primary drivers of these pathologies. AhR exerts antimicrobial, antiviral, and antiproliferative effects, emphasizing that it may alleviate psychosis by "killing" the translocated microbes before causing more damage (25). Indeed, AhR can also clear intracellular pathogens, such as *Toxoplasma gondii,* a SCZ-associated parasite, suggesting antipsychotic properties.

Antidepressant/antipsychotic drugs may alleviate pathology by drug-activated autophagy (clearing of molecular debris and damaged cells), thus lowering the overall organismal inflammatory burden (26) (27).

The antidepressant action of SSRI may be explained by the facilitation of mitochondrial transfer from astrocyte to neuron, a property mediated by 5-HT (Fig. 2.1). Furthermore, SSRIs have been shown to prevent microglial activation, highlighting another non-synaptic antidepressant mechanism (Table 1).

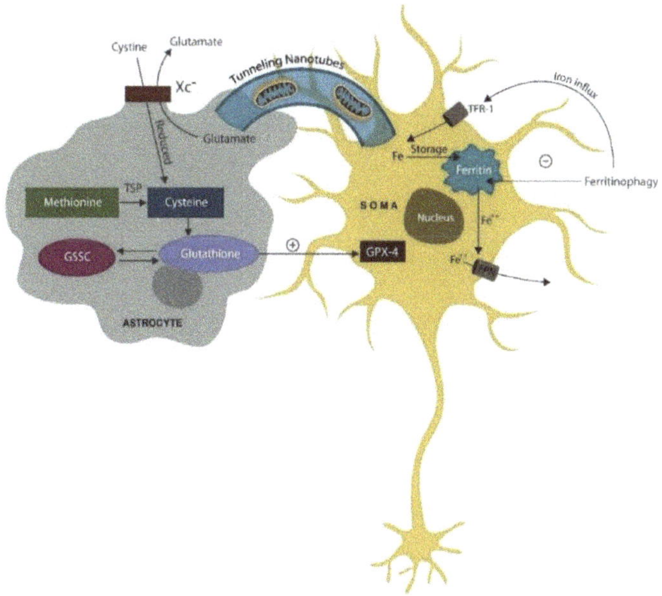

Fig. 2.1 Glial cells, including astrocytes, supply the neuron with healthy mitochondria via tunneling nanotubules (TNTs), preventing apoptosis (137) (138). In addition, astrocytes prevent neuronal ferroptosis by transferring antioxidants, including GPX-4. The astrocyte uptakes cystine via cystine/glutamate antiporter (Xc-). Cysteine can also be obtained from methionine via glutathione. Fe2+ enters the neuron through the transferrin receptor 1 (TRF-1), is stored in ferritin, and requires ferritinophagy to be released. Excess Fe2+ exits the neuron via ferroportin (FPT) channels.

Non-synaptic mechanisms	References
AhR modulation	28
Autophagy activation	29
Mitochondria trafficking	30
Antimicrobial	31
Antiviral	32
Anti-parasitic	33
Microglia deactivation	34
Altering the cell membrane	35

Table 2.1 Non-synaptic antidepressant and antipsychotic compounds identified to date.

Chapter 2 References:

1. Friedrich MJ. Depression Is the Leading Cause of Disability Around the World. JAMA. 2017 Apr 18;317(15):1517. doi: 10.1001/jama.2017.3826. PMID: 28418490.

2. Grosse, L. et al. Deficiencies of the T and natural killer cell system in major depressive disorder: T regulatory cell defects are associated with inflammatory monocyte activation. Brain Behav. Immun. 54, 38–44 (2016).

3. Sahbaz, C., Zibandey, N., Kurtulmus, A. et al. It reduced regulatory T cells with increased proinflammatory response in patients with schizophrenia. Psychopharmacology 237, 1861–1871 (2020). https://doi.org/10.1007/s00213-020-05504-0

4. Juanola O, Piñero P, Gómez-Hurtado I, Caparrós E, García-Villalba R, Marín A, Zapater P, Tarín F, González-Navajas JM, Tomás-Barberán FA, Francés R. Regulatory T Cells Restrict Permeability to Bacterial Antigen Translocation and Preserve Short-Chain Fatty Acids in Experimental Cirrhosis. Hepatol Commun. 2018 Oct 22;2(12):1610-1623. doi: 10.1002/hep4.1268.

5. Hu S, Chen Y, Chen Y, Wang C. Depression and Anxiety Disorders in Patients With Inflammatory Bowel Disease. Front Psychiatry. 2021 Oct 8;12:714057. doi: 10.3389/fpsyt.2021.714057. PMID: 34690829; PMCID: PMC8531580.

6. Sung KY, Zhang B, Wang HE, Bai YM, Tsai SJ, Su TP, Chen TJ, Hou MC, Lu CL, Wang YP, Chen MH. Schizophrenia and risk of new-onset inflammatory bowel disease: a nationwide longitudinal study. Aliment Pharmacol Ther. 2022 May;55(9):1192-1201. doi: 10.1111/apt.16856.

7. Anderson AM, Ma Q, Letendre SL, Iudicello J. Soluble Biomarkers of Cognition and Depression in Adults with HIV Infection in the

Combination Therapy Era. Curr HIV/AIDS Rep. 2021
Dec;18(6):558-568. doi: 10.1007/s11904-021-00581-y.

8. Severance EG, Gressitt KL, Stallings CR, Origoni AE, Khushalani S, Leweke FM, Dickerson FB, Yolken RH. Discordant patterns of bacterial translocation markers and implications for innate immune imbalances in schizophrenia. Schizophr Res. 2013 Aug;148(1-3):130-7. doi: 10.1016/j.schres.2013.05.018.

9. Kelly DL, Li X, Kilday C, Feldman S, Clark S, Liu F, Buchanan RW, Tonelli LH. Increased circulating regulatory T cells in medicated people with schizophrenia. Psychiatry Res. 2018 Nov;269:517-523. doi: 10.1016/j.psychres.2018.09.006

10. Ellul P, Mariotti-Ferrandiz E, Leboyer M, Klatzmann D. Regulatory T Cells As Supporters of Psychoimmune Resilience: Toward Immunotherapy of Major Depressive Disorder. Front Neurol. 2018 Mar 20;9:167. doi: 10.3389/fneur.2018.00167.

11. Maes M, Kanchanatawan B, Sirivichayakul S, Carvalho AF. In Schizophrenia, Increased Plasma IgM/IgA Responses to Gut Commensal Bacteria Are Associated with Negative Symptoms, Neurocognitive Impairments, and the Deficit Phenotype. Neurotox Res. 2019 Apr;35(3):684-698. doi: 10.1007/s12640-018-9987-y.

12. Maes M, Kubera M, Leunis JC. The gut-brain barrier in major depression: intestinal mucosal dysfunction with an increased translocation of LPS from gram negative enterobacteria (leaky gut) plays a role in the inflammatory pathophysiology of depression. Neuro Endocrinol Lett. 2008 Feb;29(1):117-24.

13. Moncrieff J, Cooper RE, Stockmann T, Amendola S, Hengartner MP, Horowitz MA. The serotonin theory of depression: a systematic umbrella review of the evidence. Mol Psychiatry. 2023;28:3243–56.

14. He B, Sheng C, Yu X, Zhang L, Chen F, Han Y. Alterations of gut microbiota are associated with brain structural changes in the spectrum of Alzheimer's disease: the SILCODE study in Hainan cohort. Front Aging Neurosci. 2023 Jul 14;15:1216509. doi: 10.3389/fnagi.2023.1216509.

15. Üçok, A.; Polat, A.; Çakır, S.; Genç, A. One year outcome in first episode schizophrenia: Predictors of relapse. Eur. Arch. Psychiatry Clin. Neurosci. 2005, 256, 37–43. [

16. Holm, M.; Taipale, H.; Tanskanen, A.; Tiihonen, J.; Mitterdorfer-Rutz, E. Employment among people with schizophrenia or bipolar disorder: A population-based study using nationwide registers. Acta Psychiatr. Scand. 2020, 143, 61–71.

17. Lévesque, I.S.; Abdel-Baki, A. Homeless youth with first-episode psychosis: A 2-year outcome study. Schizophr. Res. 2019, 216, 460–469.

18. Harrison, G.; Hopper, K.; Craig, T.; Laska, E.; Siegel, C.; Wanderling, J.; Dube, K.C.; Ganev, K.; Giel, R.; Der Heiden, W.A.; et al. Recovery from psychotic illness: A 15- and 25-year international follow-up study. Br. J. Psychiatry 2001, 178, 506–517.

19. Jääskeläinen, E.; Juola, P.; Hirvonen, N.; McGrath, J.J.; Saha, S.; Isohanni, M.; Veijola, J.; Miettunen, J. A Systematic Review and Meta-Analysis of Recovery in Schizophrenia. Schizophr. Bull. 2012, 39, 1296–1306.

20. Warner, R. Recovery from Schizophrenia Psychiatry and Political Economy, 3rd ed.; Brunner-Routledge: Hove, UK; New York, NY, USA, 1997; p. 74

21. Howes, O.D.; Cummings, C.; Chapman, G.E.; Shatalina, E. Neuroimaging in schizophrenia: An overview of findings and their

implications for synaptic changes. Neuropsychopharmacology 2022, 48, 151–167

22. Leung, M.; Cheung, C.; Yu, K.; Yip, B.; Sham, P.; Li, Q.; Chua, S.; McAlonan, G. Gray Matter in First-Episode Schizophrenia Before and After Antipsychotic Drug Treatment. Anatomical Likelihood Estimation Meta-analyses With Sample Size Weighting. Schizophr. Bull. 2009, 37, 199–211

23. Ho, B.C.; Andreasen, N.C.; Ziebell, S.; Pierson, R.; Magnotta, V. Long-term antipsychotic treatment and brain volumes: A longitudinal study of first-episode schizophrenia. Arch. Gen. Psychiatry 2011, 68, 128–137.

24. Cahn, W.; Pol HE, H.; Lems, E.B.; van Haren, N.E.; Schnack, H.G.; van der Linden, J.A.; Schothorst, P.F.; van Engeland, H.; Kahn, R.S. Brain volume changes in first-episode schizophrenia: A 1-year follow-up study. Arch. Gen. Psychiatry 2002, 59, 1002–1010

25. Boule, L.A.; Burke, C.G.; Jin, G.-B.; Lawrence, B.P. Aryl hydrocarbon receptor signaling modulates antiviral immune responses: Ligand metabolism rather than chemical source is the stronger predictor of outcome. Sci. Rep. 2018, 8, 1826.

26. Congdon, E.E.; Wu, J.W.; Myeku, N.; Figueroa, Y.H.; Herman, M.; Marinec, P.S.; Gestwicki, J.E.; Dickey, C.A.; Yu, W.H.; Duff, K.E. Methylthioninium chloride (methylene blue) induces autophagy and attenuates tauopathy in vitro and in vivo. Autophagy 2012, 8, 609–622.

27. Matteoni, S.; Matarrese, P.; Ascione, B.; Ricci-Vitiani, L.; Pallini, R.; Villani, V.; Pace, A.; Paggi, M.G.; Abbruzzese, C. Chlorpromazine induces cytotoxic autophagy in glioblastoma cells via endoplasmic reticulum stress and unfolded protein response. J. Exp. Clin. Cancer Res. 2021, 40, 347.

28. Madison CA, Hillbrick L, Kuempel J, Albrecht GL, Landrock KK, Safe S, Chapkin RS, Eitan S. Intestinal epithelium aryl hydrocarbon receptor is involved in stress sensitivity and maintaining depressive symptoms. Behav Brain Res. 2023 Feb 25;440:114256. Doi: 10.1016/j.bbr.2022.114256.

29. Gulbins, A., Schumacher, F., Becker, K.A. et al. Antidepressants act by inducing autophagy controlled by sphingomyelin–ceramide. Mol Psychiatry 23, 2324–2346 (2018). https://doi.org/10.1038/s41380-018-0090-9

30. Cardon I, Grobecker S, Jenne F, Jahner T, Rupprecht R, Milenkovic VM, Wetzel CH. Serotonin effects on human iPSC-derived neural cell functions: from mitochondria to depression. Mol Psychiatry. 2024 Mar 26. doi: 10.1038/s41380-024-02538-0.

31. Caldara M, Marmiroli N. Antimicrobial Properties of Antidepressants and Antipsychotics-Possibilities and Implications. Pharmaceuticals (Basel). 2021 Sep 10;14(9):915. doi: 10.3390/ph14090915. PMID: 34577614; PMCID: PMC8470654.

32. Girgis RR, Lieberman JA. Anti-viral properties of antipsychotic medications in the time of COVID-19. Psychiatry Res. 2021 Jan;295:113626. doi: 10.1016/j.psychres.2020.113626. Epub 2020 Nov 30. PMID: 33290940; PMCID: PMC7833567.

33. Fond G, Macgregor A, Tamouza R, Hamdani N, Meary A, Leboyer M, Dubremetz JF. Comparative analysis of anti-toxoplasmic activity of antipsychotic drugs and valproate. Eur Arch Psychiatry Clin Neurosci. 2014 Mar;264(2):179-83. doi: 10.1007/s00406-013-0413-4. Epub 2013 Jun 15. PMID: 23771405.

34. Mariani N, Everson J, Pariante CM, Borsini A. Modulating microglial activation by antidepressants. Journal of

Psychopharmacology. 2022;36(2):131-150.
doi:10.1177/02698811211069110

35. Alves I, Staneva G, Tessier C, Salgado GF, Nuss P. The interaction
of antipsychotic drugs with lipids and subsequent lipid
reorganization was investigated using biophysical methods. Biochim
Biophys Acta. 2011 Aug;1808(8):2009-18. doi:
10.1016/j.bbamem.2011.02.021

Chapter 3
The Biophysical Basis of Severe Mental Illness

Mitochondrial loss and aberrant microglial activation can kill neuronal cells, causing depression and negative symptoms of schizophrenia. Both pathologies were associated with cellular senescence and glial conversion from neuroprotective to neurotoxic. Senescent cells in the gut barrier further facilitate microbial translocation. Host immune system activation, promotes autoimmune inflammation and antibodies against microbial molecules.

It is possible that aside from the Vagus nerve, the gut-brain communication can occur by synchronized oscillations (see chapter 9). For example, whole body vibration was demonstrated to increase regulatory T cells, lymphocytes depleted in SMI as well as in inflammatory bowel disease.

Brain cells communicate with each other in many "languages". They can use calcium to convey information, extracellular vesicles, tunneling nanotubules (transport mitochondria), volume transmission (via interstitial fluid), and of course, wired communication via synapse. Any or all communication platforms can go wrong in mental illness. For example, depletion of cell battery, the mitochondrion, lowers energy, likely leading to the energy deficit, a domain of major depressive disorder.

Where have mitochondria gone?

In neurons, mitochondria are very busy organelles as these cells require a lot of energy to process the information necessary for our daily lives. Neurons live as long as we do, or at least until old age. As the brain uses 20% of the body's energy, mitochondria work very hard and wear off quickly, requiring replacement. Here comes the astrocyte, the star-shaped cell that exports fresh mitochondria to the neuronal cells to continue working. Drugs, such as Prozac and other SSRIs, enhance mitochondrial trafficking to neurons, helping many depressed people recover. However, giving these drugs for a long time may be detrimental as SSRIs often make us apathetic and careless as well as tolerant of various moral issues. Interestingly, fluoride, the halogen added to the drinking water, augments the properties of SSRIs, but it is unknown whether SSRIs also enhance fluoride toxicity. For this reason, treating depression for a long time may be preferable, but not necessarily with SSRIs (unless nothing else is helpful). Another reason not to use these drugs for too long is the "mania switch," especially in people who have bipolar diathesis but are unaware of it. Another problem is bleeding, especially if combined with aspirin or anticoagulants.

So, what is the ideal maintenance treatment for chronic depression? I like to say, "If you want to treat the brain, start with the gut." "Leaky gut," very common in depressed people, should be addressed first (see chapter 19).

Brain work requires communication among cells throughout the CNS. In many ways, nerve and glial cells, such as astrocytes and microglia, talk to each other. Like most, the "language" glia is calcium, as glial cells converse via calcium waves.

Neurons crosstalk in a "wired" and "unwired" manner. The former involves synaptic transmission, while the latter occurs by volume transmission (also called exocrine/paracrine pathway), referring to molecules released by the brain cells that flow with the interstitial fluid to reach target cells. Recently, two other communication platforms, EVs and TNT, were described. Yet another documented but rarely discussed communication modality is oscillations that can synchronize distant brain areas. Indeed, synchronization can also be accomplished with regions outside the brain, probably the molecular networks that store memory and process information. Interestingly, gray matter volume (GMV) reduction in SMI abolishes the gamma oscillations in the 30-100 HZ range associated with consciousness, awareness, and other higher-order functions.

Depression, as a mitochondrial disease

One of the hallmarks of major depressive disorder (MDD), low energy and psychomotor retardation, likely reflect mitochondrial dysfunction. These organelles were once bacteria that entered nucleated cells and became metabolic furnaces, generating energy in the form of ATP by oxidation of nutrients.

The amount of mitochondrial damage and loss can be measured by the blood level of mitochondrial DNA (mtDNA), which is higher in MDD patients compared to the general population and is considered a biomarker of this disorder (1). Aside from mitochondria, astrocytes supply the neurons with glutathione, a powerful antioxidant that defends from iron-induced damage (see the section on ferroptosis).

Besides the neurons and glial cells, the brain also contains endothelial cells (ECs), which line the inner walls of blood vessels and exchange nutrients and water with the astrocyte through processes known as end-feet. ECs protect the CNS through their specialized TJs, the molecular interdigitations that keep the cells of the BBB together. Dysfunctional BBB allows peripheral toxins and translocated gut microbes to cross into the brain, inducing inflammation and damage. This can be quantified by measuring the level of translocation markers, such as intestinal fatty acid binding protein (I-FABP), LPS-binding protein (LBP), and soluble CD14 (sCD14). These biomarkers are upregulated in several neuropsychiatric conditions, including SCZ, MDD, and Alzheimer's disease (AD), linking these conditions to migrating gut microbes into the systemic circulation (2).

Senescent brain cells, a phenotype prevalent in SMI, generate a toxic secretome, senescence-associated secretory phenotype (SASP), that spreads senescence to the neighboring healthy cells. SASP can damage mitochondria, causing a cellular "energy crisis" that may force the brain cells to burn lactate, the preferred metabolic source of cancer cells. Lactate translates into acetylation, a posttranslational modification that augments brain aging, predisposing to neurodegenerative diseases such as AD. In addition, SASP disrupts the BBB, facilitating the translocation of gut microbes.

Senescent neurons may reenter the cell cycle but often remain permanently fused as these cells lack the molecular machinery to replicate fully. A better understanding of neuronal fusion will likely clarify the etiology of many neuropsychiatric conditions and lead to novel treatments (3).

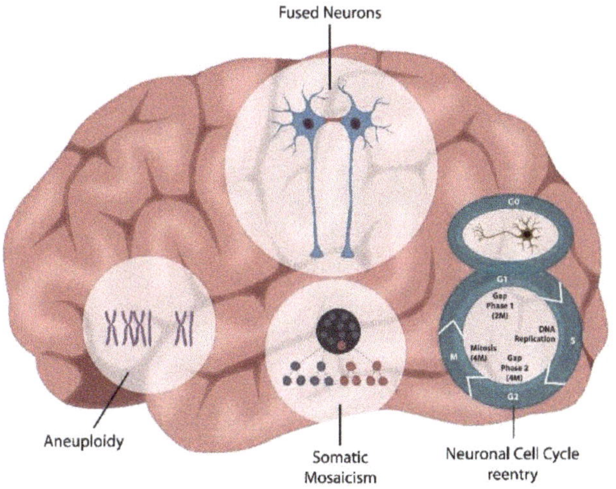

Fig. 3.1 A frequent characteristic of senescent neurons is reentering the cell cycle. However, because postmitotic neuronal cells lack the molecular machinery to complete mitosis, they may remain in a fused or aneuploid state with diverse neuronal genomes (somatic mosaicism).

Another exciting characteristic of senescent glial cells is the "cannibalization" of healthy neurons, likely engendering negative SCZ symptoms such as alogia, avolition, depression, and poverty of speech and thought (4). For example, senescent microglia may undergo aberrant activation, leading to pathologies such as MDD, SCZ, anxiety disorder, and ASD. Indeed, premature cellular senescence, a characteristic of SMI, SASP, and excessive lactate, may trigger neuropathology without synaptic involvement (5).

The Human Microbiome Project, launched in 2007, and the discovery of innate lymphoid cells (ILCs) in 2008 are significant advances that have begun to shed light on the pathogenesis of some disorders of uncertain etiology, including neuropsychiatric illnesses.

The gut microbial community is immunologically "tolerated" in the GI tract but may elicit immunogenicity and pathology upon translocation into host tissues. Indeed, numerous studies have reported the presence of intestinal microbes and their molecules in host tissues, such as the circulatory system and the brain. For example, a brain virome (viral microbiome) in Brodman area 46 was associated with SCZ (6).

Recent studies have shown that select gut microbes can synthesize serotonergic hallucinogens, such as tryptamine and N, N-dimethyltryptamine (DMT). For example, *Ruminococcus gnavus and Clostridium sporogenes* express tryptophan decarboxylase, an enzyme capable of converting dietary tryptophan into tryptamine. Furthermore, since serotonergic hallucinogens are AhR ligands, this transcription factor is further implicated in neuropathology.

The use of the psychotomimetic anesthetic, ketamine, for treatment-resistant depression has raised an interesting question: do humans possess an inbuilt antidepressant system akin to endogenous opioids? If so, do antidepressant drugs (which possess antibiotic properties) eliminate the hallucinogenic bacteria, increasing the prevalence of depression? For example, Prozac (fluoxetine) was demonstrated to kill the gut microbes and those in the environmental waters. Indeed, Prozac (and likely all SSRIs) was shown to eliminate *Escherichia coli (E. coli)* in the Great Lakes, emphasizing the antibiotic to kill properties of this drug (7). Moreover, fluoxetine degradation in environmental water produces fluoride, a halogen implicated in MDD and other neuropsychiatric conditions (8) (9). Adding fluoride to the drinking water, a practice started in 1945, roughly coincides with the increased prevalence of depression in the US. For example, people born after 1945 were ten times more likely to have a diagnosis of depression compared to the previous generation (10).

The crosstalk between oral and gut microbiomes

The commensal microbes in different body niches communicate with brain cells via AhR and Vagus nerve as well as by neurotransmitters. Indeed, gut microbes produce all the known neurotransmitters.

The interkingdom dialog maintains the delicate balance between the host and microbiome-released molecules, probably to avert overproduction. For example, in the microbial kingdom, DA is an iron chelator, but once it crosses the gut barrier, it becomes a component of the host reward system. This action requires coordination via microbe-host dialog. Under pathological circumstances, dysfunctional communication between the microbiome and the human host generates pathology, including depression and suicide.

Along this line, a recent study on university students with suicidal ideation has highlighted the connection between immune response to commensal microbes and psychopathology, especially MDD and suicidality (11) (12) (13). This study has found that the four major histocompatibility complex (MHC) alleles and the absence of oral microbe *Alloprevotella rava* increased the risk of suicidal behavior, emphasizing a microbe-gene link in this pathology.

Suicide is the second leading cause of mortality in young adults, contributing to more than 40,000 deaths per year in the US alone. Previous studies have associated suicidal behavior with several alleles of the MHC, a network of genes encoding for the human leukocyte antigen (HLA). For example, the presence of the

DQB1*02 allele was reported to increase while HLA-DQB1*05 lowered the odds of suicidal behavior, suggesting that genetics and immunity play a significant role in the pathogenesis of this disorder. The altered human microbiome was previously linked to suicidal behavior, suggesting that microbiota could be involved in this pathology (14). Indeed, the markers of bacterial translocation into the host circulatory system, including LBP, sCD14, cf-mDNA, and I-FABP, were reported to be elevated in individuals with recent suicide attempts, connecting this pathology with a dysfunctional gut barrier. This is further substantiated by the earlier studies that reported increased suicide rates in patients with IBD, further connecting microbial translocation outside the GI tract with this behavior.

Elevated circulatory LBP, sCD14, cf-mDNA, and I-FABP have established biomarkers of increased intestinal permeability. However, plasma levels of indole, short-chain fatty acids (SCFAs), such as propionate and butyrate, may comprise novel markers of microbial migration.

Communication via antibodies or autoantibodies

Commensal microbes express proteins identical or similar to those of the human host. These proteins can activate the immune system upon translocation, causing pathology. Due to molecular mimicry (resemblance), antibodies against microbial antigens can interact with host proteins, in an autoantibody-like manner. For example, *Bacteroides species* and *Pseudomonas fluorescens* produce γ-aminobutyric acid (GABA) and GABA-binding proteins that may elicit the formation of antibodies, probably explaining the pathogenesis of anti-GABA-B receptor encephalitis (15). This is significant as a recent study has associated elevated anti-GABA-B receptor antibodies in the cerebrospinal fluid (CSF) with suicidality, linking this behavior to autoimmune pathology. In addition, *E. coli*, expressing glutamate receptors B and D (GluR)-B and GluR-D, can, upon translocation, elicit the production of anti-N-methyl-d-aspartate-receptor (NMDAR) antibodies, immunoglobulins strongly correlated with suicidal behavior (16).

The study of microbiome and microbial translocation has blurred the concept of autoimmunity, begging the question: are human autoantibodies generated spontaneously, or are they conventional antibodies against microbial proteins translocated outside the GI tract? The answer to this question is significant, as regular antibodies against microbes and their proteins connect SMI with the microbial organ and open the possibility of treating what we perceive as autoimmunity with antibiotics (17).

Putting the above information together, Ahrens AP et al. is the first study to examine the interface between commensal microbes and the MHC. This system undergoes gene diversification by interacting with the human microbiome. *Alloprevotella rava*, a succinate-producing, Gram-negative bacillus, belongs to the *Prevotellaceae* family and can be found in the oral cavity. *Prevotellaceae* have been associated with the upregulation of Th17 cells known for generating interleukin 13 (IL13), a recently identified marker of suicidal behavior in patients with major depressive disorder (MDD). In addition, *Prevotellaceae* were implicated in other psychiatric disorders, including SCZ, probably accounting for the significant number of patients with this disorder who engage in suicidal behavior. Indeed, activation of IL-13 alpha one receptor (IL-13Rα1) in the dopaminergic neurons of *substantia nigra* was found to increase the vulnerability of these cells to oxidative damage, likely predisposing to Parkinson's disease (PD).

Human saliva and gut microbes were reported to undergo daily, seasonal, and geographical variations that affect gene expression, including those of the MHC. This is significant, as numerous epidemiological studies have reported a seasonal pattern of suicidal behavior (with counts peaking in the spring and declining in winter), probably coinciding with the surge of viral infections.

The oral cavity is an essential gateway to the human GI tract; thus, it affects the composition of the gut microbiome and, by extension, other organs. Several earlier studies have associated both the salivary and intestinal microbial communities with suicidal behavior, linking this pathology to the gene-microbiota interface. The translocation of microorganisms outside of the GI tract and the generation of antibodies to antigens mimicking neuronal proteins have been linked to suicidal behavior, connecting this pathology to immunity and autoimmunity. Moreover, MHC genetics was associated with the risk of suicide as well as autoimmune diseases. In the future, suicidal behavior may be reconceptualized as an infectious or immune rather than psychiatric illness. Indeed, before the discovery of *Helicobacter Pylori (H. Pylori)*, peptic ulcer disease was included among psychiatric disorders, setting a precedent for this type of pathogenetic shift. Interestingly, at a deeper level, autoimmunity and suicide have self-harm as a common denominator, while psychotropic drugs' upregulation of tolerant regulatory T cells (Tregs) attenuates this pathology.

Chapter 3 References:

1. Li, W., Zhu, L., Chen, Y. et al. Association between mitochondrial DNA levels and depression: a systematic review and meta-analysis. BMC Psychiatry 23, 866 (2023). https://doi.org/10.1186/s12888-023-05358-8

2. Stehle JR Jr, Leng X, Kitzman DW, Nicklas BJ, Kritchevsky SB, High KP. Lipopolysaccharide-binding protein, a surrogate marker of microbial translocation, is associated with physical function in healthy older adults. J Gerontol A Biol Sci Med Sci. 2012 Nov;67(11):1212-8. doi: 10.1093/gerona/gls178

3. Hilliard M, Giordano-Santini R, Li Z et al. Fusogen-mediated neuron–neuron fusion disrupts neural circuit connectivity and alters animal behavior. PNAS. 2020. doi: 10.1073/pnas.1919063117

4. Yanuck SF. Microglial Phagocytosis of Neurons: Diminishing Neuronal Loss in Traumatic, Infectious, Inflammatory, and Autoimmune CNS Disorders. Front Psychiatry. 2019 Oct 3;10:712. doi: 10.3389/fpsyt.2019.00712.

5. Zhu, H., Guan, A., Liu, J. et al. Noteworthy perspectives on microglia in neuropsychiatric disorders. J Neuroinflammation 20, 223 (2023). https://doi.org/10.1186/s12974-023-02901-

6. Mahin Ghorbani, Unveiling the Human Brain Virome in Brodmann Area 46: Novel Insights Into Dysbiosis and Its Association With Schizophrenia, Schizophrenia Bulletin Open, Volume 4, Issue 1, January 2023, sgad029, https://doi.org/10.1093/schizbullopen/sgad029

7. Rachel Kaufman, Prozac Killing E. coli in the Great Lakes. National Geographic (2011).

8. Adkins EA, Brunst KJ. Impacts of Fluoride Neurotoxicity and Mitochondrial Dysfunction on Cognition and Mental Health: A Literature Review. Int J Environ Res Public Health. 2021 Dec 7;18(24):12884. doi: 10.3390/ijerph182412884.

9. Khan MF, Murphy CD. Bacterial degradation of the antidepressant drug fluoxetine produces trifluoroacetic acid and fluoride ions. Appl Microbiol Biotechnol. 2021 Dec;105(24):9359-9369. doi: 10.1007/s00253-021-11675-3

10. Lim ICZY, Tam WWS, Chudzicka-Czupała A, McIntyre RS, Teopiz KM, Ho RC, Ho CSH. Prevalence of depression, anxiety and post-traumatic stress in war- and conflict-afflicted areas: A meta-analysis. Front Psychiatry. 2022 Sep 16;13:978703. doi: 10.3389/fpsyt.2022.978703.

11. Ahrens AP, Sanchez-Padilla DE, Drew JC, Oli MW, Roesch LFW,Triplett EW. Saliva microbiome, dietary, and genetic markers are associated with suicidal ideation in university students. Sci Rep.2022 Aug 22;12(1):14306. Doi: 10.1038/s41598-022-18020-2.

12. Nässberger L, Träskman-Bendz L. Increased soluble interleukin-2 receptor concentrations in suicide attempters. Acta PsychiatrScand. 1993 Jul;88(1):48-52. doi: 10.1111/j.1600-

13. Tonelli LH, Stiller J, Rujescu D, Giegling I, Schneider B, Maurer K,Schnabel A, Möller HJ, Chen HH, Postolache TT. She elevated cytokine expression in the orbitofrontal cortex of victims of suicide. ActaPsychiatr Scand. 2008 Mar;117(3):198-206. doi: 10.1111/j.1600-0447.2007.01128.x.

14. Cai LF, Wang SB, Hou CL, Li ZB, Liao YJ, Jia FJ. Association Between Non-Suicidal Self-Injury and Gut Microbial Characteristics in Chinese Adolescents. Neuropsychiatr Dis Treat. 2022 Jul 1;18:1315-1328. Doi: 10.2147/NDT.S360588.

15. Zhang, X., Lang, Y., Sun, L. et al. Clinical characteristics and predictive analysis of anti-gamma-aminobutyric acid-B (GABA-B)receptor encephalitis in Northeast China. BMC Neurol 20, 1(2020). https://doi.org/10.1186/s12883-019-1585-y

16. Arvola M, Keinänen K. Characterization of the ligand-binding domains of glutamate receptor (GluR)-B and GluR-D subunits expressed in Escherichia coli as periplasmic proteins. J Biol Chem.1996 Jun 28;271(26):15527-32. doi: 10.1074/jbc.271.26.15527.PMID: 8663017

17. Vangoitsenhoven R, Cresci GAM. Role of Microbiome and Antibiotics in Autoimmune Diseases. Nutr Clin Pract. 2020 Jun;35(3):406-416. doi: 10.1002/ncp.10489. Epub 2020 Apr 22. PMID: 32319703.

18. Carneiro-Filho BA, Lima IP, Araujo DH, Cavalcante MC,Carvalho GH, Brito GA, Lima V, Monteiro SM, Santos FN, RibeiroRA, Lima AA. Intestinal barrier function and secretion in methotrexate-induced rat intestinal mucositis. Dig Dis Sci. 2004Jan;49(1):65-72. doi: 10.1023/b:ddas.0000011604.45531.2c.

Chapter 4
The "Gut-Brain," Enteric Nervous System (ENS)

The enteric nervous system, containing more neurons than the spinal cord, comprises an abdominal brain in which the microbiome plays a major role by generating most neurotransmitters. For example, 90% of total body serotonin and 60% of dopamine are produced by the gut microbes. It is, therefore, not surprising that the microbiome is a major player in the pathogenesis of SMIs. In this regard, the enteric nervous system not only facilitates the brain-gut dialog but also coordinates the distribution of microbiota-generated neurotransmitters. In contrast, elimination of certain microbial species by antibiotic treatment can result in upregulation or downregulation of brain neurotransmitters, leading to pathology.

Another key role of gut microbes consists of metabolizing most drugs, including the psychotropics, modifying their pharmacodynamic properties. In fact, it could be argued that the first pass metabolism takes place in the gut rather than the liver as it was previously thought.

The communication between the insular cortex and intestinal epithelial cells is of particular interest to the psychiatrist as this circuit is indispensable for interoceptive awareness, including insight into the illness...

The brain bugs

Is there a brain microbiome? Recent studies have reported brain-inhabiting bacteria and viruses in patients with neurodegenerative disorders. Since the gut barrier and BBB are impaired in neuropsychiatric illnesses, pathogens from the body's periphery can ingress the brain. In addition, dormant microbes thrive in the CNS for a long time in an inactive state, awaiting the availability of nutrients (such as iron) to replicate.

Interleukin-22 (IL-22), the "guardian" of the gut barrier, is produced by several lymphoid cell types, including Th1, Th17, Th22, natural killer T cells (NKCs), and innate lymphoid cells (ILCs). Deficient IL-22 enables microbial translocation from the GI tract into the systemic circulation. For this reason, recombinant human IL-22 is a potential novel SCZ treatment.

This chapter examines the role of two critical organs, the gut and the microbial organ, in the etiopathogenesis of SMI.

The gut, measuring around 15 feet with approximately 400 m2 of intestinal barrier, contains over 100 million neurons, which, together with the 600 million neurons contained by the enteric nervous system (ENS), comprise a unique abdominal brain. It is, therefore, not surprising that ancient Egyptians thought of the intestine as an organ of utmost importance that deserved a particular guardian god, Qebehsenuef. In contrast, the brain was of no significance to this culture, as it was believed to be nothing more than a producer of mucus.

We are rediscovering the importance of the gut and its influence on CNS physiology and pathology. A recent study found that gut enteroendocrine cells communicate with the brain via the Vagus nerve, probably conveying local status to the CNS (1).

The ENS is the most significant component of the autonomic nervous system (ANS) known for transmitting microbial signals to the brain via the myenteric plexus. At the molecular level, AhR (directly or via the STAT pathway) promotes the release of IL-22, a significant protector of the gut barrier (2).

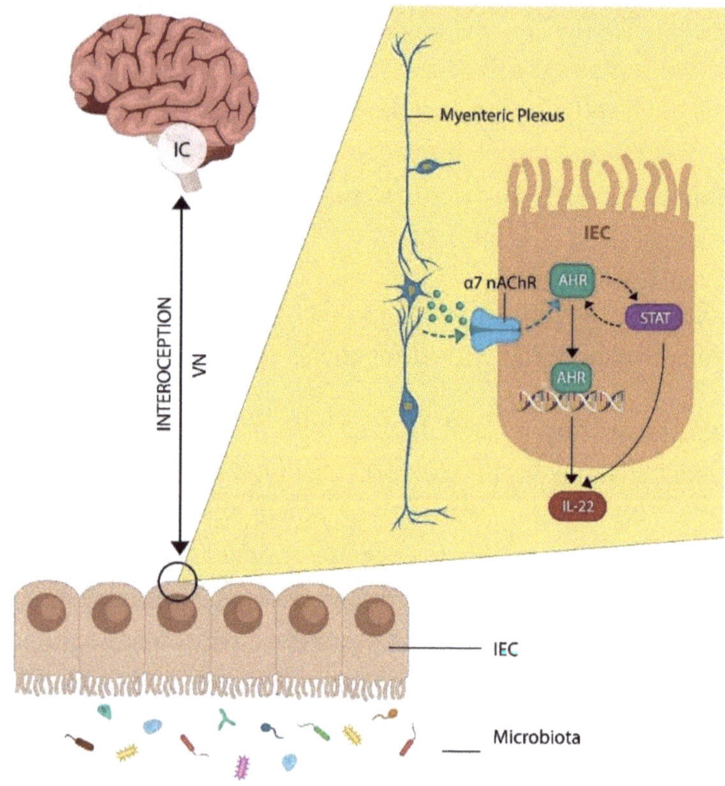

Fig. 4.1 Interoception is realized by connecting intestinal epithelial cells (IECs) to the insular cortex (IC). The AhR/STAT system in the IEC communicates via acetylcholine (ACh) with the myenteric plexus, which subsequently connects to the Vagus nerve. In the process, interleukin 22 is released to protect the gut barrier.

Another recent study found that gut inflammations are recorded in the insular cortex (IC), suggesting that the expression 'gut feeling' may be more than just a figure of speech (3). Indeed, these studies document the dialog between the brain and gut, the so-called gut-brain axis".

Interoception, awareness of the body's internal state, "dwells" in the IC and is likely realized via the intestine-brain link. This is significant as interoceptive awareness is disrupted in SMI and frontotemporal dementia (FTD), connecting these pathologies to the "leaky gut" and microbial migration out of the GI tract.

Intestinal epithelial cells (IECs) sense microbial signals and relay them to the mucosal immune cells, which defend against enteric pathogens and protect commensal flora. IECs are interspersed among enteroendocrine cells in close contact with the Vagus nerve.

The GI tract contains the most extensive immune system in the body, known as gut-associated lymphoid tissue (GALT). GALT includes 70-80% of all body immune cells and plays a significant role in the immunological tolerance (non responsiveness) to intestinal microorganisms and food proteins. In other words, GALT maintains the delicate balance between immune response to pathogens and nonresponse to food and commensal microbes.

Under pathological circumstances, loss of tolerance can trigger autoimmune inflammation directed against commensals. Microbial molecules often resemble host proteins; thus, antibodies against the former may cross-react with the latter, inducing pathology. For example, some gut microbes express adrenergic receptors, which, upon microbial migration into the host systemic circulation, can elicit antibodies directed at human adrenergic receptors, inducing pathology. This pathology can manifest as anxiety, endothelial disease, or even heart failure (5) (6) (7).

Recently, a subgroup of patients with SCZ exhibited antibodies against DA receptors, a phenomenon that can be explained by microbial translocation. Since gut microbes generate about 60% of total body DA and DA-related proteins, antibodies against these molecules may be mis conceptualized as autoantibodies. Indeed, these antibodies prove that microbial translocation is implicated in the pathogenesis of SMI. This is further substantiated by the fact that SCZ patients have a more permeable gut barrier than the general population, likely accounting for the increased levels of microbial migration. This also explains the high comorbidity of SCZ with IBD, in which a dysfunctional gut barrier is well-documented (8). Moreover, migration of bacteria outside the GI tract was previously associated with SCZ exacerbation or new onset psychosis. For example, urinary tract infections (UTIs), usually caused by *E. coli*, have been known to induce psychosis or SCZ relapse. Another example is the 2011 *E. coli* outbreak in Germany, in which cases of new-onset psychosis were identified, a pathology that subsided with infection resolution (9).

Aside from 5-HT and DA, gut microbiota produces almost all known neurotransmitters, including glutamate, gamma-aminobutyric acid (GABA), and acetylcholine (ACh), which may elicit the formation of antibodies against the associated proteins, such as receptors or transporters (10) (11). It is essential to distinguish between antibodies and autoantibodies because some medications commonly used in autoimmune disorders, such as methotrexate, increase gut permeability and may be detrimental in patients with SCZ (12). Conversely, antibiotic use may cause a deficit of these neurotransmitters by eliminating the producing commensal flora, inducing neuropsychiatric symptoms. For example, fifteen antibiotics, including penicillin, fluoroquinolones, macrolides, cephalosporins, and doxycycline, were associated with increased susceptibility to psychosis (12).

The GI tract contains trillions of microorganisms, including bacteria, viruses, fungi, archaea, and their genes. The microbiome protects the host against pathogens and generates energy and nutrients in exchange for sharing the gut microenvironment. This symbiosis led to the concept of a "microbial organ" to convey the importance of commensal flora for human physiology. Indeed, many genes the microbiome expresses generate nutrients that the host cannot manufacture, such as short-chain fatty acids (SCFAs), including butyrate, propionate, and acetate. Butyrate is an inhibitor of histone deacetylases (HDACs), facilitating epigenetically the expression of many genes. Insufficient butyrate has been associated with SMI, including MDD and SCZ. For example, a decreased abundance of butyrate-producing microbes *Ruminococcus and Roseburia* has been documented in SMI (13).

The microbial organ interacts with psychotropic drugs, metabolizing these agents before they reach the liver (Fig. 4.2). However, the antibiotic properties of antipsychotic and antidepressant drugs can alter the composition of the microbiota, potentially explaining the weight gain and increased BMI, which are common characteristics of many antipsychotic agents (Fig. 2). This interaction underscores the need for further research into the potential side effects of these drugs on the gut microbiome.

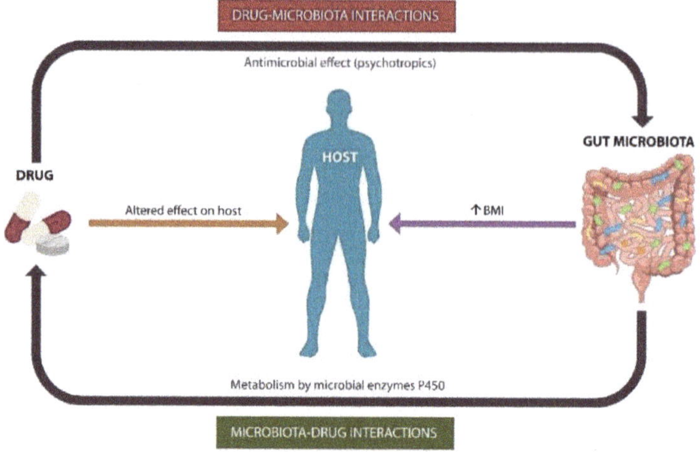

Fig. 4.2 Gut microbes initiate the metabolism of most drugs, including psychotropics, altering their properties. Conversely, these agents possess antibiotic properties and can eliminate many microbial taxa, thus influencing their metabolism. Increased BMI, a common adverse effect of many psychotropics, may be the result of antipsychotic/antidepressant-induced dysbiosis caused by these agents.

Indeed, psychotropic drug-induced weight gain may be mediated by AhR activation (14). AhR, a xenobiotic sensor, is located in the gut barrier and the BBB and regulates the gut-brain axis. In addition, 5-HT, melatonin, and DA are AhR ligands, making this receptor relevant for neuropsychiatry. This understanding of the role of AhR in mediating drug-induced weight gain provides valuable insights into the underlying mechanisms of this common side effect.

Like enteroendocrine cells, AhR is a key sensor for gut microbiota and microbial metabolites, playing a crucial role in mucosal immunity and gut barrier function. AhR is widely distributed in the brain in the cerebellum, cortex, and hippocampus, enabling dialogue for CNS-microbiota. As AhR is also a master regulator of cellular senescence, overactivation of this transcription factor triggers epithelial and endothelial senescence, further increasing the permeability of the gut barrier and BBB (14). This may be significant as SMI has been associated with premature cellular/neuronal senescence, porous biological barrier, and GMV reduction.

An emerging field, the study of gut microbes and aging, has identified several microorganisms, including *Streptococcus spp.*, as promoters of accelerated aging, linking SMI to the microbiome. Along this line, previous studies have associated streptococcal throat infection with elevated risks of mental illness, primarily obsessive-compulsive and tic disorders, emphasizing further the microbe-mental illness link. Moreover, preclinical studies have shown that transplantation of *Streptococcus vestibularis* induced deficits in social behaviors, further connecting this bacterium to SMI (15). Along this line, recent studies with graphene drums found that gut microbes exhibit oscillatory activity, forming an interkingdom communicating platform (16). This is significant as Neural Synchrony Theory has proposed that the same frequency of brain waves may engender cognition and consciousness.

The GI tract and the microbiome communicate with the brain, enabling many physiological functions, including interoceptive awareness. Impaired gut barrier permeability may lead to pathology, including autoimmune diseases and SMI.

Chapter 4 References:

1. Yu CD, Xu QJ, Chang RB. Vagal sensory neurons and gut-brain signaling. Curr Opin Neurobiol. 2020 Jun;62:133-140. doi: 10.1016/j.conb.2020.03.006.

2. Mar, J.S., Ota, N., Pokorzynski, N.D. et al. IL-22 alters gut microbiota composition and function, increasing aryl hydrocarbon receptor activity in mice and humans. Microbiome 11, 47 (2023). https://doi.org/10.1186/s40168-023-01486-1

3. Koren T, Yifa R, Amer M, Krot M, Boshnak N, Ben-Shaanan TL, Azulay-Debby H, Zalayat I, Avishai E, Hajjo H, Schiller M, Haykin H, Korin B, Farfara D, Hakim F, Kobiler O, Rosenblum K, Rolls A. Insular cortex neurons encode and retrieve specific immune responses. Cell. 2021 Nov 24;184(24):5902-5915.e17. doi: 10.1016/j.cell.2021.10.013.

4. Zheng L, Wen XL. Gut microbiota and inflammatory bowel disease: The current status and perspectives. World J Clin Cases. 2021 Jan 16;9(2):321-333. Doi: 10.12998/wjcc.v9.i2.321. PMID: 33521100

5. Zhang, X., Norton, J., Carrière, I. et al. Preliminary evidence for a role of the adrenergic nervous system in generalized anxiety disorder. Sci Rep 7, 42676 (2017). https://doi.org/10.1038/srep42676

6. Karczewski P, Pohlmann A, Wagenhaus B, Wisbrun N, Hempel P, Lemke B, Kunze R, Niendorf T, Bimmler M. Antibodies to the α1-adrenergic receptor cause vascular impairments in rat brain as demonstrated by magnetic resonance angiography. PLoS One. 2012;7(7):e41602. doi: 10.1371/journal.pone.0041602.

7. Gurguis, G., Antai-Otong, D., Vo, S. et al. Adrenergic Receptor Function in Panic Disorder: I. Platelet α2 Receptors Gi Protein Coupling, Effects of Imipramine, and Relationship to Treatment

Outcome. Neuropsychopharmacol 20, 162–176 (1999). https://doi.org/10.1016/S0893-133X(98)00062-1

8. Bernstein CN, Hitchon CA, Walld R, Bolton JM, Sareen J, Walker JR, Graff LA, Patten SB, Singer A, Lix LM, El-Gabalawy R, Katz A, Fisk JD, Marrie RA; CIHR Team in Defining the Burden and Managing the Effects of Psychiatric Comorbidity in Chronic Immunoinflammatory Disease. Increased Burden of Psychiatric Disorders in Inflammatory Bowel Disease. Inflamm Bowel Dis. 2019 Jan 10;25(2):360-368. doi: 10.1093/ibd/izy235.

9. Kleimann A, Toto S, Eberlein CK, Kielstein JT, Bleich S, Frieling H, Sieberer M. Psychiatric symptoms in patients with Shiga toxin-producing E. coli O104:H4 induced haemolytic-uraemic syndrome. PLoS One. 2014 Jul 9;9(7):e101839. doi: 10.1371/journal.pone.0101839.

10. Xue R, Zhang H, Pan J, Du Z, Zhou W, Zhang Z, Tian Z, Zhou R, Bai L. Peripheral Dopamine Controlled by Gut Microbes Inhibits Invariant Natural Killer T Cell-Mediated Hepatitis. Front Immunol. 2018 Oct 17;9:2398. doi: 10.3389/fimmu.2018.02398.

11. Le Dréan, G., Blottière, H.M. Glutamate from the microbiome controls host metabolism. Nat Metab (2024). https://doi.org/10.1038/s42255-024-01050-7

12. Essali N, Miller BJ. Psychosis is an adverse effect of antibiotics. Brain Behav Immun Health. 2020 Sep 19;9:100148. doi: 10.1016/j.bbih.2020.100148. PMID: 34589893; PMCID: PMC8474525.

13. Beutheu Youmba S, Belmonte L, Galas L, Boukhettala N, Bôle-Feysot C, Déchelotte P, Coëffier M. Methotrexate modulates tight junctions through NF-κB, MEK, and JNK pathways. J Pediatr

Gastroenterol Nutr. 2012 Apr;54(4):463-70. doi:
10.1097/MPG.0b013e318247240d.

14. Li, S., Song, J., Ke, P. et al. The gut microbiome is associated with
brain structure and function in schizophrenia. Sci Rep 11, 9743
(2021). https://doi.org/10.1038/s41598-021-89166-8

15. Fehsel K, Schwanke K, Kappel BA, Fahimi E, Meisenzahl-Lechner
E, Esser C, Hemmrich K, Haarmann-Stemmann T, Kojda G, Lange-
Asschenfeldt C. Activation of the aryl hydrocarbon receptor by
clozapine induces preadipocyte differentiation and contributes to
endothelial dysfunction. J Psychopharmacol. 2022 Feb;36(2):191-
201. doi: 10.1177/02698811211055811

16. Kawamoto S, Hara E. Crosstalk between gut microbiota and cellular
senescence: a vicious cycle leading to the aging gut. Trends Cell
Biol. 2024 Jan 13:S0962-8924(23)00254-4. Doi:
10.1016/j.tcb.2023.12.004. Epub ahead of print. PMID: 38220548.

17. Rosłoń, I.E., Japaridze, A., Steeneken, P.G. et al. Probing nano
motion of single bacteria with graphene drums. Nat. Nanotechnol.
17, 637–642 (2022). https://doi.org/10.1038/s41565-022-01111-6

Chapter 5
Cholesterol: Putting the Brake on Aggression

Most medical discipline, except psychiatry, badmouth cholesterol for causing atherosclerosis. In contrast, the brain needs all the cholesterol it can get and contains more cholesterol than any other organ in the body. Indeed, this lipid is indispensable for preventing aggressive and violent behaviors, as well as to avert brain volume loss.

Brain cholesterol is made locally and contributes to the integrity of myelin sheath, cellular and mitochondrial membranes as well as brain parenchyma.

Most statins cross the blood brain barrier and enter the brain, lowering local cholesterol. Despite several industry-sponsored studies that found statins neuroprotective, most data are negative, linking low cholesterol to aggression, violence, and cortical thinning.

During the 20th century, people became obsessed with cholesterol and weight gain; however, the two are not identical. Dietary cholesterol contributes very little, if at all, to the blood levels of this lipid as the liver produces much more cholesterol than people can consume. Moreover, brain cholesterol is the key to lowering aggression and maintaining the integrity of brain parenchyma. For this reason, it is essential not only for the neuropsychiatrists but also for the society at large, as violence has been increasing over the past four decades.

The BBB prevents the brain's uptake of cholesterol from the peripheral circulation. However, in patients with SCZ and dementia, the BBB is often dysfunctional, allowing peripheral cholesterol and statins to ingress into the brain. Moreover, in patients with SCZ or dementia, oxidized cholesterol, such as 24-hydroxycholesterol, can cross from the brain into the systemic circulation, frequently triggering aggressive behavior.

Several statins cross the BBB and lower the CNS cholesterol, which may lead to violent behaviors as well as suicide in patients with SMI (1) (2) (3). The CNS contains 23% of the total body cholesterol and, in humans, is the wealthiest organ in this lipid. As peripheral cholesterol does not cross the BBB, the brain must generate its own. In addition, some cholesterol metabolites, including 27-hydroxycholesterol and 24S-hydroxycholesterol, can cross from the peripheral circulation into the brain,

The link between cholesterol and aggression appears to be enacted at the level of the SSRI target, the serotonin transporter (SERT), which expresses a cholesterol-binding site. Interestingly, statins upregulate SERT, potentially exacerbating aggressive behaviors, while SSRIs inhibit this transporter (4).

Statins were first marketed in the US on September 1st, 1987, less than a year before Prozac. Interestingly, despite the availability of Prozac, the number of people receiving treatment for depression tripled between 1987 and 1997, likely implicating statins (3) (4) (5)

The situation is further compounded by the fact that L-tryptophan was taken off the market shortly after Prozac was released, suggesting that people who used L-tryptophan as a treatment for depression may have switched to Prozac, swelling the number of individuals medicated with this drug (5).

AhR is a ligand-activated transcription factor of growing importance for the pathophysiology of mental illness. It is found predominantly at the biological barriers, including the gut and BBB, where it interacts directly with endogenous and exogenous molecules, xenobiotics, and intestinal microorganisms. Moreover, AhR is the master regulator of cellular senescence and activates this phenotype in response to various ligands. The AhR connection to SMI involves premature cellular senescence induced by AhR overactivation (6) (7). Interestingly, decreased levels of low-density lipoprotein (LDLs) were shown to activate AhR, connecting this receptor to aggressive behaviors (8). Moreover, as AhR is activated by oxidized lipids, including 7-ketocholesterol (7KCl), a dysfunction of this transcription factor could lead to premature brain aging and SMI (9) (7).

Most patients with SMI do not exhibit violent behaviors and are more likely to be victims of aggressive acts perpetrated by others. However, a subgroup of individuals with low cholesterol and decreased vitamin D3 engage in criminal violations, linking oxidized membrane lipids to aggression and violence (10) (11) (12) (8) (9). Indeed, cholesterol level is considered a biological marker of psychiatric aggression as it likely reflects dysfunctional serotonergic signaling (13) (10).

Cholesterol is transported across the cell membranes and other lipids, including phosphoinositides, phosphatidylserine (PS), and sphingolipids. Impaired cholesterol transport can lead to violent behavior due to GMV reduction and downregulation of neuronal dendritic spines (14) (11). For example, a recent systematic review of patients with SCZ found a correlation between low serum cholesterol and aggression toward self or others (12) (15). Another study in women with SCZ found an inverse correlation between cholesterol HDL levels and aggressive behavior (16) (13).

Cholesterol is a precursor of both vitamin D and 7KCl. The latter, generated via 7-dehydrocholesterol reductase, is highly toxic and disrupts neurotransmission when incorporated into neuronal membranes. In addition, 7KCl promotes premature cellular senescence, a phenotypic marker of SMI (17). Vitamin D3 (calcitriol) inhibits 7-dehydrocholesterol reductase, averting the formation of 7KCh and protecting against senescence. In contrast, low vitamin D3 leads to 7KCh accumulation and activation of AhR, a key driver of cellular senescence (Fig. 5.1).

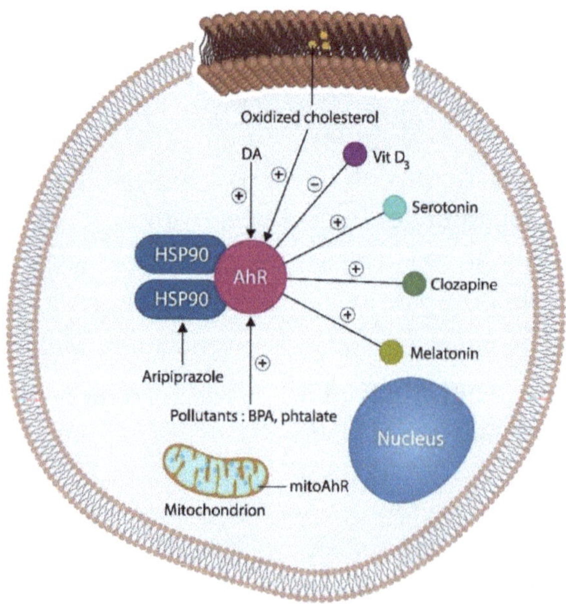

Fig. 5.1 AhR and HSP90 ligands. AhR, a key player in mental health disorders, is stabilized in the cytosol by two chaperone molecules of HSP90. AhR activation

separates this protein from its chaperones. Active AhR enters the nucleus and acts as a transcription factor. Several neurotransmitters, including DA and 5-HT, activate AhR. Clozapine and carbidopa are also AhR ligands. Pollutants can activate AhR, explaining their link to SCZ pathogenesis. Low cholesterol and vitamin D3 are AhR activators. Aripiprazole binds HSP90, strengthening its bond with AhR, therefore keeping this transcription factor in the cytosol.

Recent studies have shown that 7KCl can increase intracellular iron (Fe^{2+}), promoting AhR-mediated oxidative stress and ferroptosis, a non-apoptotic cell death, demonstrated in MDD and SCZ (18) (14). Moreover, cholesterol oxides were shown to decrease the fluidity of neuronal and mitochondrial membranes, disrupting neurotransmission. Furthermore, accumulation of intracellular Ca^{2+} enhances neuronal senescence, promoting SMI (19) (15) (Fig. 1). In contrast, treatment with membrane lipid replacement (MLR) offers a comprehensive approach to mental health care, as it may avert not only aggression but also metabolic pathology (20).

Taken together, SCZ has been associated with dysmetabolism, premature cellular senescence, and early brain aging. Senescence contributes to gray matter loss, predisposing to aggressive behaviors. 7KCl promotes brain aging via AhR overactivation, Fe^{2+}, and Ca^{2+} accumulation.

In the CNS, vitamin D3 functions as a neurohormone/transcription factor that controls the expression of several genes, including tyrosine hydroxylase (TyrH) and tryptophan hydroxylase 2 (TPH2), instrumental for the DA and 5-HT biosynthesis. For example, dopaminergic neurons in *Substantia nigra, nucleus basalis of Meynert, and Purkinje cells* in the cerebellum express vitamin D receptors (VDRs), highlighting the role of calcitriol in maintaining the integrity of DA signaling.

Under pathological circumstances, microglia, the CNS-resident macrophages, were shown to promote neuroinflammation, contributing to aggression associated with suicide, bipolar disorder, SCZ, and ASD. Moreover, activated microglia were shown to selectively target the dopaminergic neurons in *Substantia nigra*, contributing to Parkinson's disease (PD) (21) (16). Consequently, vitamin D3 is therapeutic for PD as it averts DA depletion and microglial activation (22). Furthermore, aberrantly activated microglia may engage in the phagocytosis of healthy neurons and synapses, likely explaining the GMV reduction in patients with SMI (23) (17).

The role of AhR-calcitriol crosstalk

AhR regulates the expression of human cytochrome P450 1A1 (CYP1A1), an enzyme involved in cholesterol metabolism, while oxidized cholesterol activates AhR via a feedback mechanism (24).

Polyphenols, both natural and synthetic, are AhR inhibitors that can reverse the effects of oxidized lipids on this receptor, alleviating depression and psychosis (18) (25) (Table 5.1). Indeed, AhR overactivation was strongly associated with cardiovascular diseases (CVD), including atherosclerosis, myocarditis, coronary artery disease, and pulmonary hypertension, highlighting a link between heart disease and neuropsychiatric disorders.

Exogenous agonists	Endogenous agonists	Dietary antagonists	Synthetic antagonists
Benzotriazole UV stabilizer	Tryptophan photo metabolites and FICZ	Quercetin	Salicylamide
Plasticizers (Bisphenol)	Indoles	Apigenin	1,3-diketone
Clozapine	D3 hydroxyderivatives	Luteolin	IK-175
Carbidopa	DA	Alstonine	HBU651

Table 5.1 AhR agonists and antagonists

Multiple studies over the past four decades have associated low levels of vitamin D3 with SMI, while VDRs were found in the brain areas relevant to these disorders. In addition, during early development, vitamin D3 participates in the neurogenesis of DA neurons, suggesting that aberrant activation of this process later in life may lead to the development of PD. For example, vitamin D has been implicated in DA dysregulation syndrome (DDS), an iatrogenic condition occurring in PD patients treated with DA replacement therapy (26).

Akt-GSK3 axis drives violence and suicide.

Protein kinase B or Akt is a serine-threonine kinase involved in multiple cellular processes, including the homeostasis of cell membrane lipids.

Akt pathway is activated by phosphoinositide 3-kinases (Pi3K) in response to cell surface receptor occupancy. For example, brain-derived neurotrophic factor (BDNF) binding to its receptor tyrosine kinases (RTKs) can activate the Akt pathway via Pi3K phosphorylation. GSK3 beta (GSK-3β) is a downstream kinase negatively regulated by Akt. This kinase is implicated in numerous physiological and pathological processes, including MDD, SCZ, and aggressive/suicidal behavior.

The link between GSK-3β and aggression originated with the realization that mood stabilizers, such as lithium and valproic acid, suppress this enzyme, modulating dopaminergic and serotonergic signaling (27) (20).

Novel studies have found that the Akt/GSK-3β pathway interacts with the plasma lipid bilayer when recruited to the cell membrane, which assumes an inactive conformation. For example, oxidized low-density lipoproteins (ox-LDL), including phospholipids, inactivate Akt, disinhibiting GSK-3β.

Taken together, physiological levels of brain cholesterol prevent aggressive, including suicidal, behaviors in patients with SMI. Although cholesterol does not cross the BBB, its metabolites and cholesterol-lowering drugs do, enhancing neuropathology. Low cholesterol also means low vitamin D3, a risk factor for SMI.

Chapter 5 References:

1. Saheki A, Terasaki T, Tamai I, Tsuji A. In vivo and in vitro blood-brain barrier transport of 3-hydroxy-3-methylglutaryl coenzyme A (HMG-CoA) reductase inhibitors. Pharm Res. 1994;11:305–11.

2. Leppien E, Mulcahy K, Demler TL, Trigoboff E, Opler L. Effects of Statins and Cholesterol on Patient Aggression: Is There a Connection? Innov Clin Neurosci. 2018 Apr 1;15(3-4):24-27. PMID: 29707423; PMCID: PMC5906086.

3. Cham S, Koslik HJ, Golomb BA. Mood, Personality, and Behavior Changes During Treatment with Statins: A Case Series. Drug Saf Case Rep. 2016 Dec;3(1):1. Doi: 10.1007/s40800-015-0024-2. PMID: 27747681; PMCID: PMC5005588.

4. Deveau CM, Rodriguez E, Schroering A, Yamamoto BK. Serotonin transporter regulation by cholesterol-independent lipid signaling. Biochem Pharmacol. 2021 Jan;183:114349. doi: 10.1016/j.bcp.2020.114349.

5. Olfson M, Marcus SC, Druss B, Elinson L, Tanielian T, Pincus HA. National trends in the outpatient treatment of depression. JAMA. 2002 Jan 9;287(2):203-9. doi: 10.1001/jama.287.2.203. PMID: 11779262.

6. Salminen A. Aryl hydrocarbon receptor (AhR) reveals evidence of antagonistic pleiotropy in regulating the aging process. Cell Mol Life Sci. 2022 Aug 20;79(9):489. doi: 10.1007/s00018-022-04520-x. PMID: 35987825; PMCID: PMC9392714.

7. Moyer BJ, Rojas IY, Kerley-Hamilton JS, Hazlett HF, Nemani KV, Trask HW, West RJ, Lupien LE, Collins AJ, Ringelberg CS, Gimi B, Kinlaw WB 3rd, Tomlinson CR. Inhibition of the aryl hydrocarbon receptor prevents Western diet-induced obesity. Model for AHR activation by kynurenine via oxidized-LDL, TLR2/4, TGFβ, and

IDO1. Toxicol Appl Pharmacol. 2016 Jun 1;300:13-24. doi: 10.1016/j.taap.2016.03.011. Epub 2016 Mar 25. PMID: 27020609; PMCID

8. Golomb BA, Stattin H, Mednick S. Low cholesterol and violent crime. J Psychiatr Res. 2000 Jul-Oct;34(4-5):301-9. doi: 10.1016/s0022-3956(00)00024-8. PMID: 11104842.

9. Choy O. Nutritional factors associated with aggression. Front Psychiatry. 2023 Jun 21;14:1176061. doi: 10.3389/fpsyt.2023.1176061. PMID: 37415691; PMCID: PMC10320003.

10. Mascitelli L, Pezzetta F, Goldstein MR. Low cholesterol, delinquency, and suicidality. Prim Care Companion J Clin Psychiatry. 2008;10(5):413-4. doi: 10.4088/pcc.v10n0511c.

11. Hering H, Lin CC, Sheng M. Lipid rafts in maintaining synapses, dendritic spines, and surface AMPA receptor stability. J Neurosci. 2003 Apr 15;23(8):3262-71. doi: 10.1523/JNEUROSCI.23-08-03262.2003.

12. Mufti RM, Balon R, Arfken CL. Low cholesterol and violence. Psychiatr Serv. 1998 Feb;49(2):221-4. doi: 10.1176/ps.49.2.221. PMID: 9575009.

13. Herceg D, Mimica N, Herceg M, Puljić K. Aggression in Women with Schizophrenia Is Associated with Lower HDL Cholesterol Levels. Int J Mol Sci. 2022 Oct 6;23(19):11858. doi: 10.3390/ijms231911858.

14. Miyajima H, Adachi J, Kohno S, Takahashi Y, Ueno Y, Naito T. Increased oxysterols associated with iron accumulation in the brains and visceral organs of acaeruloplasminaemia patients. QJM. 2001 Aug;94(8):417-22. doi: 10.1093/qjmed/94.8.417.

15. Martin N, Zhu K, Czarnecka-Herok J, Vernier M, Bernard D. Regulation and role of calcium in cellular senescence. Cell Calcium. 2023 Mar;110:102701. doi: 10.1016/j.ceca.2023.102701.

16. Gao C, Jiang J, Tan Y, Chen S. Microglia in neurodegenerative diseases: mechanism and potential therapeutic targets. Signal Transduct Target Ther. 2023 Sep 22;8(1):359. doi: 10.1038/s41392-023-01588-0.

17. Villani A, Peri F. Microglia: Picky Brain Eaters. Dev Cell. 2019 Jan 7;48(1):3-4. doi: 10.1016/j.devcel.2018.12.013. PMID: 30620901.

18. Vauzour D. Dietary polyphenols as modulators of brain functions: biological actions and molecular mechanisms underpinning their beneficial effects. Oxid Med Cell Longev. 2012;2012:914273.

19. Beaulieu JM, Zhang X, Rodriguiz RM, Sotnikova TD, Cools MJ, Wetsel WC, Gainetdinov RR, Caron MG. Role of GSK3 beta in behavioral abnormalities induced by serotonin deficiency. Proc Natl Acad Sci U S A. 2008 Jan 29;105(4):1333-8. doi: 10.1073/pnas.0711496105.

20. Jaworski T, Banach-Kasper E, Gralec K. GSK-3β at the Intersection of Neuronal Plasticity and Neurodegeneration. Neural Plast. 2019 May 2;2019:4209475. doi: 10.1155/2019/4209475. PMID: 31191636; PMCID: PMC6525914.

Chapter 6
Saving Face in the Time of COVID

Patients with severe mental illness exhibit cognitive deficits which resemble but are not identical with the ones encountered in dementias, such as Alzheimer's disease. A cognitive inability to recognize objects is called agnosia. The agnosia most often present in schizophrenia is anosognosia or impaired insight into illness. In contrast, patients with right hemispheric stroke may have left hemineglect, being unaware of the left side of their body.

Face blindness or prosopagnosia is discussed here because it is a new area of interest in neuropsychiatry and is often present in depression and schizophrenia. Prosopagnosia and anosognosia for cognitive deficit were reported in COVID-19. In fact, the pandemic brought prosopagnosia back into the research focus, suggesting that viruses may have higher affinity for a particular, face-recognizing, brain region, the fusiform gyrus.

Prosopagnosia in mood and anxiety disorders is well-documented. At the same time, SSRIs have been shown to decrease vigilance to fearful facial expressions, suggesting that these drugs are negative regulators of facial perception. Moreover, SSRIs affect people's sense of right and wrong, indicating a likely affinity for the insular cortex (IC).

The draconic infection control measures implemented by most countries during COVID-19, including mandatory surgical masks, are likely to affect facial recognition in children as they require constant practice to avoid prosopagnosia.

The fusiform gyrus, located on the basal surface of the occipital and temporal lobes, is a brain structure involved in processing visual information, facial recognition, and perceiving stimuli with high spatial frequencies, such as facial threat cues. Dysfunctional fusiform gyrus was implicated in MDD, anxiety, SCZ, and ASD.

In 1985, the neurologist and author Oliver Sacks wrote a book, "The Man Who Mistook His Wife for a Hat". This is a real story about Dr. P, a musician and painter with severe visual agnosia who could not identify facial expressions or recognize himself in the mirror, a condition known as prosopagnosia or face blindness. In addition, Dr. P could not name or place objects in categories. For example, he could not describe the shape of an orange but could identify it by smell or taste. To educate the public about prosopagnosia, Oliver Sacks, who suffered from this fusiform gyrus dysfunction, lectured and wrote extensively on this subject.

Face recognition is essential for the social functioning of human beings, who often need to identify familiar faces in large crowds. One of my patients with prosopagnosia once said: " It is embarrassing when people tell you that you looked them in the eyes and did not say a word". Another middle-aged gentleman stated: "Doctor, I don't have a problem recognizing you in your office, but if I see you on the street, I probably could not recall your face".

Developmental prosopagnosia (DP) is a lifelong face recognition defect that remains unchanged throughout the years, although patients may adapt, learning to identify people by their mannerisms or voice. On the other hand, acquired prosopagnosia (AP) occurs after head trauma, tumors, or strokes that involve the fusiform gyrus. Interestingly, sporadic cases of prosopagnosia were encountered after COVID-19, suggesting that the virus can alter the fusiform cortex (1).

The unintended consequences of surgical masks

"We speak with the left hemisphere," exclaimed Paul Broca in 1865 after locating the motoric word center in the left frontal lobe. However, it took another eight decades until Joachim Brodamer 1947 identified the face recognition area of the brain and coined the term prosopagnosia. This happened after one of Brodamer's patients sustained a stroke and became unable to recognize his family members (2). After seeing similar cases and performing autopsies, Brodamer discovered a small area in the right visual association cortex that responded to faces more than other stimuli, making him proudly state: "We recognize faces with the right hemisphere" (3).

The COVID-19 pandemic brought unique challenges, including mouth and nose-covering masks, rendering facial recognition more difficult (4). Indeed, several studies have found that surgical face masks significantly impair facial identification to the extent that prosopagnosia patients, aware of their deficits, learn to avoid people (5-8). In this regard, a novel neuroimaging study of brain activity has correlated the pre-COVID fusiform gyrus resting state with the development of social anxiety, emphasizing that prosopagnosia patients are prone to this disorder (9).

Other research on facial regions conveying social cues found that some areas are more informative than others. For example, the nose and mouth provide more clues on approachability and trustworthiness than the hair, ears, or chin (10). Mask-wearing may disrupt the estimation of other peoples' intentions, thrust, or friendliness, leading to more reserved and guarded attitudes toward peers. Indeed, the term "pandemic paranoia" has been coined to illustrate the heightened level of human mistrust and suspicion during the COVID-19 pandemic (11-12).

Masks and the development

Faces are vital for the psychosocial development of infants who can recognize some facial features as early as birth (13). At two months and a half, babies respond to smiling mother's face by smiling back thus, establishing an early nonverbal interaction that builds trust and significance (14). By six months, infants can recognize many individual faces, including those of other races however, in the absence of exposure, this plasticity disappears by the age of 12 (15-16). Indeed, neuroimaging studies found that children with less out-group experience activate the fusiform gyrus differently in response to own vs. other races (5). Interestingly, a novel study revealed that treatment with propranolol can diminish the negative racial bias, indicating that noradrenergic pathways likely drive the fusiform gyrus (17). This may be significant for child development as lockdowns and isolation during the COVID-19 pandemic likely diminished the inter- racial contact, possibly increasing the out-group bias.

The pathophysiology of facial recognition

In the 1970s, Charlic Gross identified neurons in the inferior temporal cortex of macaque monkeys that responded selectively to faces (18). In human infants, the "face cells," which fire in response to people previously seen, have been identified, indicating that the fusiform gyrus requires "experience" to develop (19) fully.

In 2005, during brain surgery for intractable seizure, a surgeon found that single neurons can react to the faces of specific people. These so-called "grandmother cells", a term coined by Jerome Lettvin, have been called different names by different groups, including Jennifer Aniston neurons, Luke Skywalker, or the Tower of Pisa neurons (20-21). Individual neuronal cells responding to specific faces may explain hallucinatory palinopsia, a hallucination of face identity generated by intracerebral stimulation of the right lateral fusiform gyrus (22). Palinopsia differs from Capgras Syndrome, a delusional misidentification disorder, in which faces are recognized but do not generate a sense of emotional familiarity, prompting the patient to think of close family members as impostors (24). In contrast, hyper-familiarity for faces (HFF) is a syndrome in which unfamiliar people appear familiar, prompting the patient to treat strangers as close friends (25).

Novel studies have found that visual mental imagery engages the left rather than the right fusiform gyrus, suggesting that imagination dwells in the left hemisphere (26). This is significant as antisocial tendencies and psychotic hallucinations are lateralized to the left hemisphere, linking imagery with the subjective perception of reality (27-28).

Interestingly, actively hallucinating patients with SCZ have shown less right fusiform gyrus activity compared to controls, probably emphasizing a right hemisphere compensatory mechanism (29).

Fusiform gyrus and severe mental illness

Although the fusiform gyrus is rarely considered in the pathogenesis of neuropsychiatric disorders, developmental prosopagnosia has been associated with depression, anxiety, SCZ, and ASD. Neuroimaging studies found GMV loss in many brain areas, including the fusiform gyrus, anterior cingulate cortex (ACC), insula, amygdala, and hippocampus, in patients with SCZ and MDD (30) (31).

At the molecular level, DA mediates face recognition via dopamine receptor 1 (DA1R), a neurotransmitter decreased in aging and chronic antipsychotic use, suggesting that prosopagnosia can be iatrogenic.

Gut microbes can alter the structural–functional connectivity in the fusiform gyrus, influencing face recognition (32). In addition to gut microbes, several viruses, including SARS-CoV-2, were associated with prosopagnosia and social anxiety (33). Indeed, the SARS-CoV-2 virus exploits DA receptors to enter host cells, probably accounting for the face recognition defects in SCZ (34).

Chapter 6 References:

1. Marie-Luise Kieseler, Brad Duchaine; Persisting Prosopagnosia due to COVID-19. Journal of Vision 2021;21(9):2408. doi: https://doi.org/10.1167/jov.21.9.2408.

2. Wegrzyn M, Garlichs A, Heß RWK, Woermann FG, Labudda K. The hidden identity of faces: a case of lifelong prosopagnosia. BMC Psychol. 2019 Jan 22;7(1):4. doi: 10.1186/s40359-019-0278-z

3. De Renzi E, Perani D, Carlesimo GA, Silveri MC, Fazio F. Prosopagnosia can be associated with damage confined to the right hemisphere--an MRI and PET study and a review of the literature. Neuropsychologia. 1994 Aug;32(8):893-902. doi: 10.1016/0028-3932(94)90041-8.

4. Tabish SA. COVID-19 pandemic: Emerging perspectives and future trends. J Public Health Res. 2020 Jun 4;9(1):1786. doi 10.4081/jphr.2020.1786.

5. Carragher DJ, Hancock PJB. Surgical face masks impair human face-matching performance for familiar and unfamiliar faces. Cogn Res Princ Implic. 2020 Nov 19;5(1):59. doi: 10.1186/s41235-020-00258-x.

6. Freud E, Di Giammarino D, Camilleri C. Mask-wearing selectivity alters observers' face perception. Cogn Res Princ Implic. 2022 Nov 16;7(1):97. doi: 10.1186/s41235-022-00444-z.

7. Tsantani M, Gray KLH, Cook R. New evidence of impaired expression recognition in developmental prosopagnosia. Cortex. 2022 Sep;154:15-26. doi: 10.1016/j.cortex.2022.05.008.

8. Carbon CC. Wearing Face Masks Strongly Confuses Counterparts in Reading Emotions. Front Psychol. 2020 Sep 25;11:566886. Doi: 10.3389/fpsyg.2020.566886.

9. Gong Q, Li Q, Zhang X, et al. Pre-COVID resting-state brain activity in the fusiform gyrus prospectively predicts social anxiety alterations during the pandemic. Research Square; 2022. DOI: 10.21203/rs.3.rs-2177845/v1.

10. Stanbouly D, Chuang SK. What are the Psychosocial Consequences of Chronic Mask-Wearing in the COVID-19 Pandemic? J Oral Maxillofac Surg. 2021 Sep;79(9):1815-1816. doi: 10.1016/j.joms.2021.04.014.

11. Ellett L, Schlier B, Kingston JL, Zhu C, So SH, Lincoln TM, Morris EMJ, Gaudiano BA. Pandemic paranoia in the general population: international prevalence and sociodemographic profile. Psychol Med. 2022 Sep 6:1-8. doi: 10.1017/S0033291722002975.

12. Lyons M, Bootes E, Brewer G, Stratton K, Centifanti L. "COVID-19 spreads round the planet, and so do paranoid thoughts". A qualitative investigation into personal experiences of psychosis during the COVID-19 pandemic. Curr Psychol. 2021 Oct 12:1-10. doi: 10.1007/s12144-021-02369-0.

13. Pascalis O, de Haan M, Nelson CA. Is face processing species-specific during the first year of life? Science. 2002 May 17;296(5571):1321-3. doi: 10.1126/science.1070223.

14. Ellinwood, E.H. Perception of faces: Disorders in organic and psychopathological states. Psych Quar 43, 622–646 (1969). https://doi.org/10.1007/BF01564275

15. Żochowska A, Jakuszyk P, Nowicka MM, Nowicka A. Are covered faces eye-catching for us? The impact of masks on attentional processing of self and other faces during the COVID-19 pandemic. Cortex. 2022 Apr;149:173-187. doi: 10.1016/j.cortex.2022.01.015. Epub 2022 Feb 10. PMID: 35257944; PMCID: PMC8830153.

16. McKone E, Wan L, Pidcock M, Crookes K, Reynolds K, Dawel A, Kidd E, Fiorentini C. A critical period for faces: Other-race face recognition is improved by childhood but not adult social contact. Sci Rep. 2019 Sep 6;9(1):12820. doi: 10.1038/s41598-019-49202- 0. PMID: 31492907

17. Farmer H, Hewstone M, Spiegler O, Morse H, Saifullah A, Pan X, Fell B, Charlesford J, Terbeck S. Positive intergroup contact modulates fusiform gyrus activity to black and white faces. Sci Rep. 2020 Feb 14;10(1):2700. doi: 10.1038/s41598-020-59633-9.

18. Terbeck S, Kahane G, McTavish S, McCutcheon R, Hewstone M, Savulescu J, Chesterman LP, Cowen PJ, Norbury R. β- Adrenoceptor blockade modulates fusiform gyrus activity to black versus white faces. Psychopharmacology (Berl). 2015 Aug;232(16):2951-8. doi: 10.1007/s00213-015-3929-7.

19. Taubert J, Wardle SG, Ungerleider LG. What does a "face cell" want?'. Prog Neurobiol. 2020 Dec;195:101880. doi: 10.1016/j.pneurobio.2020.101880.

20. Mash C, Bornstein MH, Arterberry ME. Brain dynamics in young infants' recognition of faces: EEG oscillatory activity in response to mother and stranger. Neuroreport. 2013 May 8;24(7):359-63. doi: 10.1097/WNR.0b013e32835f6828

21. Gross CG. Genealogy of the "grandmother cell". Neuroscientist. 2002 Oct;8(5):512-8. doi: 10.1177/107385802237175.

22. Quiroga RQ. Concept cells: the building blocks of declarative memory functions. Nat Rev Neurosci. 2012 Jul 4;13(8):587-97. doi: 10.1038/nrn3251.

23. Gersztenkorn D, Lee AG. Palinopsia revamped: a systematic review of the literature. Surv Ophthalmol. 2015 Jan-Feb;60(1):1- 35. doi: 10.1016/j.survophthal.2014.06.003.

24. Barrelle A, Luauté JP. Capgras Syndrome and Other Delusional Misidentification Syndromes. Front Neurol Neurosci. 2018;42:35-43. doi: 10.1159/000475680.

25. Devinsky O, Davachi L, Santchi C, Quinn BT, Staresina BP, Thesen T. Hyperfamiliarity for faces. Neurology. 2010 Mar 23;74(12):970-4. doi: 10.1212/WNL.0b013e3181d5dc22.

26. Spagna A, Hajhajate D, Liu J, Bartolomeo P. Visual mental imagery engages the left fusiform gyrus, not the early visual cortex: A meta-analysis of neuroimaging evidence. Neurosci Biobehav Rev. 2021 Mar;122:201-217. doi: 10.1016/j.neubiorev.2020.12.029.

27. Hugdahl K, Løberg EM, Jørgensen HA, Lundervold A, Lund A, Green MF, Rund B. Left hemisphere lateralization of auditory hallucinations in schizophrenia: a dichotic listening study. Cogn Neuropsychiatry. 2008 Mar;13(2):166-79. doi: 10.1080/13546800801906808.

28. Hecht D. Cerebral lateralization of pro- and anti-social tendencies. Exp Neurobiol. 2014 Mar;23(1):1-27. doi: 10.5607/en.2014.23.1.1. Epub 2014 Mar 27. PMID: 24737936; PMCID: PMC3984952.

29. Katharina Kunzelmann, Matthias Grieder, Claudia van Swam, Philipp Homan, Stephanie Winkelbeiner, Daniela Hubl, Thomas Dierks. Am I hallucinating, or is my fusiform cortex activated? Functional activation differences in schizophrenia patients with and without hallucinations, The European Journal of Psychiatry, Volume 33, Issue 1, 2019, Pages 1-7, https://doi.org/10.1016/j.ejpsy.2018.06.002.

30. Zhang X, Yao S, Zhu X, Wang X, Zhu X, Zhong M. Gray matter volume abnormalities in individuals with cognitive vulnerability to depression: a voxel-based morphometry study. J Affect Disord. 2012 Feb;136(3):443-52. doi: 10.1016/j.jad.2011.11.005.

31. Harrington A, Oepen G, Spitzer M. Disordered recognition and perception of human faces in acute schizophrenia and experimental psychosis. Compr Psychiatry. 1989 Sep- Oct;30(5):376-84. doi: 10.1016/0010-440x(89)9000

32. Zhang S, Xu X, Li Q, Chen J, Liu S, Zhao W, Cai H, Zhu J, Yu Y. Brain Network Topology and Structural-Functional Connectivity Coupling Mediate the Association Between Gut Microbiota and Cognition. Front Neurosci. 2022 Mar 29;16:814477. doi: 10.3389/fnins.2022.814477. PMID: 35422686; PMCID: PMC9002058.

33. Kindred R, Bates GW. The Influence of the COVID-19 Pandemic on Social Anxiety: A Systematic Review. Int J Environ Res Public Health. 2023 Jan 29;20(3):2362. doi: 10.3390/ijerph20032362.

34. Khalefah MM, Khalifah AM. It is determining the relationship between SARS-CoV-2 infection, dopamine, and COVID-19 complications. J Taibah Univ Med Sci. 2020 Dec;15(6):550-553. doi: 10.1016/j.jtumed.2020.10.006.

Chapter 7
Dopamine and Schizophrenia

Dopamine is certainly implicated in schizophrenia but is it the main character in this drama? Probably not. Excessive dopamine in the brain would generate mania, increased energy, wakefulness, and reward-seeking behavior, rather than delusions, hallucinations, and negative symptoms. In addition, increased prevalence of schizophrenia at higher latitude, association with *Escherichia coli* infections and inflammatory bowel disease, the presence of autoantibodies, or antibodies against microbial components, as well as link to plasticizers and pollutants may not fit the dopamine model.

If not dopamine, then what?

The candidate for the main role in schizophrenia would need to be:

1. Capable of sensing both endogenous and exogenous stimuli

2. Capable of sensing dopamine, dopamine agonists and antagonists as well as environmental pollutants and toxicants.

3. Capable of binding vitamin D, the key latitude sensor,

4. Capable of sensing microbial metabolites, and

5. Possess antiviral/antimicrobial properties.

The only candidate meeting these five criteria is aryl hydrocarbon receptor. Moreover, AhR is also expressed in the intestinal barrier and the blood brain barrier, where it maintains the integrity of tight junctions, therefore regulating barrier permeability.

The antiviral properties of AhR, including anti-SARS-CoV-2, drew the attention of researchers and clinicians to this receptor, implicated in intoxications, infections, and endogenous/exogenous sensing. Moreover, AhR is activated by the oxidized lipids in cell and mitochondrial membrane, previously implicated in psychosis and mood disorders. Furthermore, AhR has the capability of shifting the tryptophan catabolism from serotonin to kynurenine pathway that can lead to the formation of quinolinic acid, a toxin involved in psychopathology.

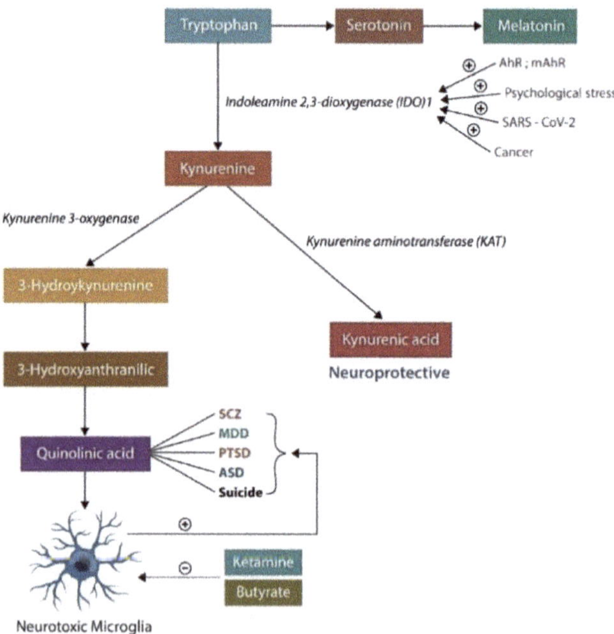

Fig. 7.1 Indoleamine 2,3 dioxygenase is an AhR ligand, an enzyme that shifts tryptophan catabolism from the 5-HT/melatonin pathway to kynurenine. The neurotoxic branch of the kynurenine pathway leads to toxic quinolinic acid formation. Coversely, butyrate generated in the gut by the microbial fermentation of fiber, opposes quinolinic acid-activated microglia and the subsequent pathology.

Like butyrate, ketamine also inhibits quinolonic acid, alleviating the symptoms of depression.

When the DA hypothesis was developed in the 1950s, many characteristics of SCZ were poorly defined. For example, autoantibodies, comorbidity with inflammatory bowel disease (IBD), higher prevalence in northern regions, and association with pollutants and plasticizers were unknown. Over time, the DA hypothesis was revised twice to consider genetic and epigenetic factors. However, the role of microbes and viruses in SMI pathogenesis was never adequately explored.

Studies during the COVID-19 pandemic found that the SARS-CoV-2 virus can induce cognitive deficits, of which the patients themselves were unaware, demonstrating impaired insight (anosognosia). In addition, these patients exhibited peripheral monocytosis (defined as 7.35% or more of the total number of leukocytes). The correlation between monocytes and anosognosia is not limited to COVID-19, as it was reported earlier in the context of HIV-associated neurocognitive disorder (HAND) (1). This is significant as monocyte levels are also elevated in SCZ, where most patients exhibit anosognosia (2) (3). Indeed, a recent study found that during the preclinical phase of SCZ, patients demonstrate monocytosis and increased microbial translocation markers, further linking gut microbes to this pathology (4). Moreover, upregulated blood monocytes were documented during the transition phase from mild cognitive impairment (MCI) to Alzheimer's disease (AD), connecting bacterial translocation with neurodegenerative disorders (5) (6). In this regard, microbes and LPS were found in AD brains, further linking bacteria to cognition and insight (7) (8). Peripheral monocytes can infiltrate the CNS and differentiate into microglia, cells that, under pathological circumstances, can engage in the aberrant phagocytosis of healthy neurons, leading to neurodegeneration. SCZ-related cognitive deficit, probably including anosognosia, may be explained by this pathology (9) (10).

The cholinergic anti-inflammatory pathway (CAP) is a brain-to-periphery neural loop mediated by alpha7 nicotinic acetylcholine receptors (α7nAChRs) expressed by neurons, immune cells, and IECs (Figure 7.2). CAP likely participates in interoceptive awareness and regulates intestinal permeability, reporting gut status to the insula (11) (12). Interoceptive awareness, or simply interoception, refers to directing attention to the clues inside the body, including respiration, heartbeat beat, or pain. It is believed that von Economo neurons (VENS) in the IC (insular cortex) and ACC (anterior cingulate cortex) are master regulators of interoceptive awareness.

Patients with SMI often do not feel pain the way other people do. Throughout my career, I came in contact, usually in the emergency room, with SCZ patients with self-injurious behavior, who mutilated themselves intentionally yet seemed unaware of their injuries or the pain they must elicit. For example, I recall a young man who frequently put his fingers under the door hinges and then slammed the door, fracturing his fingers. When asked about pain, he denied it and replied: "Angels feel no pain." Although he was kept in locked door seclusion, he tried to engage in the same behavior each time he was released.

Addiction medicine studies have found that acetylcholine (ACh) and nicotine can activate IC, ameliorating anosognosia and suggesting a link between insight and cholinergic pathways (13) (14). Moreover, CAP likely mediates "cholinergic behavior" (addiction, emotion, and motivation) induced by ACh or nicotine, probably explaining the excessive smoking in patients with SCZ (15) (16). Indeed, nicotine was also demonstrated to improve spatial neglect in stroke patients, suggesting that anosognosia is driven, at least in part, by the cholinergic pathways (17) (18). (Figure 7.2).

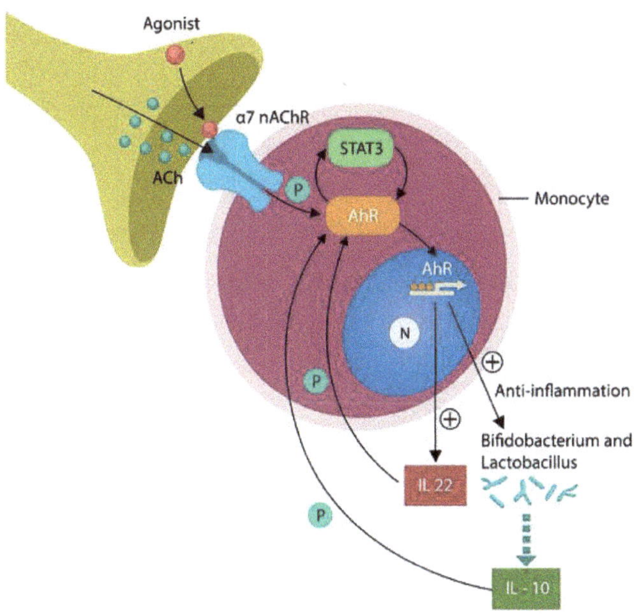

Fig. 7.2 shows interoceptive awareness. At the molecular level, insight is likely driven by α7nAChRs, which connect CAP to the AhR/STAT3/IL-22 axis. Beneficial gut microbes, such as Bifidobacterium and Lactobacillus, release IL-10, a cytokine that provides feedback to the IC via STAT3 phosphorylation. IL-22 (related to IL-10) also phosphorylates STAT3, closing the feedback loop.

AhR, discovered in the 1970s, has been known as the dioxin receptor, a protein expressed in many tissues, including the gut barrier and BBB. It was later revealed that several AhR ligands are molecules involved in neurodegeneration and SMI. For example, gut microbes and their metabolites, vitamin D3, pollutants, DA, clozapine, 5HT, melatonin, and carbidopa are AhR ligands. On the other hand, aripiprazole binds the heat shock protein 90 (HSP90), a chaperone that prevents AhR entry into the nucleus to promote the expression of many genes, probably including SCZ risk genes.

5-HT activates AhR in IECs, shifting tryptophan catabolism to the kynurenine pathway. Indeed, SSRIs were demonstrated to activate indoleamine 2,3-dioxygenase 1 (IDO1) directly (Fig. 7.1).

AhR also regulates TJs and cellular senescence, a phenotype characterizing SCZ, PTSD, and neurodegenerative disorders. Senescence affects the neuronal cells and the peripheral tissues, emphasizing the systemic nature of SMI. Indeed, the senescent intestinal barrier has been associated with microbial migration from the GI tract (where microbiota is immunologically tolerated) into the systemic circulation (where the host immune system vehemently attacks microbes) (20).

The immune reaction to translocated microbes and their molecules is marked by the release of proinflammatory cytokines and antibodies against microbial receptors that may trigger neuropsychiatric pathology. For example, microbiota-derived lipopolysaccharide (LPS), an antigen of Gram-negative bacteria, was detected in the brains of patients with AD and SCZ. This is significant as it highlights the role of microbial translocation in the etiopathogenesis of these disorders (21) (22). Another example of microbial involvement in mental illness is urinary tract infection (UTI)-associated psychosis. This condition is usually triggered by *Escherichia coli (E. coli),* further emphasizing this specific bacterium's role in neuropathology (23). Indeed, this pathogen was connected to the 2011 outbreak in Germany in which some patients experienced first psychotic episode.

The following section will discuss several potential antipsychotic strategies, including non-DA agents and microbiota-derived compounds.

Muscarinic antipsychotic drugs

From the discovery of chlorpromazine in the 1950s to the present, antipsychotic drugs were designed to block primarily dopaminergic transmission at the level of postsynaptic neurons. Currently, muscarinic cholinergic receptor agonists, such as xanomeline, comprise a novel class of DA-independent antipsychotic drugs, indicating that blocking DA neurotransmission is not the only mechanism that can avert psychosis. Indeed, cholinergic antipsychotic properties have been previously known.

Plasmalogens replacement therapy

Plasmalogens are glycerophospholipids found in cell membranes and serum lipoproteins. Dysfunctional plasmalogen was demonstrated in several neuropsychiatric disorders, including SCZ (24)

Plasmalogens affect the biophysical properties of membranes as they lower fluidity, optimizing receptor alignment and neurotransmission. Approximately 20% of all phospholipids in the human body are plasmalogens, which contain ethanolamine or choline. Plasmalogen replacement therapy (PRT) restores the physiological plasmalogen levels, facilitating disease progression. Decreased plasmalogen content has also been reported in normal aging, SMI, neurodegenerative, and metabolic disorders (25) (26).

Garth L Nicolson started membrane lipid replacement (MLR) to treat veterans with Gulf War Illness (27). Replacement therapy refers to the oral administration of natural glycerophospholipids to restore physiological levels of lipids in cell/neuronal membranes. Lately, this strategy has attracted increased interest as potentially valuable for a variety of pathologies, including neuropsychiatric disorders, cancer, neurological, and metabolic conditions.

Plasmalogen replacement therapy (PRT) is a specialized form of MLR that relies on small molecules to increase membrane plasmalogen levels, aiming to improve disease outcomes. Another advantage of PRT is the ability to lower cholesterol levels naturally. Indeed, plasmalogens have earned the name of "natural statins" and should be used instead of statins in psychiatric patients.

Butyrate

Butyrate, a SCFA, is the product of gut microbiota fiber fermentation in the colon. Butyrate crosses the BBB and reaches the brain, positively affecting SCZ and MDD. It is currently in clinical trials for cognitive and negative symptoms of SCZ (28) (29). More details on the progress of these studies can be found at ClinicalTrials.gov under the identifier NCT03010865.

Butyrate is now available as a dietary supplement, marketed by BodyBio as sodium butyrate. Of course, dietary fiber can help generate more butyrate in the GI tract; however, in the presence of dysbiosis, the fibrinolytic, butyrate-producing microbes, such as *Roseburia intestinalis, Faecalibacterium prasunitzi, and Eubacterium* may be unavailable. Since dietary fiber and fermenting microbes are necessary for generating SCFA, 35–50 g of fiber daily is required to synthesize sufficient butyrate (30). In general, the population of Western countries consumes an average of 10–20 g per day, requiring butyrate supplementation.

Propionate

Propionate is another SCFA produced primarily by the *Bacteroidetes phylum.* Interestingly, the second-generation antipsychotic drugs may selectively eliminate this species, likely leading to weight gain by propionate depletion (31). Since both butyrate and propionate act on intestinal G protein-coupled receptors (GPCRs), including GPR41 and GPR43, expressed by intestinal L-cells, they promote the release of anorexigenic hormones, glucagon-like peptide-1 (GLP-1), and peptide YY (PYY) (32). Indeed, SCFA induces weight loss by acting on the hypothalamic POMC/CART neurons, indicating that the antipsychotic and metabolic actions of SCFA are highly intertwined.

Taken together, as opposed to the AhR model, the DA hypothesis remains unable to explain certain aspects of SCZ, such as high comorbidity with IBD, association with *E. coli infections, prevalence at higher latitudes*, and link with pollutants and plasticizers. Moreover, DA protects the brain against both parenchymal loss and depletion of gamma oscillations; therefore, chronic blockade of brain DA pathways may lead to iatrogenic cortical thinning, decreasing the chance of sustained recovery.

Chapter 7 References:

1. Juengst, S.; Skidmore, E.; Pramuka, M.; McCue, M.; Becker, J. Factors contributing to impaired self-awareness of cognitive functioning in an HIV positive and at-risk population. Disabil. Rehabil. 2011, 34, 19–25

2. Zhu, X.; Zhou, J.; Zhu, Y.; Yan, F.; Han, X.; Tan, Y.; Li, R. Neutrophil/lymphocyte, platelet/lymphocyte and monocyte/lymphocyte ratios in schizophrenia. Australas Psychiatry 2022, 30, 95–99. [Google Scholar] [CrossRef] [PubMed]

3. Melbourne, J.K.; Rosen, C.; Chase, K.A.; Feiner, B.; Sharma, R.P. Monocyte Transcriptional Profiling Highlights a Shift in Immune Signatures Throughout Illness in Schizophrenia. Front. Psychiatry 2021, 12, 649494.

4. Weber, N.S.; Gressitt, K.L.; Cowan, D.N.; Niebuhr, D.W.; Yolken, R.H.; Severance, E.G., Monocyte activation detected before a diagnosis of schizophrenia in the US Military New Onset Psychosis Project (MNOPP). Schizophr. Res. 2018, 197, 465–469

5. Munawara, U.; Catanzaro, M.; Xu, W.; Tan, C.; Hirokawa, K.; Bosco, N.; Dumoulin, D.; Khalil, A.; Larbi, A.; Lévesque, S.; et al. Hyperactivation of monocytes and macrophages in MCI patients contributes to the progression of Alzheimer's disease. Immun. Aging 2021, 18, 29. [Google Scholar] [CrossRef]

6. Migliorelli, R.; Tesón, A.; Sabe, L.; Petracca, G.; Petracchi, M.; Leiguarda, R.; E Starkstein, S. Anosognosia in Alzheimer's disease: A study of associated factors. J. Neuropsychiatry 1995, 7, 338–344

7. Kim, H.S.; Kim, S.; Shin, S.J.; Park, Y.H.; Nam, Y.; Kim, C.W.; Lee, K.W.; Kim, S.-M.; Jung, I.D.; Yang, H.D.; et al. Gram-negative bacteria and their lipopolysaccharides in Alzheimer's disease:

Pathologic roles and therapeutic implications. Transl. Neurodegener. 2021, 10, 49. [Google Scholar] [CrossRef]

8. Zhao, Y.; Cong, L.; Lukiw, W.J. Lipopolysaccharide (LPS) Accumulates in Neocortical Neurons of Alzheimer's Disease (AD) Brain and Impairs Transcription in Human Neuronal-Glial Primary Co-cultures. Front. Aging Neurosci. 2017, 9, 407.

9. Kim, H.S.; Kim, S.; Shin, S.J.; Park, Y.H.; Nam, Y.; Kim, C.W.; Lee, K.W.; Kim, S.-M.; Jung, I.D.; Yang, H.D.; et al. Gram-negative bacteria and their lipopolysaccharides in Alzheimer's disease: Pathologic roles and therapeutic implications. Transl. Neurodegener. 2021, 10, 49. [Google Scholar] [CrossRef]

10. Zhao, Y.; Cong, L.; Lukiw, W.J. Lipopolysaccharide (LPS) Accumulates in Neocortical Neurons of Alzheimer's Disease (AD) Brain and Impairs Transcription in Human Neuronal-Glial Primary Co-cultures. Front. Aging Neurosci. 2017, 9, 407.

11. Borovikova, L.V.; Ivanova, S.; Zhang, M.; Yang, H.; Botchkina, G.I.; Watkins, L.R.; Wang, H.; Abumrad, N.; Eaton, J.W.; Tracey, K.J. Vagus nerve stimulation attenuates the systemic inflammatory response to endotoxin. Nature 2000, 405, 458–462. [Google Scholar] [CrossRef]

12. Yang, X.; Zhao, C.; Chen, X.; Jiang, L.; Su, X. Monocytes primed with GTS-21/α7 nAChR (nicotinic acetylcholine receptor) agonist develop anti-inflammatory memory. QJM Int. J. Med. 2017, 110, 437–445

13. Sha Paciorek, A.; Skora, L. Vagus Nerve Stimulation as a Gateway to Interoception. Front. Psychol. 2020, 11, 1659.

14. Karczmar, A.G. Cholinergic Behaviors, Emotions, and the "Self." J. Mol. Neurosci. 2013, 53, 291–297. [Google Scholar] [CrossRef]

15. Critchley, H.D.; Wiens, S.; Rotshtein, P.; Öhman, A.; Dolan, R.J. Neural systems supporting interoceptive awareness. Nat. Neurosci. 2004, 7, 189–195. [Google Scholar] [CrossRef] [Green Version]

16. Damasio, A.; Damasio, H.; Tranel, D. Persistence of Feelings and Sentience after Bilateral Damage of the Insula. Cereb. Cortex 2012, 23, 833–846. [Google Scholar] [CrossRef] [Green Version]

17. Devue, C.; Collette, F.; Balteau, E.; Degueldre, C.; Luxen, A.; Maquet, P.; Brédart, S. Here I am: The cortical correlates of visual self-recognition. Brain Res. 2007, 1143, 169–182.

18. Lucas, N.; Saj, A.; Schwartz, S.; Ptak, R.; Schnider, A.; Thomas, C.; Conne, P.; Leroy, R.; Pavin, S.; Diserens, K.; et al. Effects of Pro-Cholinergic Treatment in Patients Suffering from Spatial Neglect. Front. Hum. Neurosci. 2013, 7, 574. [Google Scholar] [CrossRef] [Green Version]

19. Rus, C.P., de Vries, B.E.K., de Vries, I.E.J. et al. Treatment of 95 post-Covid patients with SSRIs. Sci Rep 13, 18599 (2023). https://doi.org/10.1038/s41598-023-45072-9

20. Sharma R. Emerging Interrelationship Between the Gut Microbiome and Cellular Senescence in the Context of Aging and Disease: Perspectives and Therapeutic Opportunities. Probiotics Antimicrob Proteins. 2022 Aug;14(4):648-663. doi: 10.1007/s12602-021-09903-3.

21. Kim, H.s., Kim, S., Shin, S.J. et al. Gram-negative bacteria and their lipopolysaccharides in Alzheimer's disease: pathologic roles and therapeutic implications. Transl Neurodegener 10, 49 (2021). https://doi.org/10.1186/s40035-021-00273-y

22. Severance EG, Yolken RH. From Infection to the Microbiome: An Evolving Role of Microbes in Schizophrenia. Curr Top Behav Neurosci. 2020;44:67-84. doi: 10.1007/7854_2018_84.

23. Mostafa S, Miller BJ. Antibiotic-associated psychosis during treatment of urinary tract infections: a systematic review. J Clin Psychopharmacol. 2014 Aug;34(4):483-90. doi: 10.1097/JCP.0000000000000150.

24. Kaddurah-Daouk R, McEvoy J, Baillie R, Zhu H, K Yao J, Nimgaonkar VL, Buckley PF, Keshavan MS, Georgiades A, Nasrallah HA. Impaired plasmalogens in patients with schizophrenia. Psychiatry Res. 2012 Aug 15;198(3):347-52. doi: 10.1016/j.psychres.2012.02.019. Epub 2012 Apr 16. PMID: 22513041.

25. Ginsberg L., Rafique S., Xuereb J.H., Rapoport S.I., Gershfeld N.L. Disease and Anatomic Specificity of Ethanolamine Plasmalogen Deficiency in Alzheimer's Disease Brain. Brain Res. 1995;698:223–226. doi: 10.1016/0006-8993(95)00931-F. [PubMed] [CrossRef] [Google Scholar]

26. Olanow C.W., Stern M.B., Sethi K. The Scientific and Clinical Basis for the Treatment of Parkinson Disease (2009) Neurology. 2009;72:S1–S136. doi: 10.1212/WNL.0b013e3181a1d44c.

27. Nicolson G. Continuing research into Gulf War illness. Science. 2001 May 4;292(5518):853. PMID: 11341275.

28. Li X, Fan X, Yuan X, Pang L, Hu S, Wang Y, Huang X, Song X. The Role of Butyric Acid in Treatment Response in Drug-Naïve First Episode Schizophrenia. Front Psychiatry. 2021 Aug 23;12:724664. doi: 10.3389/fpsyt.2021.724664.

29. Caspani G, Kennedy S, Foster JA, Swann J. Gut microbial metabolites in depression: understanding the biochemical mechanisms. Microb Cell. 2019 Sep 27;6(10):454-481. doi: 10.15698/mic2019.10.693.

30. Slavin J. Fiber and prebiotics: mechanisms and health benefits. Nutrients. (2013) 5:1417–35. 10.3390/nu5041417

31. Prior TI, Baker GB. Interactions between the cytochrome P450 system and the second-generation antipsychotics. J Psychiatry Neurosci. (2003) 28:99–112

32. Chambers ES, Preston T, Frost G, Morrison DJ. Role of gut microbiota-generated short-chain fatty acids in metabolic and cardiovascular health. Curr Nutr Rep. (2018) 7:198–206. 10.1007/s13668-018-0248-8

Chapter 8
Serotonin and Morality

It is generally accepted that the human brain possesses an inbuilt moral system independent of individual beliefs, ethnicity, or religion. For example, taking someone's life or property is negatively sanctioned in every culture or belief system, while social fairness, empathy, and pro-social behaviors are viewed in a positive light (1). C.G. Jung believed that morality is not imposed from outside (society) but is endogenous and inbuilt: "We have it in ourselves from the start." Neuroimaging studies have shown that the human moral compass is probably located in the insula and driven by the von Economo neurons (VENS) signaling via 5-HT.

VENS are large, spindle-shaped projection neurons that are more numerous in the right hemisphere than in the left. These cells are believed to process moral dilemmas, pro-social information, empathy, interoception, and free will (2) (3).

VENS also processes stimulus anticipation, an anticipatory wave originating in IC and ACC that occurs up to 15 seconds before the actual action (4). This is significant as machines can sense and translate stimulus anticipation into action, opening the possibility of thought-operated devices. These tools would be handy for patients with poor mobility, such as stroke and spinal cord injury.

Excessive activation of IC and ACC occurs in anxiety and MDD and can be reversed by SSRIs, suggesting once more that these drugs interfere with the function of VENS (5). Other studies found that 5-HT promotes prosocial behavior and enhances harm aversion (6). In this study, a single dose of citalopram altered the moral judgment of volunteers playing the Ultimatum Game. Ultimatum Game consists of dividing a fixed amount of money into two parts; individuals taking SSRIs showed a likelihood of accepting unfair offers to avoid harming the other player, suggesting that with upregulated 5HT, emotion overrides morality (6) (7).

VENS are believed to process moral dilemmas in situations that require morally unacceptable actions for a greater good.

Below are some examples of moral dilemmas:

1. You are at the wheel of a runaway trolley, quickly approaching a fork in the tracks. On the tracks going to the left is a group of five railway workmen. On the tracks going to the right is a single railway workman. If you do nothing, the trolley will proceed to the left, causing the deaths of the five workmen. The only way to avoid the deaths of these workmen is to hit a switch on your dashboard that will cause the trolley to proceed to the right, causing the death of the single workman. Would you hit the switch to avoid the deaths of the five workmen?

2. Enemy soldiers have taken over your village. They have orders to kill everyone. You have hidden in the basement of a large house along with other people. Outside, you hear the voices of soldiers who have come to search the house. Your baby begins to cry loudly. You cover his mouth to block the sound. If you remove your hand from his mouth, the soldiers will hear his crying and will kill you, your baby, and the other people hiding in the basement. To save yourself and the others, you must smother your child to death. Would you smother your child in order to save yourself and other people?

3. A working individual is the caregiver for their mother, who has cancer. On the one hand, they want to provide proper care and miss work, but on the other, they fear losing their job. The individual is torn between two responsibilities. If they lose their job, they will not have the resources to care for the mother, while if they miss work less, they will not be able to provide quality care.

Table 1. Examples of moral dilemmas

This SSRI-induced emotional bias is problematic as these agents may increase the susceptibility to societal manipulation or exploitation. In general, people exposed to these drugs avoid confrontation even when witnessing injustice. Moreover, SSRIs can also induce apathy, which, along with harm aversion and willingness to accept unfair scenarios, may lead to iatrogenic self-deprecation and tolerance of social unfairness, processes that could manipulate the behavior of a population (8). Furthermore, upregulated 5-HT may increase the behavioral adverse effects of fluoride, a halogen added to drinking water since 1945 (9). Moreover, the bacterial degradation of 5-HT in environmental waters generates more fluoride, impacting aquatic life and the water consumed by humans (10).

Von Economo neurons (VENS)

Constantin von Economo was born in 1876 in Braila, Romania, but grew up in Trieste, a city in Italy which at that time belonged to Austria. He studied neurology, histology, and psychiatry in Paris and Munich, where he worked with Emil Kraepelin and Alois Alzheimer. In 1925, von Economo described a distinct group of large neurons known today as VENS. Over the past 100 years, VENS have been found in several superior mammals, including apes, elephants, and dolphins, and play a key role in self-awareness, interoception, and empathy.

Frontotemporal dementia behavioral variant (bvFTD) is a unique neurodegenerative disorder that "kills" VENs preferentially without affecting the other brain cells, presenting an opportunity to study what happens in the absence of these neurons.

In bvFTD, young onset dementia (YOD) that starts before the age of 65, memory can remain intact for many years, making it difficult to differentiate this disorder from SCZ, antisocial personality disorder (APD), or bipolar pathology.

Criminal behavior, a hallmark of bvFTD, was demonstrated in over 50% of patients and occurs later in life, taking the family and friends by surprise. Indeed, families are facing an unusual situation as their loved ones, usually described as caring, friendly, and pleasant throughout their lives, have become careless, calloused, selfish, and remorseless. Usually, bvFTD patients had regular and successful careers, with no history of mental illness, drugs, or lawbreaking. The personality change occurs slowly over several years, and family members rarely consider this condition an illness.

A criminal violation followed by incarceration is often the first symptom alerting the family that there may be more than meets the eye. Moreover, as bvFTD patients exhibit no cognitive impairment, they are usually convicted or admitted to psychiatric hospitals.

At the cellular level, there is a selective loss of VENS, the "empathy cells" known for processing self-awareness, social cognition, morality, and emotional intelligence. Selective VENS loss in bvFTD with subsequent criminal behavior usually brings these individuals into the criminal justice system.

The selective elimination of VENs in bvFTD may be due to their large size, which makes them more susceptible to plasma membrane lipid oxidation and mitochondrial loss. The discovery of VENS and their link to criminal violations indicates that developmental psychopathy likely involves the same cells in IC and ACC.

I am presenting four cases from Patton State Hospital in San Bernardino County, California, and the surrounding communities to help you better understand bvFTD and VENS pathology.

Case #1 The teacher who shot her neighbor

Ms. KS (initials changed), a Caucasian female, age 68, divorced, retired elementary school teacher, lived alone before admission to Patton State Hospital. Ms. KS did not have a psychiatric history until the age of 56 when she purchased a gun and shot her neighbor in the shoulder. She stated that she attacked the man because he was spying on her and intruded into her house during the night. She was convicted of attempted murder and sent to prison, where her condition deteriorated, prompting her transfer to our forensic institution. KS was diagnosed with SCZ and admitted as a forensic detainee.

During her hospital stay, KS was treated with various antipsychotic drugs with minimal symptomatic relief. She was unaware that she did anything wrong, and her poor insight and impulsivity were documented during her six years at this hospital. Because of poor insight, KS never met the criteria for the conditional release program (CONREP).

In 2014, KS became more forgetful, required assistance with most activities of daily living (ADLs), and changed her dietary preferences. For example, she asked for ice cream daily, although earlier in her life, she had detested ice cream. In time, KS became more apathetic and often refused to get out of bed. The internal medicine consultant performed a dementia workup, but the laboratory studies came back normal, except for mild anemia and a vitamin D level of 29.3 nmol/L. KS scored 25/30 on the Mini Mini-Mental Status Exam (MMSE), and when a Montreal Cognitive Assessment (MoCA) was administered, the score was 23/30, consistent with executive dysfunction. At this point, a neuropsychology consult was called, and after a battery of tests, bvFTD was diagnosed.

With this information, the treatment team petitioned the Court, arguing that KS did not benefit from hospitalization in a forensic institution as she was not expected to recover. The judge agreed with the treating clinicians and ordered placement in a facility specialized in dementia.

Due to the numerous clinical and legal ramifications, this case was featured in the media at the time:

https://www.reuters.com/article/us-crime-dementia-idUSKBN0KE1Q020150105/

https://www.foxnews.com/health/breaking-the-law-may-be-a-sign-of-dementia

https://clbb.mgh.harvard.edu/when-frontotemporal-dementia-leads-to-crime-prosecution-or-protection/

Case #2 The attorney with a sweet tooth

An outpatient we treated in 2013 was 72 years -72-year-old retired attorney arrested because he stole chocolate from a grocery store while casually conversing with the owner. When confronted, he replied: "What's the problem? I have a sweet tooth?". According to the family, the patient came across as careless and indifferent to his children and the spouse, being either apathetic or angry and irritable. For example, when he learned that his son-in-law died unexpectedly, he responded by saying, "Let's go out to eat." According to his wife, his eating habits had changed dramatically, mainly consuming sweets he had previously avoided. When told to eat more nutritious food, he often became angry.

Case #3 The psychiatrist turned a drug dealer

Dr. Joel Stanley Dreyer was a well-respected psychiatrist who practiced in Riverside, California. In the 1990s, Dr. Dreyer was diagnosed with bvFTD but continued to practice psychiatry, and in 2010 was convicted for prescribing, selling, and distributing large amounts of addictive painkillers. As a result of careless prescribing, one person died of an overdose, and Dr. Dreyer was convicted and served ten years in prison despite having been diagnosed with bvFTD before his crime. This case emphasizes that some jurisdictions do not recognize bvFTD as an attenuating circumstance. The court ruling was based on the testimony of the prison psychiatrist, who did not challenge the diagnosis of bvFTD but stated that since not all individuals with this disorder engage in criminal behavior, "direct causality" between Dr. Dreyer's crime and bvFTD could not be established. A detailed history of this case can be found at the link below:

https://story.californiasunday.com/joel-dreyer-criminal-psychiatrist/.

Case #4 The Buick murderer

On July 16, 2003, Mr. GRW, an 83-year-old man, crashed his Buick LeSabre in an open-air market in Santa Monica, California, killing ten and injuring 63 individuals. Despite the catastrophic event he caused, GRW did not express remorse and showed indifference, callousness, and lack of empathy. In the court, he appeared numb, angry, and unapologetic, stating that he was sorry the dead and injured could not "enjoy the value of their purchases." No psychiatric evaluation was ordered because there was no previous history. However, criminal behavior may often represent the first symptom of bvFTD. Despite never being diagnosed with a neurodegenerative disorder, people who knew GRW noticed a drastic personality change in the years before this event, indicative of bvFTD. His neighbors, friends, and pastor described GRW as caring, pleasant, and friendly. He had been married for over 60 years, was compassionate, involved in people's lives, and, after retirement, volunteered with various civic organizations. Although GRW was never officially diagnosed with bvFTD, this case illustrates the difficulty clinicians encounter because this neurodegenerative disorder affects executive function, leaving memory intact for many years. Indeed, shortly before his crime, GRW was able to pass his DMV license renewal test, suggesting that his memory was unaffected. Since in California, drivers who are 70 or older must renew their driver's license in person, GRW did not raise a dementia red flag with the DMV worker.

Taken together, it appears that human morality is driven by 5-HT signaling with VENS. SSRI-upregulated 5-HT alters the function of this neuro-moral network, predisposing it to empathy and altruism at the expense of self-deprecation. Conversely, loss of VENS in bvFTD results in danger to others due to the absence of 5-HT target cells.

Chapter 8 References:

1. Mendez MF. The neurobiology of moral behavior: review and neuropsychiatric implications. CNS Spectr. 2009 Nov;14(11):608-20. Doi: 10.1017/s1092852900023853.

2. Hallett M. Volitional control of movement: the physiology of free will. Clin Neurophysiol. 2007 Jun;118(6):1179-92. doi: 10.1016/j.clinph.2007.03.019.

3. Lavazza A. Free Will and Neuroscience: From Explaining Freedom Away to New Ways of Operationalizing and Measuring It. Front Hum Neurosci. 2016 Jun 1;10:262. doi: 10.3389/fnhum.2016.00262.

4. Lovero KL, Simmons AN, Aron JL, Paulus MP. Anterior insular cortex anticipates impending stimulus significance. Neuroimage. 2009 Apr 15;45(3):976-83. doi: 10.1016/j.neuroimage.2008.12.070.

5. Alan N Simmons, Estibaliz Arce, Kathryn L Lovero, Murray B Stein, Martin P Paulus, Subchronic SSRI administration reduces insula response during affective anticipation in healthy volunteers, International Journal of Neuropsychopharmacology, Volume 12, Issue 8, September 2009, Pages 1009–1020, https://doi.org/10.1017/S1461145709990149

6. Crockett MJ, Clark L, Hauser MD, Robbins TW. Serotonin selectively influences moral judgment and behavior through effects on harm aversion. Proc Natl Acad Sci U S A. 2010 Oct 5;107(40):17433-8. doi: 10.1073/pnas.1009396107.

7. Tost H, Meyer-Lindenberg A. I fear for you: a role for serotonin in moral behavior. Proc Natl Acad Sci U S A. 2010 Oct 5;107(40):17071-2. doi: 10.1073/pnas.1012545107.

8. Masdrakis VG, Markianos M, Baldwin DS. Apathy associated with antidepressant drugs: a systematic review. Acta Neuropsychiatr. 2023 Aug;35(4):189-204. doi: 10.1017/neu.2023.6.

9. Lu F, Zhang Y, Trivedi A, Jiang X, Chandra D, Zheng J, Nakano Y, Abduweli Uyghurturk D, Jalai R, Onur SG, Mentes A, DenBesten PK. Fluoride-related changes in behavioral outcomes may be related to increased serotonin. Physiol Behav. 2019 Jul 1;206:76-83. doi: 10.1016/j.physbeh.2019.02.017.

10. Khan MF, Murphy CD. Bacterial degradation of the anti-depressant drug fluoxetine produces trifluoroacetic acid and fluoride ions. Appl Microbiol Biotechnol. 2021 Dec;105(24):9359-9369. doi: 10.1007/s00253-021-11675-3

Chapter 9
Ironing Out the Gray Matter

Iron is a crucial nutrient for the human body but can also be toxic as it forms reactive oxygen species (ROS). For this reason, iron metabolism is tightly regulated both at the organismal and cellular levels. Senescent cells upregulate intracellular iron, probably due to impaired ferritin breakdown. Ferritin is an iron-storing protein that prevents toxicity by sequestering this metal.

There is a growing body of evidence that iron accumulation in senescent microglia activates these cells, converting them to neurotoxicity, a phenotype known for eliminating viable neurons and synapses (1) (2) (3). Indeed, neurotoxic microglia engage in "eating" live neurons and convert astrocytes into neurotoxic cells, further contributing to GMV reduction.

Lactate, the metabolic fuel preferred by cancer cells, is a product of glycolysis, a cellular metabolism that does not require mitochondrial participation.

Excessive lactate can activate lactylation of histone proteins, an epigenetic modification associated with behavioral disturbances (4) (5). Lactate modulates iron metabolism via hepcidin, a liver hormone in charge of iron exit from cells, including the neurons (6).

Lactylation plays a major role in disseminating neurotoxicity from senescent microglia to astrocytes (7) (8). For example, iron, as well as lactylation of histone three lysine 18 (H3K18), can trigger astrocytic neurotoxicity and subsequent GMV reduction.

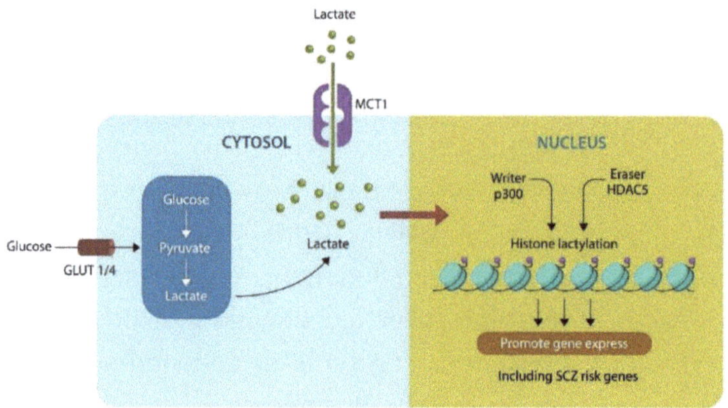

Fig.9.1 Lactate is derived from glucose metabolism or brought into the cell by lactate transporter MCT1. The nucleus histone proteins are lactylated, promoting gene expression, including the SCZ-risk genes. Lactylation of histone three lysine 18 (H3K18) can trigger neurotoxicity in astrocytes, leading to neuronal loss by the absence of support from this glia.

Microglia are hypervigilant resident brain macrophages that surveil the CNS microenvironment for debris and pathogens while facilitating neurogenesis. Novel studies have shown that specific microglial phenotypes may become neurotoxic, engaging not only in the elimination of synapses and intact neurons but also driving neurotoxicity in astrocytes.

Cellular senescence is a phenotype adopted by cells in distress to avoid apoptosis (cell death), malignant transformation, or irreparable DNA damage. Cellular senescence averts cancer; however, the inflammation promoted by SASP can paradoxically promote tumorigenesis (9). In addition, SASP has been shown to hasten gray matter depletion, promoting cortical thinning, a pathology associated with aggressive behavior. In addition, senescent cells inhibit rapid brain oscillations, especially the gamma waves related to consciousness (30-100 HZ).

In the brain, senescent neurons can undergo ferroptosis if astrocytes are neurotoxic or senescence if astrocytes are healthy and capable of supplying the neurons with the necessary antioxidants, such as glutathione peroxidase 4 (GPX-4) and ferritin, as well as "fresh" mitochondria. As SSRIs can facilitate this process, it suggests a non-synaptic mechanism for combating depression (10). In other words, depression may improve, especially energy, due to the transfer of healthy mitochondria from astrocytes.

Cellular senescence was believed to be irreversible; however, newer studies have demonstrated that aging cells can be rejuvenated via phosphatidylinositol-dependent kinase 1 (PDK1) inhibitors, including the BBB-crossing OSU-03012 (11). Aside from PDK1 inhibitors, blocking the downstream protein kinase B (Akt)/ glycogen synthase kinase three β (GSK3 β) pathway may accomplish the same effect (12). Indeed, many drugs, including some antipsychotics and lithium, inhibit GSK3 β, suggesting that natural compounds exerting this effect may be beneficial against affective and psychotic disorders. For example, kaempferol, a polyphenol, berberine, and membrane lipid replacement (MLR) may exhibit antipsychotic properties (13).

Brain oscillations and gray matter volume loss

Iron-activated microglia and subsequent aberrant neuronal phagocytosis contribute to GMV depletion, a phenomenon closely associated with losing gamma-band oscillations on EEG. In addition, GMV reduction predisposes aggressive behavior, linking together cortical thinning, loss of rapid oscillations, and risk of violence, suggesting a biological triad for predicting violence.

Oscillations or vibrations are fundamental properties of all matter, including biological systems (14) (15) (16). For example, simple organisms, including yeast, were shown to communicate with their counterparts via synchronized glycolytic oscillations, indicating that this is a highly conserved mechanism (17). Indeed, specific frequencies may be ideal for encoding and transmitting information, suggesting that oscillations may play a key role in neurotransmission, functioning along with synaptic and volume transmission (18) (19).

How brain oscillatory frequencies relate to neuronal network information processing is unclear. However, a growing body of evidence has demonstrated that neurons can function as oscillators, making cognition possible by synchronizing (bringing to the same frequency) various oscillators in other brain areas (20) (21). Adaptive resonance theory (ART) and communication through coherence (CTC) are two neurophysiological models that utilize inter-region synchronization to explain information processing (22) (23). For example, the auditory cortex generates spontaneous oscillations in response to the exogenous oscillatory input, synchronizing with the environment (24).

Synchronized oscillations may engender a body-wide communication platform, connecting structures inside and outside the CNS. For example, GI tract microbes entrain "brain-like" oscillations, contributing to the gut-brain axis (25) (26) (27) (28) (29) (30). This is in line with another novel discovery that oscillations drive the expression of microbial genes, cell cycle progression, and antibiotic resistance (31) (32) (33). Furthermore, the GI tract microbiota oscillations are driven by metabolism, suggesting that the enteric nervous system (ENS) may function as an oscillatory sensor, conveying this information to the CNS.

Interoceptive awareness and oscillations

Synchronization of oscillatory activity is believed to drive human awareness, while desynchronization and inhibition of inter-regional signaling induce unconsciousness as observed during general anesthesia (34) (35) (36). For example, gamma oscillations promote connectivity between different brain regions, which is essential for body movement, memory, and emotion (37) (38). Gamma waves drive interoceptive awareness, emotion, and cognition, contributing to emotional intelligence, the ability to comprehend events from the point of view of another person (39) (40). Moreover, awareness of one's limbs, body parts, pain, or well-being constitutes insight (interoceptive awareness). In psychopathology, including SCZ, anosognosia (poor insight) is a marker of aggressive behaviors (41).

Insight, the role of local hormones and inhibitory neurons

Like GMV reduction, insight is rarely studied by neuropsychiatry, although poor insight is the most consistent symptom of SCZ. It is believed that local γ -aminobutyric acid (GABA) neurons generating somatostatin (SST) produce gamma oscillations associated with higher brain functions, including insight (42) (43). In contrast, dysfunctional gamma oscillations were linked to CNS pathology, including AD, PD, and SCZ, connecting illness insight with the loss of GABA interneurons (44) (45) (46) (47) (Fig 2).

The brain on death row

Several studies have examined EEG oscillations in the perpetrators of violent crimes on death row. Diminished or absent gamma frequencies were demonstrated in the inmates with SCZ and violent behaviors, suggesting that impaired cognition and deficient insight increase the odds of violent crime (48). Low EEG activity in the right prefrontal cortex and increased in the striatum reflect cortico-subcortical desynchronization, a hallmark of criminal behavior (49) (50) (51). Altered information processing in the frontal lobe or hypofrontality, likely leads to dysfunctional synchronization with subcortical stimuli and inability to distinguish reality from imaginary content (52).

Together, gamma frequencies facilitate the synchronization of various brain areas, increasing insight and lowering violent behavior. Loss of the gamma band promotes aggression as desynchronization blurs the distinction between reality and imagined scenarios.

Lowering criminal behaviors by enhancing gamma band

Since decreased or absent high-frequency gamma oscillations promote violent crime, is it possible to lower crime by entraining gamma frequencies?

Along this line, noninvasive stimulatory techniques, such as low-level laser therapy (LLLT), transcranial alternating current stimulation (tACS), or transcranial magnetic stimulation (TMS), may enhance the gamma band, facilitating synchronization to improve insight and prevent criminal behavior (53) (54) (55) (56). Indeed, a 40 Hz auditory steady-state response (ASSR) was shown to promote gamma waves, opening novel therapeutic avenues of noninvasive treatments for anosognosia and negative symptoms of SCZ (57) (58) (59) (60). In addition, local SST has been implicated in CNS synchronization and brain plasticity, suggesting that loss of this hormone may promote negative and cognitive symptoms in SCZ (61) (62). Indeed, aging downregulates SST and upregulates the non-pituitary growth hormone (npGH), inducing premature neuronal senescence, which decreases the gamma band (63) (64).

Since SST-generating GABAergic interneurons are depleted in SCZ, stimulation at 40 Hz may entrain this frequency in the cortex.

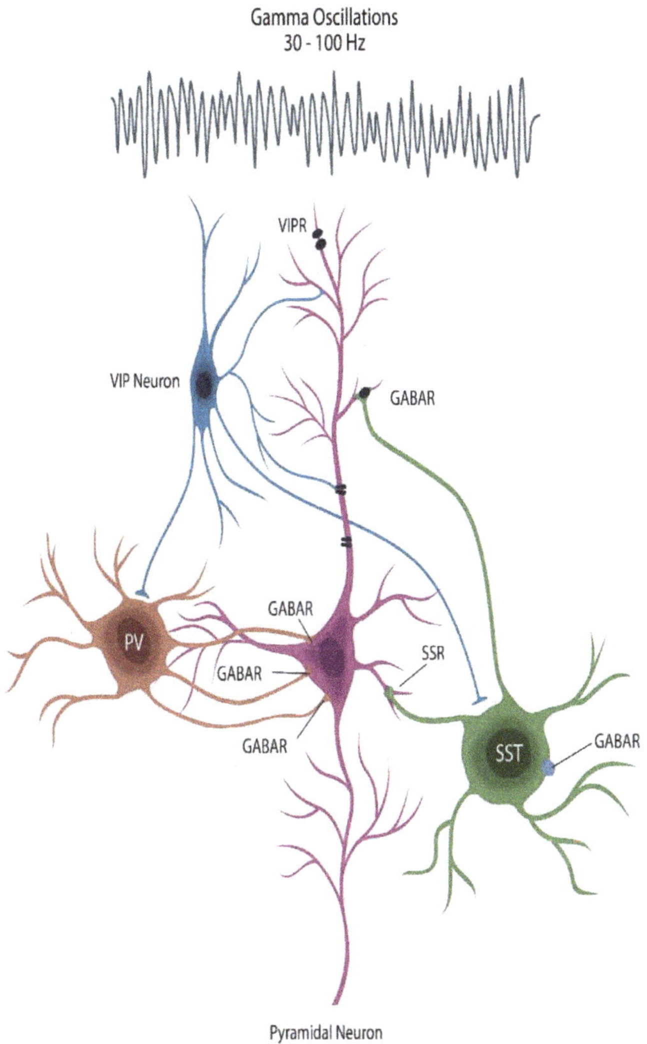

Fig. 9.2 <u>The mechanism of gamma oscillations</u>: Gamma oscillations comprise a rapid brain rhythm believed to be generated by the synaptic "chatter" of inhibitory GABAergic interneurons, such as parvalbumin (PV)—and somatostatin (SST)-expressing cells that signal via GABA receptors. Loss of inhibitory neurons

disinhibits pyramidal cells, leading to psychosis. Vasoactive intestinal peptide (VIP) neurons counteract inhibition by inhibiting the inhibitory neurons, which leads to the disinhibition of pyramidal neurons.

Taken together, SMI is characterized by premature cellular senescence and GMV reduction. Lowering the effects of senescence to avoid aberrant microglia activation could avert brain atrophy and restore the gamma band. This can be accomplished via natural biochemical approaches, such as MLR, Berberine, and Kaempferol, or biophysical interventions, including entraining gamma waves via LLLT, tACS, TMS, or ASSR.

Chapter 9 References:

1. Hu Y, Fryatt GL, Ghorbani M, Obst J, Menassa DA, Martin-Estebane M, Muntslag TAO, Olmos-Alonso A, Guerrero-Carrasco M, Thomas D, Cragg MS, Gomez-Nicola D. Replicative senescence dictates the emergence of disease-associated microglia and contributes to Aβ pathology. Cell Rep. 2021 Jun 8;35(10):109228. doi: 10.1016/j.celrep.2021.109228.

2. Ng PY, McNeely TL, Baker DJ. Untangling senescent and damage-associated microglia in the aging and diseased brain. FEBS J. 2023 Mar;290(5):1326-1339. doi: 10.1111/febs.16315.

3. Donley DW, Realing M, Gigley JP, Fox JH. Iron activates microglia and directly stimulates indoleamine-2,3-dioxygenase activity in the N171-82Q mouse model of Huntington's disease. PLoS One. 2021 May 14;16(5):e0250606. doi: 10.1371/journal.pone.0250606.

4. Hagihara H, Shoji H, Otabi H, Toyoda A, Katoh K, Namihira M, Miyakawa T. Protein lactylation induced by neural excitation. Cell Rep. 2021 Oct 12;37(2):109820. doi: 10.1016/j.celrep.2021.109820. PMID: 34644564.

5. Zhang D, Tang Z, Huang H, Zhou G, Cui C, Weng Y, et al. Metabolic regulation of gene expression by histone lactylation. Nature. 2019;574(7779):575–80.

6. Gregory J Anderson, David M Frazer, Lactate as a regulator of iron homeostasis, Life Metabolism, Volume 2, Issue 5, October 2023, load033, https://doi.org/10.1093/lifemeta/load033

7. Wei L, Yang X, Wang J, Wang Z, Wang Q, Ding Y, Yu A. H3K18 lactylation of senescent microglia potentiates brain aging and Alzheimer's disease through the NFκB signaling pathway. J Neuroinflammation. 2023 Sep 11;20(1):208. doi: 10.1186/s12974-023-02879-7

8. Galle, E., Wong, CW., Ghosh, A., et al. H3K18 lactylation marks tissue-specific active enhancers. Genome Biol 23, 207 (2022). https://doi.org/10.1186/s13059-022-02775-y

9. Coppé JP, Desprez PY, Krtolica A, Campisi J. The senescence-associated secretory phenotype: the dark side of tumor suppression. Annu Rev Pathol. 2010;5:99-118. doi: 10.1146/annurev-pathol-121808-102144.

10. Wang Y, Ni J, Gao T, Gao C, Guo L, Yin X. Activation of astrocytic sigma-1 receptor exerts antidepressant-like effect via facilitating CD38-driven mitochondria transfer. Glia. 2020 Nov;68(11):2415-2426. doi: 10.1002/glia.23850.

11. Ding L, Ren C, Yang L, Wu Z, Li F, Jiang D, Zhu Y, Lu J. OSU-03012 Disrupts Akt Signaling and Prevents Endometrial Carcinoma Progression in vitro and in vivo. Drug Des Devel Ther. 2021 Apr 30;15:1797-1810. doi: 10.2147/DDDT.S304128

12. Emamian ES. AKT/GSK3 signaling pathway and schizophrenia. Front Mol Neurosci. 2012 Mar 15;5:33. doi: 10.3389/fnmol.2012.00033.

13. Ren J, Lu Y, Qian Y, Chen B, Wu T, Ji G. Recent progress regarding kaempferol for treating various diseases. Exp Ther Med. 2019 Oct;18(4):2759-2776. doi: 10.3892/etm.2019.7886.

14. Rose MF, Ahmad KA, Thaller C, Zoghbi HY. Excitatory neurons of the proprioceptive, interoceptive, and arousal hindbrain networks share a developmental requirement for Math1. Proc Natl Acad Sci U S A. 2009 Dec 29;106(52):22462-7. doi: 10.1073/pnas.0911579106.

15. Fujimoto H, Matsuoka T, Kato Y, Shibata K, Nakamura K, Yamada K, Narumoto J. Brain regions associated with anosognosia for memory disturbance in Alzheimer's disease: a magnetic resonance

imaging study. Neuropsychiatr Dis Treat. 2017 Jul 5;13:1753-1759. doi: 10.2147/NDT.S139177.

16. Einstein, Albert (1905). "Über die von der molekularkinetischen Theorie der Wärme geforderte Bewegung von in ruhenden Flüssigkeiten suspendierten Teilchen" [On the Movement of Small Particles Suspended in Stationary Liquids Required by the Molecular-Kinetic Theory of Heat] (PDF). Annalen der Physik (in German). 322 (8): 549-560. Bibcode:1905AnP...322..549E. doi:10.1002/andp.19053220806. We have archived (PDF) from the original on 9 October 2022.

17. Bazargani N, Attwell D. Astrocyte calcium signaling: the third wave. Nat Neurosci. 2016 Feb;19(2):182-9. doi: 10.1038/nn.4201. PMID: 26814587.

18. Rulands S, Lee HJ, Clark SJ, Angermueller C, Smallwood SA, Krueger F, Mohammed H, Dean W, Nichols J, Rugg-Gunn P, Kelsey G, Stegle O, Simons BD, Reik W. Genome-Scale Oscillations in DNA Methylation during Exit from Pluripotency. Cell Syst. 2018 Jul 25;7(1):63-76.e12. doi: 10.1016/j.cels.2018.06.012.

19. Heltberg MS, Lucchetti A, Hsieh FS, Minh Nguyen DP, Chen SH, Jensen MH. Enhanced DNA repair through droplet formation and p53 oscillations. Cell. 2022 Nov 10;185(23):4394-4408.e10. doi: 10.1016/j.cell.2022.10.004

20. Stiefel, K. M., and Ermentrout, G. B. (2016). Neurons as oscillators. J. Neurophysiol. 116, 2950–2960. doi: 10.1152/jn.00525.2015

21. Lin, H. R., Wang, C. H., Deng, Q. L., Xu, C., Deng, Z. K., and Zhou, C. (2021). Review on chaotic dynamics of memristive neuron and neural network. Nonlinear Dyn. 106, 959–973. doi: 10.1007/s11071-021-06853-x

22. Grossberg, S. (2013). Adaptive Resonance Theory: how a brain learns to attend, learn, and recognize a changing world consciously. Neural. Netw. 37, 1–47. doi: 10.1016/j.neunet.2012.09.017

23. Pérez-Cervera, A., Seara, T. M., and Huguet, G. (2020). Phase-locked states in oscillating neural networks and their role in neural communication. Commun. Nonlinear. Sci. Numer. Simul. 80, 104992. doi: 10.1016/j.cnsns.2019.104992

24. Cao L, Thut G, Gross J. The role of brain oscillations in predicting self-generated sounds. Neuroimage. 2017 Feb 15;147:895-903. doi: 10.1016/j.neuroimage.2016.11.001. Epub 2016 Nov 3. PMID: 27818209; PMCID: PMC5315057.

25. Hussain T, Murtaza G, Kalhoro DH, Kalhoro MS, Metwally E, Chughtai MI, Mazhar MU, Khan SA. Relationship between gut microbiota and host-metabolism: Emphasis on hormones related to reproductive function. Anim Nutr. 2021 Mar;7(1):1-10. doi: 10.1016/j.aninu.2020.11.005.

26. Martinez-Corral R, Liu J, Prindle A, Süel GM, Garcia-Ojalvo J. Metabolic basis of brain-like electrical signaling in bacterial communities. Philos Trans R Soc Lond B Biol Sci. 2019 Jun 10;374(1774):20180382. doi: 10.1098/rstb.2018.0382.

27. Martinez-Corral R, Liu J, Süel GM, Garcia-Ojalvo J. Bistable emergence of oscillations in growing Bacillus subtilis biofilms. Proc Natl Acad Sci U S SA. 2018 Sep 4;115(36): E8333-E8340. doi: 10.1073/pnas.1805004115.

28. Prindle A, Liu J, Asally M, Ly S, Garcia-Ojalvo J, Süel GM. Ion channels enable electrical communication in bacterial communities. Nature. 2015 Nov 5;527(7576):59-63. doi: 10.1038/nature15709.

29. Liu J, Prindle A, Humphries J, Gabalda-Sagarra M, Asally M, Lee DY, Ly S, Garcia-Ojalvo J, Süel GM. Metabolic co-dependence

gives rise to collective oscillations within biofilms. Nature. 2015 Jul 30;523(7562):550-4. doi: 10.1038/nature14660.

30. Lenz P, Søgaard-Andersen L. Temporal and spatial oscillations in bacteria. Nat Rev Microbiol. 2011 Aug 15;9(8):565-77. doi: 10.1038/nrmicro2612.

31. Erkin Şeker , Bacterial Vibrations.Sci. Transl. Med.5,196ec126-196ec126(2013).DOI:10.1126/scitranslmed.3007046

32. Raskin DM, de Boer PA. Rapid pole-to-pole oscillation of a protein required for directing division to the middle of Escherichia coli. Proc Natl Acad Sci U S A. 1999 Apr 27;96(9):4971-6. doi: 10.1073/pnas.96.9.4971.

33. Mojica-Benavides M, van Niekerk DD, Mijalkov M, Snoep JL, Mehlig B, Volpe G, Goksör M, Adiels CB. Intercellular communication induces glycolytic synchronization waves between individually oscillating cells. Proc Natl Acad Sci U S SA. 2021 Feb 9;118(6):e2010075118. doi: 10.1073/pnas.2010075118.

34. Weber A, Prokazov Y, Zuschratter W, Hauser MJ. Desynchronisation of glycolytic oscillations in yeast cell populations. PLoS One. 2012;7(9):e43276. doi: 10.1371/journal.pone.0043276

35. Aggarwal A, Brennan C, Shortal B, Contreras D, Kelz MB, Proekt A. Coherence of Visual-Evoked Gamma Oscillations Is Disrupted by Propofol but Preserved Under Equipotent Doses of Isoflurane. Front Syst Neurosci. 2019 May 8;13:19. doi: 10.3389/fnsys.2019.00019.

36. Dipoppa, M., Ranson, A., Krumin, M., Pachitariu, M., Carandini, M., and Harris, K. D. (2018). Vision and Locomotion Shape the Interactions between Neuron Types in Mouse Visual Cortex. Neuron 98, 602–615.e8. doi: 10.1016/j.neuron.2018.03.037

37. Amir, A., Headley, D. B., Lee, S.-C., Haufler, D., and Paré, D. (2018). Vigilance-Associated Gamma Oscillations Coordinate the Ensemble Activity of Basolateral Amygdala Neurons. Neuron 97, 656–669.e7. doi: 10.1016/j.neuron.2017.12.035

38. Besserve M, Lowe SC, Logothetis NK, Schölkopf B, Panzeri S. Shifts of Gamma Phase across Primary Visual Cortical Sites Reflect Dynamic Stimulus-Modulated Information Transfer. PLOS Biology. 2015;13:e1002257. doi: 10.1371/journal.pbio.1002257.

39. Davis ZW, Muller L, Martinez-Trujillo J, Sejnowski T, Reynolds JH. Spontaneous travelling cortical waves gate perception in behaving primates. Nature. 2020;587:432–436. doi: 10.1038/s41586-020-2802-y.

40. Gallotto S, Sack AT, Schuhmann T, de Graaf TA. Oscillatory Correlates of Visual Consciousness. Front Psychol. 2017 Jul 7;8:1147. doi: 10.3389/fpsyg.2017.01147.

41. Başar E. A review of gamma oscillations in healthy subjects and in cognitive impairment. Int J Psychophysiol. 2013 Nov;90(2):99-117. doi: 10.1016/j.ijpsycho.2013.07.005

42. Pelkey, K. A., Chittajallu, R., Craig, M. T., Tricoire, L., Wester, J. C., and McBain, C. J. (2017). Hippocampal GABAergic Inhibitory Interneurons. Physiol. Rev. 97, 1619–1747. doi: 10.1152/physrev.00007.2017

43. Murueta-Goyena, A., Ortuzar, N., Lafuente, J.V. et al. Enriched Environment Reverts Somatostatin Interneuron Loss in MK-801 Model of Schizophrenia. Mol Neurobiol 57, 125–134 (2020). https://doi.org/10.1007/s12035-019-01762-y

44. Petrie KA, Schmidt D, Bubser M, Fadel J, Carraway RE, Deutch AY. Neurotensin activates GABAergic interneurons in the prefrontal

cortex. J Neurosci. 2005 Feb 16;25(7):1629-36. doi: 10.1523/JNEUROSCI.3579-04.2005.

45. Chen CM, Stanford AD, Mao X, Abi-Dargham A, Shungu DC, Lisanby SH, Schroeder CE, Kegeles LS. GABA level, gamma oscillation, and working memory performance in schizophrenia. Neuroimage Clin. 2014 Mar 20;4:531-9. doi: 10.1016/j.nicl.2014.03.007

46. Antonoudiou P, Tan YL, Kontou G, Upton AL, Mann EO. Parvalbumin and Somatostatin Interneurons Contribute to the Generation of Hippocampal Gamma Oscillations. J Neurosci. 2020 Sep 30;40(40):7668-7687. doi: 10.1523/JNEUROSCI.0261-20.2020.

47. Vendemia JMC, Caine KE, Evans JR. Quantitative EEG Findings in Convicted Murderers (2005), Vol 9 No 3. DOI: https://doi.org/10.1300/J184v09n03_02

48. James R. Evans, Ph.D. & Nan-Sook Park M.A. (1997) Quantitative EEG Findings Among Men Convicted of Murder, Journal of Neurotherapy: Investigations in Neuromodulation, Neurofeedback and Applied Neuroscience, 2:2, 31-39, DOI: 10.1300/J184v02n02_05

49. Raine A, Meloy JR, Bihrle S, Stoddard J, LaCasse L, Buchsbaum MS. Reduced prefrontal and increased subcortical brain functioning assessed using positron emission tomography in predatory and affective murderers. Behav Sci Law. 1998 Summer;16(3):319-32. doi: 10.1002/(sici)1099-0798(199822)16:3<319::aid-bsl311>3.0.co;2-g.

50. Schug RA, Yang Y, Raine A, Han C, Liu J, Li L. Resting EEG deficits in accused murderers with schizophrenia. Psychiatry Res. 2011 Oct 31;194(1):85-94. doi: 10.1016/j.pscychresns.2010.12.017.

51. J. R. Evans, Quantitative EEG findings in a group of death row inmates, Archives of Clinical Neuropsychology, Volume 12, Issue 4, 1997, Pages 315–316, https://doi.org/10.1093/arclin/12.4.315a

52. Zomorrodi, R., Loheswaran, G., Pushparaj, A., et al. Pulsed Near Infrared Transcranial and Intranasal Photobiomodulation Significantly Modulates Neural Oscillations: a pilot exploratory sA Pilot Exploratory Study. Sci Rep 9, 6309 (2019). https://doi.org/10.1038/s41598-019-42693-x

53. Dompe C, Moncrieff L, Matys J, Grzech-Leśniak K, Kocherova I, Bryja A, Bruska M, Dominiak M, Mozdziak P, Skiba THI, Shibli JA, Angelova Volponi A, Kempisty B, Dyszkiewicz-Konwińska M. Photobiomodulation-Underlying Mechanism and Clinical Applications. J Clin Med. 2020 Jun 3;9(6):1724. doi: 10.3390/jcm9061724. PMID: 32503238; PMCID: PMC7356229.

54. Liu J, Prindle A, Humphries J, Gabalda-Sagarra M, Asally M, Lee DY, Ly S, Garcia-Ojalvo J, Süel GM. Metabolic co-dependence gives rise to collective oscillations within biofilms. Nature. 2015 Jul 30;523(7562):550-4. doi: 10.1038/nature14660.

55. Pathak H, Sreeraj VS, Venkatasubramanian G. Transcranial Alternating Current Stimulation (tACS) and Its Role in Schizophrenia: A Scoping Review. Clin Psychopharmacol Neurosci. 2023 Nov 30;21(4):634-649. doi: 10.9758/cpn.22.1042.

56. Koshiyama, D. et al. Auditory gamma oscillations predict global symptomatic outcome in the early stages of psychosis: a longitudinal investigation. Clin. Neurophysiol. 129, 2268–2275 (2018).

57. Griskova-Bulanova I, Dapsys K, Melynyte S, Voicikas A, Maciulis V, Andruskevicius S, Korostenskaja M. 40Hz auditory steady-state response in schizophrenia: Sensitivity to stimulation type (clicks

versus flutter amplitude-modulated tones). Neurosci Lett. 2018 Jan 1;662:152-157. doi: 10.1016/j.neulet.2017.10.025.

58. Zhang Y, Zhang Z, Luo L, Tong H, Chen F, Hou ST. 40 Hz Light Flicker Alters Human Brain Electroencephalography Microstates and Complexity Implicated in Brain Diseases. Front Neurosci. 2021 Dec 13;15:777183. doi: 10.3389/fnins.2021.777183.

59. Chan D, Suk HJ, Jackson BL, Milman NP, Stark D, Klerman EB, Kitchener E, Fernandez Avalos VS, de Weck G, Banerjee A, Beach SD, et al. Gamma frequency sensory stimulation in mild probable Alzheimer's dementia patients: Results of feasibility and pilot studies. PLoS One. 2022 Dec 1;17(12):e0278412. doi: 10.1371/journal.pone.0278412.

60. Jang HJ, Chung H, Rowland JM, Richards BA, Kohl MM, Kwag J. Distinct roles of parvalbumin and somatostatin interneurons in gating the synchronization of spike times in the neocortex. Sci Adv. 2020 Apr 22;6(17):eaay5333. Doi: 10.1126/sciadv.aay5333.

61. Liguz-Lecznar M, Urban-Ciecko J, Kossuth M. Somatostatin and Somatostatin-Containing Neurons in Shaping Neuronal Activity and Plasticity. Front Neural Circuits. 2016 Jun 30;10:48. doi: 10.3389/fncir.2016.00048.

62. Murty DVPS, Manikandan K, Kumar WS, Ramesh RG, Purokayastha S, Javali M, Rao NP, Ray S. Gamma oscillations weaken with age in healthy elderly in human EEG. Neuroimage. 2020 Jul 15;215:116826. doi: 10.1016/j.neuroimage.2020.116826

63. Chesnokova V, Zonis S, Apostolou A, Estrada HQ, Knott S, Wawrowsky K, Michelsen K, Ben-Shlomo A, Barrett R, Gorbunova V, Karalis K, Melmed S. Local non-pituitary growth hormone is induced with aging and facilitates epithelial damage. Cell Rep. 2021

Dec 14;37(11):110068. doi: 10.1016/j.celrep.2021.110068. PMID: 34910915

64. Nelson Espinosa, Alejandra Alonso, Cristian Morales, Pedro Espinosa, Andrés E Chávez, Pablo Fuentealba, Basal Forebrain Gating by Somatostatin Neurons Drives Prefrontal Cortical Activity, Cerebral Cortex, Volume 29, Issue 1, January 2019, Pages 42–53, https://doi.org/10.1093/cercor/bhx302

Chapter 10
Psychotropic Drugs Interaction with COVID-19 "Vaccine"

Very little is known about the drug-drug interaction between COVID-19 "vaccine" and psychotropic agents. However, the adverse effects of COVID-19 therapeutics, including myocarditis and infertility, can be explained by examining the components of lipid nanoparticle (LNP), polyethylene glycol (PEG) and polyamines, likely spermine.

For example, PEG is an established fusogen that can form multinucleated large cells like those encountered in giant cell myocarditis.

Polyamines, including spermine, likely used as ionizable lipids, play a key role in infertility, probably accounting for the low birth rate in countries that were the most adherent with the vaccination program.

The messenger RNA (mRNA) vaccines for COVID-19, Pfizer-BioNTech and Moderna, were authorized in the US on an emergency basis in December of 2020. The rapid distribution of these therapeutics around the country and the world led to millions of people being vaccinated in a short time span, an action that decreased hospitalization and death but also heightened the concerns about adverse effects and drug-vaccine interactions (1). The COVID-19 mRNA vaccines are of particular interest as they form the vanguard of a range of other mRNA therapeutics that are currently in the development pipeline, focusing both on infectious diseases as well as oncological applications (2).

The Vaccine Adverse Event Reporting System (VAERS) has gained additional attention during the COVID-19 pandemic, specifically regarding the rollout of mRNA therapeutics. However, the absence of a reporting platform for drug-vaccine interactions left these events poorly defined. For example, chemotherapy, anticonvulsants, and antimalarials were documented to interfere with the mRNA vaccines, but much less is known about the other drugs that could interact with these agents, causing adverse events or decreased efficacy (3-6). In addition, SARS-CoV-2 exploitation of host cytochrome P450 enzymes, reported in COVID-19 critical illness, highlights viral interference with drug metabolism (7-8). For example, patients with SMI in treatment with clozapine often displayed elevated drug levels, emphasizing drug-vaccine interaction (11).

Background

In 2021, the Centers for Disease Control and Prevention prioritized vaccination for mentally ill individuals as psychiatric illness was added to the list of COVID-19 risk factors (9). Currently, there are very few studies on mRNA vaccine efficacy in patients with SMI in treatment with psychotropic drugs. However, increased breakthrough infections and limited vaccine responses were reported by a recent epidemiological study on veterans with SMI, highlighting possible drug-vaccine interaction (10). This study aligns with earlier data, showing that, in general, patients with SMI exhibit suboptimal vaccine efficacy, a phenomenon also documented in the geriatric population (11-15). Indeed, immunological similarities and differences exist between SMI patients and older individuals. For example, persons with SMI exhibit a shorter-than-average lifespan and high comorbidity with age-related diseases due to premature cellular senescence (16-18).

In addition, SMIs were associated with lower counts of regulatory T cells (Tregs) that are often reversed by the treatment with psychotropic drugs (19-24). On the other hand, unlike older individuals, SMI patients display an increased number of natural killer cells (NKC) that are unaffected by the psychotropic medication, probably explaining the low prevalence of malignancies as well as COVID-19 critical illness in this population (25-27). Indeed, immune malfunction may account for both limited vaccine responses and protection from COVID-19 critical illness in medicated SMI patients (10) (28) (29). For example, upregulated NKCs may promptly eliminate both virus-infected and mRNA-transfected cells, disrupting translation at the ribosomal level and antibody production (30-32). In addition, psychotropic drugs' anti-inflammatory and immunosuppressant actions may protect against virus-induced "cytokine storm" while lowering the immune reactivity necessary for adequate vaccine responses (33-34).

Messenger RNA vaccines

The similarity between EVs and liposomes inspired the novel mRNA COVID-19 vaccines. Similar therapeutics have been used to treat hereditary transthyretin-mediated amyloidosis, with small interfering ribonucleic acids (siRNAs) embedded in LNPs (35-36). Replacing siRNA content with mRNA led to the concept of LNP therapeutics with nucleic acid encoding for the SARS-CoV-2 spike (S) protein to elicit neutralizing antibodies (37-38). Compared to other exogenous nucleic acid introduction methods into cells, such as viral vectors, LNPs are better tolerated, although their transfection efficacy is less robust (39).

To effectively deliver the synthetic mRNA to host ribosomes, LNPs must avoid several obstacles, including hydrolysis by extracellular RNases, activation of intracellular immune sensors, and degradation by the enzymes of the endosomal lysosomal system (ELS) (40) (41-42). Modifying and hiding mRNAs in LNPs can overcome the first two barriers, while ionizable lipids SM-102 (Moderna) and ALC-0315 (Pfizer BioNTech) may conquer the last one (43).

The mRNA-containing LNPs are comprised of four lipids: 1,2-distearoyl-sn-glycero-3-phosphocholine (DSPC), PEG, an alternative cholesterol, and ionizable lipids SM-102 or ALC-0315 (44-45). The SM-102, ALC-0315, and the alternative cholesterol are proprietary molecules and have not been released up to the present time. However, interrogating siRNA platforms, it is reasonable to conclude that ionizable lipids may resemble DLin-MC3-DMA and that a phytosterol may replace the cholesterol (46-47).

LNPs enter cells by endocytosis or phagocytosis (immune cell uptake) (48) (49). Entry by the endocytic pathway (EP) can take place via clathrin-dependent or independent routes. Regardless of the ingress modality, LNPs travel from the early to late endosomes and can withstand an environmental pH of 5.5 or higher (50-51). As exposure to the lysosomal pH of 4.5–5.0 could degrade the LNPs, exit from the endosomal-lysosomal system (ELS) must occur in the late endosomes (50). However, as late endosomes can also release their cargo via EVs, LNPs may be expulsed into the extracellular space instead of the cytosol (52) (Fig.1). Indeed, studies with split green fluorescence proteins (GFPs) have found that endosomal escape, in general, is an inefficient process as only about 2% of ELS content reaches the cytosol (53). This ratio can be increased with the help of negatively charged phospholipids, such as phosphatidylserine (PS) or analogs. For example, externalized PS (ePS) on ELS membranes generates an electrostatic imbalance between the cationic lipids and anionic phospholipids, enabling the LNP to escape (54-56).

Taken together, the successful delivery of LNP to the host translational machinery depends on overcoming several key obstacles. A significant bottleneck that must be successfully negotiated to ensure cargo delivery involves LNP lysosomal evasion and premature expulsion into the extracellular compartment.

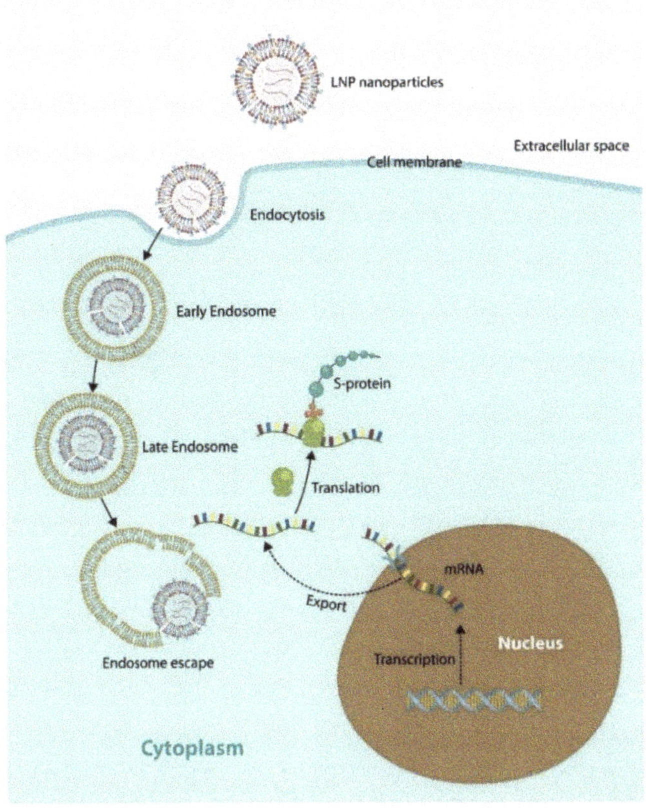

Fig. 10.1 LNPs enter host cells via endocytosis or phagocytosis (immune cell endocytosis). LNP is trafficked through the ELS, traveling from early to late endosomes. Progressing from late endosomes to lysosomes would risk LNP degradation by the hydrolyzing enzymes; therefore, ELS escape must occur in late endosomes. However, late endosomes may expulse their cargo into the extracellular compartment via EVs (not shown). This is a significant hurdle that LNPs must negotiate. Under ideal circumstances, ribosomes translate the exogenous mRNA into

the S protein. For this to occur, it must be assumed that the human translation machinery does not differentiate between endogenous (nucleus-derived) and exogenous mRNA.

The LNPs in the cytosol and potential drug- interactions

There is a lack of studies discussing the fate of LNP-mRNA in the cytosol. It is generally assumed that once released from the liposome, mRNA can find its way to the ribosomes where the S antigen is translated (57) (Fig.1). However, the modified vaccine mRNA may be perceived by the cell as defective or damaged, holding back translation by ribosomal stalling (58-60). Interestingly, several psychotropic drugs, including aripiprazole, clozapine, and lithium, were demonstrated to alter ribosomal function and protein synthesis, highlighting possible interference with the vaccine mRNA (61).

Single-molecule tracking studies have found that the cytosolic mRNA can access the cellular cytoskeleton and travel throughout the cytosol, from where it can diffuse into cytoplasmic organelles, including the nucleus (62) (63) (64) (65). For example, a recent study found that upon entering the host nuclear compartment, Pfizer BioNTech mRNA could be retrotranscribed into DNA by the long interspersed nuclear element-1 (LINE-1), emphasizing vaccine-genome interactions (66-67). Interestingly, upregulated LINE-1, a marker of SMI, can be lowered by psychotropic drugs (which increase DNA methylation), likely reducing or averting the transcription of RNA to DNA (68-69).

In the following sections, I take a closer look at the four LNP lipids and their interaction with psychotropic drugs. Why are mRNA therapeutics relevant for neuropsychiatry? LNPs can be utilized as transfer vehicles for psychotropic drugs' delivery directly to the

CNS neuronal networks. However, for that to happen, the structure of LNPs needs improvement.

1. **PEGylated lipids**

PEGylated lipids extend the duration of mRNA action and facilitate LNP endocytosis while lowering aggregation and opsonization during circulation (70-71). However, despite these advantages, PEGylation raises the so-called "PEG dilemma": prolongation of both LNP uptake and ELS escape, risking vaccine-mRNA degradation by the lysosomal enzymes (72). Given that the LNP composition is proprietary, it is unknown how the mRNA-based vaccines overcome the "PEG dilemma"; however, linking PEG oxygen to the head group of SM-102 or ALC-0315 is a previously documented solution (73). In addition, CHARMM-GUI membrane builder (http://www.charmm-gui.org/input/membrane), an in-silico lipid simulation platform, highlights the PEG oxygen bond as the likely overcomer of the "PEG dilemma" (74).

Psychotropic drugs and PEGylated lipids

Several classes of psychotropic drugs, including phenothiazines, were demonstrated to inhibit the EP by binding to the adaptor protein 2 (AP2), a cell membrane protein that plays a crucial role in clathrin-mediated endocytosis (CME) (75-76). As CME is a central LNP intake mechanism, psychotropic drugs-inhibited AP2 likely disrupts vaccine transfection (77-78). Moreover, psychotropic medications were demonstrated to accumulate in lysosomes (lysosomotropism) and increase the ELS pH, likely delaying LNP escape, thus lowering the vaccine efficacy (79-80). Along this line, the antipsychotic drug pimozide was shown to disrupt the LNP exit from ELS, emphasizing a drug-vaccine interaction that can inactivate the mRNA vaccines (81-82). Interestingly, PEGylated liposomes were previously shown to induce cytochrome P450, especially CYP3A1, CYP2C6, and CYP1A2, causing accelerated blood clearance (ABC), a phenomenon that reduces the efficacy of PEGylated nanocarriers, emphasizing a less discussed LNP weakness (83-84).

DSPC

DSPC is a non-pyrogenic, neutral phospholipid that plays a crucial role in cell apoptosis and immune regulation (85). DSPC was added to the LNP to prevent immune detection by the cytosolic sensors, including toll-like receptors (TLRs) and retinoic acid-inducible gene I (RIG-I) (86). DSPC plays a significant role in stealthy LNP entry into the cells without alerting the host's immune defenses. This is accomplished by altering the lipid asymmetry of plasma membranes, mimicking ePS, a global immunosuppressive signal (48). In addition, DSPC increases regulatory T cells (Tregs), further lowering host immune surveillance (87-88). Tregs upregulation is a double-edged sword as these lymphocytes can lower both virus-mediated inflammation (cytokine storm) and vaccine-evoked neutralizing antibodies, emphasizing that antiviral and pro-viral actions are highly intertwined (89-90).

The question that remains unanswered is why vaccine designers would utilize LNP/EP, a method with only a 2% chance of transcribing the mRNA into a neutralizing antibody.

Potential interaction with psychotropic drugs

Psychotropic drugs may lower the robustness of vaccine responses by direct mechanisms, interaction with LNPs, or indirectly by the anti-inflammatory and anti-immunogenic properties of these agents

(33) (91). For example, the immunosuppressant properties of clozapine, haloperidol, risperidone, and antidepressant drugs are well-established, emphasizing likely interference with the vaccine-associated immunogenicity (34) (92-94). Indeed, biophysical studies show that antipsychotic medications can insert themselves between the lipid molecules of the plasma membrane, triggering anti-inflammatory responses that can impair vaccine efficacy (95-98). Moreover, leukopenia and decreased immunoglobulins, well-established properties of psychotropic drugs, may directly lower the neutralizing antibodies (92) (99-101). Interestingly, chlorpromazine inhibited mRNA expression in human thymocytes, likely disrupting vaccine efficacy at the translation level (102) (103). Vaccine effectiveness can be further decreased by antipsychotic drugs-upregulated Tregs, an established defense mechanism against autoimmunity (104) (105).

Ionizable lipids

Ionizable lipids added to the LNP, SM-102, and ALC-0315 are pH-sensitive molecules, positively charged in an acidic environment and neutral at physiological pH (106). This characteristic supports protonation, facilitating LNP escape from the late endosomes (42) (107-108).

Ionizable lipids likely contain synthetic polyamines as amine groups accumulate in the ELS, increasing membrane permeability that, in turn, promotes LNP transport into the cytosol (Fig. 1) (109-111). In addition, as polyamines play a crucial role in mRNA translation and stability, they may be critical components of SM-102/ALC-0315 lipids (112). Among the polyamines, spermine has demonstrated superior cellular uptake and endosomal escape ability, suggesting that LNPs may contain this molecule (113). In addition, spermine increased vaccine efficacy by upregulating autophagy in human T cells and enhancing antigen responses (114-115).

Novel studies attributed antipsychotic properties to spermine, while its dysfunction was associated with the pathogenesis of SMI, particularly suicidal behavior (116-117). Moreover, as spermine plays a significant role in male and female reproductive physiology, disruption of this polyamine may contribute to infertility and decreased birth rates (118). Indeed, epidemiological studies from several countries have reported lower 2021 natality rates compared to the previous year, as demonstrated by Italy (-9.1%), Spain (-8.4%), Portugal (-6.6%), and New York (-19.8%) that might reflect dysfunctional polyamine signaling (119-120). Although it is difficult to trace the source of any potential infertility to mRNA vaccines, as dysfunctional polyamines were also documented in SARS-CoV-2 infection and several psychiatric disorders, it is essential to investigate these biomolecules further (121-125).

<u>Potential interference with psychotropic drugs</u>

Several psychotropic drugs were shown to alter the integrity of membrane phospholipids, suggesting possible interference with the LNP ingress and ELS escape (80). In addition, psychotropic drugs were demonstrated to alkalinize the ELS, which in turn could disrupt the pH-dependent polyamines (79). Moreover, accumulating evidence suggests that polyamines, including putrescine, spermidine, and spermine, are not only involved in the pathogenesis of SMI but are also modulated by the antipsychotic drugs, suggesting possible interference with the mRNA vaccines (116) (123). For example, spermidine, a spermine derivative, was found to protect the GABAergic and dopaminergic systems, suggesting that LNPs may interfere with this signaling (117). This is significant as DA is not only involved in psychiatric disorders but is also an established fertility promoter, and DA agonists are frequently prescribed as part of assisted reproduction technology (ART) (126-127).

Cholesterol analog

The cholesterol analog utilized in LNP is likely a phytosterol, as these molecules display high transfection capability by binding to apolipoprotein E (ApoE), followed by rapid endocytosis (128-129). However, phytosterols have a significant disadvantage as they suppress phagocytosis, probably limiting the LNP uptake in immune cells and, therefore, mRNA translation (130-131). In addition, unlike cholesterol, phytosterols cross the blood-brain barrier (BBB) and accumulate in the brain, where their oxidation may precipitate the development of neurodegenerative disorders (132-133).

Several sterols, including desmosterol, were associated with both MDD and antidepressant medication, possibly accounting for the rare post-vaccination psychiatric symptoms recorded in VAERs (134) (135-136). Moreover, cholesterol and other sterols can interact directly with dopamine transporters (DAT), possibly accounting for the post-vaccination dyskinesia noted in some patients with PD (132) (137-138).

Potential interference with psychotropic drugs

Several psychotropic drugs, including clozapine, olanzapine, haloperidol, and imipramine, were shown to up-regulate ApoE, a cholesterol transporter disrupted in SPI, suggesting possible interference with LNP transfection (139-141). As psychotropic medications upregulate the ATP-binding cassette transporter A1 (ABCA1), increasing cholesterol egress from cells, a process that may compromise vaccine efficacy by flushing LNPs into the extracellular compartment before mRNA release (142). In addition, several psychotropic drugs, including aripiprazole, haloperidol, and trazodone, were reported to increase the levels of cholesterol precursor, desmosterol, that in turn upregulates the expression of cholesterol efflux genes, likely removing LNPs from cells prematurely (143).

LNP component	Cellular effects	Psychotropic drugs	Interactions	References
PEG	Entry via EP BBB permeability increase (LNP CNS entry)	Entry by EP, alter pH (Phenothiazines, pimozide)	-Delayed LNP cellular uptake -Lower LNP endosomal escape	75-82
DSPC	Lower immunity and inflammation	Lower immunity and inflammation	Lower neutralizing antibody formation	33-34; 89-90;92-94; 99-101; 102-103
Ionizable lipids	Alter membrane asymmetry Alter polyamine homeostasis	Alter membrane asymmetry (Chlorpromazine, Risperidone)	-Lower formation of antibodies -Polyamines exhibit antidepressant and anxiolytic effects.	79; 107-111; 118; 123; 126-127
Cholesterol analogs	Transport by ApoE Phytosterols connected to neurodegeneration	Upregulate ApoE Promote cholesterol egress	May compromise vaccine efficacy by increased cholesterol egress	132-133;139-143

Table 10.1. Psychotropic drugs compound some LNP effects, altering cell entry, endosomal release, and exit of mRNA vaccines and their responses.

Legend: EP, endosomal pathway; LNP, lipid nanoparticle; ApoE, apolipoprotein E; PEG, polyethylene glycol; DSPC, 1,2-distearoyl-sn-glycero-3-phosphocholine.

Limitations

This study has potential limitations. Firstly, it refers to a new technology within the clinical standard of care, which, even though it has a considerable body of literature in the scientific and preparatory phases, is still developing the breadth of scientific observations from a clinical perspective. Secondly, some of the potential drug-immunization interactions in the latest pandemics might likely be masked by the vaccine escape properties attributed to newly emerging SARS-CoV-2 variants. As such, an even more careful approach of the subject would be required to distinguish these compounding factors of lower than anticipated immune efficacy. Thirdly, it is presumed that some of the above-observed interactions would have similarities in the future provision of mRNA therapeutics for non-communicable diseases, such as different cancer types. However, this remains a working hypothesis that requires further testing.

Discussion and conclusion

More studies are needed to assess the interaction between the major classes of psychotropic drugs, including antipsychotics, antidepressants, mood stabilizers, and mRNA therapeutics. As the PEG component of LNPs increases the permeability of BBB for a short interval, neuropsychiatry will rapidly adopt it as a vehicle for drug transport and delivery to select CNS networks. For this reason, it is important to develop a VAERS-like system for recording the interaction of psychotropic drugs with current and future mRNA therapeutics.

The exact LNP composition has not been released yet; therefore, I analyze earlier data and virtual screening research, attempting to "fill in" the blanks. For this reason, my assumptions and evidence may seem circumstantial; however, I believe they provide a foundation worth further investigation.

LNPs are crucial for transporting exogenous mRNA to the host translational machinery, where the S antigen is synthesized, eliciting neutralizing antibodies. The four LNP lipids guide the mRNA-loaded particle through the maze of extra and intracellular compartments, releasing its cargo into the cytosol. However, several bottlenecks on this journey, including ingress failure, delayed ELS escape, or premature expulsion from cells, may lower vaccine efficacy.

Treatment with psychotropic drugs may decrease the effectiveness of the mRNA vaccine by lowering inflammation/immunogenicity, inhibiting virus/LNP endocytosis, delaying ELS escape, or directly downregulating neutralizing antibodies.

Chapter 10 References:

1. Lin DY, Gu Y, Wheeler B, Young H, Holloway S, Sunny SK, Moore Z, Zeng D. Effectiveness of Covid-19 Vaccines over 9 months in North Carolina. N Engl J Med. 2022 Mar 10;386(10):933-941. doi: 10.1056/NEJMoa2117128.

2. Wei, Jiao, and Ai-Min Hui. "The paradigm shift in treatment from Covid-19 to oncology with mRNA vaccines." Cancer Treatment Reviews (2022): 102405.

3. Miatmoko A, Nurjannah I, Nehru NF, Rosita N, Hendradi E, Sari R, Ekowati J. Interactions of primaquine and chloroquine with PEGylated phosphatidylcholine liposomes. Sci Rep. 2021 Jun 14;11(1):12420. doi: 10.1038/s41598-021-91866-0.

4. Barroso RP, Basso LG, Costa-Filho AJ. Interactions of the antimalarial amodiaquine with lipid model membranes. Chem Phys Lipids. 2015 Feb;186:68-78. doi: 10.1016/j.chemphyslip.2014.12.003.

5. Brest P, Mograbi B, Hofman P, Milano G. COVID-19 vaccination and cancer immunotherapy: should they stick together? Br J Cancer. 2022 Jan;126(1):1-3. doi: 10.1038/s41416-021-01618-0.

6. Kow CS, Hasan SS. Potential interactions between COVID-19 vaccines and antiepileptic drugs. Seizure. 2021 Mar;86:80-81. doi: 10.1016/j.seizure.2021.01.021.

7. Deb S, Arrighi S. Potential Effects of COVID-19 on Cytochrome P450-Mediated Drug Metabolism and Disposition in Infected Patients. Eur J Drug Metab Pharmacokinet. 2021 Mar;46(2):185-203. doi: 10.1007/s13318-020-00668-8.

8. Bayraktar İ, Yalçın N, Demirkan K. The potential interaction between COVID-19 vaccines and clozapine: A novel approach for

clinical trials. Int J Clin Pract. 2021 Aug;75(8):e14441. doi: 10.1111/ijcp.14441. PMID: 34289643; PMCID: PMC8420459.

9. Mazereel V, Van Assche K, Detraux J, De Hert M. COVID-19 vaccination for people with severe mental illness: why, what, and how? Lancet Psychiatry. 2021 May;8(5):444-450. doi: 10.1016/S2215-0366(20)30564-2.

10. Nishimi K, Neylan TC, Bertenthal D, Seal KH, O'Donovan A. Association of Psychiatric Disorders With Incidence of SARS-CoV-2 Breakthrough Infection Among Vaccinated Adults. JAMA Netw Open. 2022 Apr 1;5(4):e227287. doi: 10.1001/jamanetworkopen.2022.7287. PMID: 35420660; PMCID: PMC9011123.

11. Hussar AE, Cradle JL, Beiser SM. A study of the immunologic and allergic responsiveness of chronic schizophrenics. Br J Psychiatry. 1971 Jan;118(542):91-2. doi: 10.1192/bjp.118.542.91. PMID: 5576273.

12. Solomon GF, Rubbo SD, Batchelder E. Secondary immune response to tetanus toxoid in psychiatric patients. J Psychiatr Res. 1970 Feb;7(3):201-7. doi: 10.1016/0022-3956(70)90007-5. PMID: 5440860.

13. Wang Y, Yu L, Zhou H, Zhou Z, Zhu H, Li Y, Zheng Z, Li X, Dong C. Serologic and molecular characteristics of hepatitis B virus infection in vaccinated schizophrenia patients in China. J Infect Dev Ctries. 2016 Apr 28;10(4):427-31. doi: 10.3855/jidc.7377. PMID: 27131009.

14. Della Bella S, Bierti L, Presicce P, Arienti R, Valenti M, Saresella M, Vergani C, Villa ML. Peripheral blood dendritic cells and monocytes are differently regulated in the elderly. Clin Immunol. 2007 Feb;122(2):220-8. doi: 10.1016/j.clim.2006.09.012.

15. Derhovanessian E, Pawelec G. Vaccination in the elderly. Microb Biotechnol. 2012 Mar;5(2):226-32. doi: 10.1111/j.1751-7915.2011.00283.x. Epub 2011 Aug 31. PMID: 21880118; PMCID: PMC3815782.

16. Lindqvist, D.; Epel, E.S.; Mellon, S.H.; Penninx, B.W.; Révész, D.; Verhoeven, J.E.; Reus, V.I.; Lin, J.; Mahan, L.; Hough, C.M.; et al. Psychiatric disorders and leukocyte telomere length: Underlying mechanisms linking mental illness with cellular aging. Neurosci. Biobehav. Rev. 2015, 55, 333–364.

17. Pousa, P.; Souza, R.; Melo, P.; Correa, B.; Mendonça, T.; Simões-E-Silva, A.; Miranda, D. Telomere Shortening and Psychiatric Disorders: A Systematic Review. Cells 2021, 10, 1423.

18. Lee S, Yu Y, Trimpert J, Benthani F, Mairhofer M, Richter-Pechanska P, Wyler E, et al. Virus-induced senescence is a driver and therapeutic target in COVID-19. Nature. 2021 Nov;599(7884):283-289. doi: 10.1038/s41586-021-03995-1.

19. Solana C, Pereira D, Tarazona R. Early Senescence and Leukocyte Telomere Shortening in SCHIZOPHRENIA: A Role for Cytomegalovirus Infection? Brain Sci. 2018 Oct 18;8(10):188. doi: 10.3390/brainsci8100188.

20. Papanastasiou E, Gaughran F, Smith S. Schizophrenia as segmental progeria. J R Soc Med. 2011 Nov;104(11):475-84. doi: 10.1258/jrsm.2011.110051. PMID: 22048679; PMCID: PMC3206717.

21. Laursen TM. Life expectancy among persons with schizophrenia or bipolar affective disorder. Schizophr Res. 2011 Sep;131(1-3):101-4. doi: 10.1016/j.schres.2011.06.008.

22. Hwang KA, Kim HR, Kang I. Aging and human CD4(+) regulatory
    T cells. Mech Ageing Dev. 2009 Aug;130(8):509-17. doi:
    10.1016/j.mad.2009.06.003.

23. Kelly DL, Li X, Kilday C, Feldman S, Clark S, Liu F, Buchanan
    RW, Tonelli LH. Increased circulating regulatory T cells in
    medicated people with schizophrenia. Psychiatry Res. 2018
    Nov;269:517-523. doi: 10.1016/j.psychres.2018.09.006.

24. Corsi-Zuelli F, Deakin B, de Lima MHF, Qureshi O, Barnes NM,
    Upthegrove R, Louzada-Junior P, Del-Ben CM. T regulatory cells as
    a potential therapeutic target in psychosis? Current challenges and
    future perspectives. Brain Behav Immun Health. 2021 Aug
    19;17:100330. doi: 10.1016/j.bbih.2021.100330.

25. Yovel G, Sirota P, Mazeh D, Shakhar G, Rosenne E, Ben-Eliyahu S.
    Higher natural killer cell activity in schizophrenic patients: the
    impact of serum factors, medication, and smoking. Brain Behav
    Immun. 2000 Sep;14(3):153-69. doi: 10.1006/brbi.1999.0574.
    PMID: 10970677.

26. Tarantino N, Leboyer M, Bouleau A, Hamdani N, Richard JR,
    Boukouaci W, Ching-Lien W, et al. Natural killer cells in first-
    episode psychosis: an innate immune signature? Mol Psychiatry.
    2021 Sep;26(9):5297-5306. doi: 10.1038/s41380-020-01008-7.

27. Bao, C., Tao, X., Cui, W. et al. Natural killer cells associated with
    SARS-CoV-2 viral RNA shedding, antibody response and mortality
    in COVID-19 patients. Exp Hematol Oncol 10, 5 (2021).
    https://doi.org/10.1186/s40164-021-00199-1

28. Nemani K, Williams SZ, Olfson M, Leckman-Westin E, Finnerty M,
    Kammer J, et al. Association Between the Use of Psychotropic
    Medications and the Risk of COVID-19 Infection Among Long-term
    Inpatients With Serious Mental Illness in a New York State-wide

Psychiatric Hospital System. JAMA Netw Open. 2022 May 2;5(5):e2210743. doi: 10.1001/jamanetworkopen.2022.10743.

29. Sfera A, Osorio C, Afzaal J, Del Campo, Z-M, Kozlakidis Z. COVID-19: A Catalyst for Novel Psychiatric Paradigms May 2021 DOI: 10.5772/intechopen.96940. In book: Biotechnology to Combat COVID-19

30. Arai S, Yamamoto H, Itoh K, Kumagai K. Suppressive effect of human natural killer cells on pokeweed mitogen-induced B cell differentiation. J Immunol. 1983 Aug;131(2):651-7. PMID: 6223088.

31. Mason PD, Weetman AP, Sissons JG, Borysiewicz LK. Suppressive role of NK cells in pokeweed mitogen-induced immunoglobulin synthesis: effect of depletion/enrichment of Leu 11b+ cells. Immunology. 1988 Sep;65(1):113-8. PMID: 3053423; PMCID: PMC1385028.

32. Brieva JA, Targan S, Stevens RH. NK and T cell subsets regulate antibody production by human in vivo antigen-induced lymphoblastoid B cells. J Immunol. 1984 Feb;132(2):611-5. PMID: 6228592.

33. Baumeister D, Ciufolini S, Mondelli V. Effects of psychotropic drugs on inflammation: consequence or mediator of therapeutic effects in psychiatric treatment? Psychopharmacology (Berl). 2016 May;233(9):1575-89. doi: 10.1007/s00213-015-4044-5.

34. Gobin V, Van Steendam K, Denys D, Deforce D. Selective serotonin reuptake inhibitors as a novel class of immunosuppressants. Int Immunopharmacol. 2014 May;20(1):148-56. doi: 10.1016/j.intimp.2014.02.030.

35. Urits I, Swanson D, Swett MC, Patel A, Berardino K, Amgalan A, Berger AA, Kassem H, Kaye AD, Viswanath O. A Review of

Patisiran (ONPATTRO®) for the Treatment of Polyneuropathy in People with Hereditary Transthyretin Amyloidosis. Neurol Ther. 2020 Dec;9(2):301-315. doi: 10.1007/s40120-020-00208-1. Epub 2020 Aug 12. Erratum in: Neurol Ther. 2021 Jun;10(1):407. PMID: 32785879; PMCID: PMC7606409.

36. Antimisiaris SG, Mourtas S, Marazioti A. Exosomes and Exosome-Inspired Vesicles for Targeted Drug Delivery. Pharmaceutics. 2018 Nov 6;10(4):218. doi: 10.3390/pharmaceutics10040218.

37. Suzuki Y, Ishihara H. Difference in the lipid nanoparticle technology employed in three approved siRNA (Patisiran) and mRNA (COVID-19 vaccine) drugs. Drug Metab Pharmacokinet. 2021 Dec;41:100424. doi: 10.1016/j.dmpk.2021.100424.

38. Manjunath K, Reddy JS, Venkateswarlu V. Solid lipid nanoparticles as drug delivery systems. Methods Find Exp Clin Pharmacol. 2005 Mar;27(2):127-44. doi: 10.1358/mf.2005.27.2.876286.

39. Settanni G, Brill W, Haas H, Schmid F. pH-Dependent Behavior of Ionizable Cationic Lipids in mRNA-Carrying Lipoplexes Investigated by Molecular Dynamics Simulations. Macromol Rapid Commun. 2022 Jun;43(12):e2100683. doi: 10.1002/marc.202100683.

40. Cullis PR, Hope MJ. Lipid Nanoparticle Systems for Enabling Gene Therapies. Mol Ther. 2017 Jul 5;25(7):1467-1475. doi: 10.1016/j.ymthe.2017.03.013

41. Sahay G, Querbes W, Alabi C, Eltoukhy A, Sarkar S, Zurenko C, et al. Efficiency of siRNA delivery by lipid nanoparticles is limited by endocytic recycling. Nat Biotechnol. 2013 Jul;31(7):653-8. doi: 10.1038/nbt.2614

42. Maugeri, M., Nawaz, M., Papadimitriou, A. et al. Linkage between endosomal escape of LNP-mRNA and loading into EVs for transport

to other cells. Nat Commun 10, 4333 (2019).
https://doi.org/10.1038/s41467-019-12275-6

43. Hou, X., Zaks, T., Langer, R. et al. Lipid nanoparticles for mRNA delivery. Nat Rev Mater 6, 1078–1094 (2021).
https://doi.org/10.1038/s41578-021-00358-0

44. Aldosari BN, Alfagih IM, Almurshedi AS. Lipid Nanoparticles as Delivery Systems for RNA-Based Vaccines. Pharmaceutics. 2021 Feb 2;13(2):206. doi: 10.3390/pharmaceutics13020206.

45. Benne N, van Duijn J, Lozano Vigario F, Leboux RJT, van Veelen P, Kuiper J, et al. Anionic 1,2-distearoyl-sn-glycero-3-phosphoglycerol (DSPG) liposomes induce antigen-specific regulatory T cells and prevent atherosclerosis in mice. J Control Release. (2018) 291:135-146. doi: 10.1016/j.jconrel.2018.10.028.

46. Patel, S. Ashwanikumar N. Robinson E. et al. Naturally-occurring cholesterol analogues in lipid nanoparticles induce polymorphic shape and enhance intracellular delivery of mRNA. Nat Commun 11, 983 (2020). https://doi.org/10.1038/s41467-020-14527-2

47. Tam YY, Chen S, Cullis PR. Advances in Lipid Nanoparticles for siRNA Delivery. Pharmaceutics. 2013 Sep 18;5(3):498-507. doi: 10.3390/pharmaceutics5030498. PMID: 24300520; PMCID: PMC3836621.

48. Birge RB, Boeltz S, Kumar S, Carlson J, Wanderley J, Calianese D, et al. Phosphatidylserine is a global immunosuppressive signal in efferocytosis, infectious disease, and cancer. Cell Death Differ. 2016 Jun;23(6):962-78. doi: 10.1038/cdd.2016.11.

49. Battistelli M, Falcieri E. Apoptotic Bodies: Particular Extracellular Vesicles Involved in Intercellular Communication. Biology (Basel). 2020 Jan 20;9(1):21. doi: 10.3390/biology9010021. PMID: 31968627; PMCID: PMC7168913.

50. Paliwal SR, Paliwal R, Vyas SP. A review of mechanistic insight and application of pH-sensitive liposomes in drug delivery. Drug Deliv. 2015 May;22(3):231-42. doi: 10.3109/10717544.2014.882469.

51. Baranov MV, Olea RA, van den Bogaart G. Chasing Uptake: Super-Resolution Microscopy in Endocytosis and Phagocytosis. Trends Cell Biol. 2019 Sep;29(9):727-739. doi: 10.1016/j.tcb.2019.05.006.

52. Gurung, S., Perocheau, D., Touramanidou, L. et al. The exosome journey: from biogenesis to uptake and intracellular signalling. Cell Commun Signal 19, 47 (2021). https://doi.org/10.1186/s12964-021-00730-1

53. Teo, S.L.Y., Rennick, J.J., Yuen, D. et al. Unravelling cytosolic delivery of cell penetrating peptides with a quantitative endosomal escape assay. Nat Commun 12, 3721 (2021). https://doi.org/10.1038/s41467-021-23997-x

54. Brock DJ, Kondow-McConaghy HM, Hager EC, Pellois JP. Endosomal Escape and Cytosolic Penetration of Macromolecules Mediated by Synthetic Delivery Agents. Bioconjug Chem. 2019 Feb 20;30(2):293-304. doi: 10.1021/acs.bioconjchem.8b00799.

55. ur Rehman Z, Hoekstra D, Zuhorn IS. Mechanism of polyplex- and lipoplex-mediated delivery of nucleic acids: real-time visualization of transient membrane destabilization without endosomal lysis. ACS Nano. 2013 May 28;7(5):3767-77. doi: 10.1021/nn3049494.

56. Wojnilowicz M, Glab A, Bertucci A, Caruso F, Cavalieri F. Super-resolution Imaging of Proton Sponge-Triggered Rupture of Endosomes and Cytosolic Release of Small Interfering RNA. ACS Nano. 2019 Jan 22;13(1):187-202. doi: 10.1021/acsnano.8b05151.

57. Wu Z, Li T. Nanoparticle-Mediated Cytoplasmic Delivery of Messenger RNA Vaccines: Challenges and Future Perspectives.

Pharm Res. 2021 Mar;38(3):473-478. doi: 10.1007/s11095-021-03015-x

58. Karamyshev AL, Karamysheva ZN. Lost in Translation: Ribosome-Associated mRNA and Protein Quality Controls. Front Genet. 2018 Oct 4;9:431. doi: 10.3389/fgene.2018.00431.

59. Chandrasekaran V, Juszkiewicz S, Choi J, Puglisi JD, Brown A, Shao S, Ramakrishnan V, Hegde RS. Mechanism of ribosome stalling during translation of a poly(A) tail. Nat Struct Mol Biol. 2019 Dec;26(12):1132-1140. doi: 10.1038/s41594-019-0331-x.

60. Baker KE, Coller J. The many routes to regulating mRNA translation. Genome Biol. 2006;7(12):332. doi: 10.1186/gb-2006-7-12-332. PMID: 17176455; PMCID: PMC1794424.

61. Liu ZSJ, Truong TTT, Bortolasci CC, Spolding B, Panizzutti B, Swinton C, et al. Effects of Psychotropic Drugs on Ribosomal Genes and Protein Synthesis. Int J Mol Sci. 2022 Jun 28;23(13):7180. doi: 10.3390/ijms23137180.

62. Yamagishi M, Shirasaki Y, Funatsu T. Single-molecule tracking of mRNA in living cells. Methods Mol Biol. 2013;950:153-67. doi: 10.1007/978-1-62703-137-0_10. PMID: 23086875.

63. Vargas DY, Raj A, Marras SA, Kramer FR, Tyagi S. Mechanism of mRNA transport in the nucleus. Proc Natl Acad Sci U S A. 2005 Nov 22;102(47):17008-13. doi: 10.1073/pnas.0505580102.

64. Fusco D, Accornero N, Lavoie B, Shenoy SM, Blanchard JM, Singer RH, Bertrand E. Single mRNA molecules demonstrate probabilistic movement in living mammalian cells. Curr Biol. 2003 Jan 21;13(2):161-167. doi: 10.1016/s0960-9822(02)01436-7.

65. Siwaszek A, Ukleja M, Dziembowski A. Proteins involved in the degradation of cytoplasmic mRNA in the major eukaryotic model

systems. RNA Biol. 2014;11(9):1122-36. doi: 10.4161/rna.34406. PMID: 25483043; PMCID: PMC4615280.

66. Aldén M, Olofsson Falla F, Yang D, Barghouth M, Luan C, Rasmussen M, De Marinis Y. Intracellular Reverse Transcription of Pfizer BioNTech COVID-19 mRNA Vaccine BNT162b2 In Vitro in Human Liver Cell Line. Curr Issues Mol Biol. 2022 Feb 25;44(3):1115-1126. doi: 10.3390/cimb44030073.

67. Zhang L, Richards A, Barrasa MI, Hughes SH, Young RA, Jaenisch R. Reverse-transcribed SARS-CoV-2 RNA can integrate into the genome of cultured human cells and can be expressed in patient-derived tissues. Proc Natl Acad Sci U S A. 2021 May 25;118(21):e2105968118. doi: 10.1073/pnas.2105968118.

68. Doyle GA, Crist RC, Karatas ET, Hammond MJ, Ewing AD, Ferraro TN, Hahn CG, Berrettini WH. Analysis of LINE-1 Elements in DNA from Postmortem Brains of Individuals with Schizophrenia. Neuropsychopharmacology. 2017 Dec;42(13):2602-2611. doi: 10.1038/npp.2017.115.

69. Houtepen LC, van Bergen AH, Vinkers CH, Boks MP. DNA methylation signatures of mood stabilizers and antipsychotics in bipolar disorder. Epigenomics. 2016 Feb;8(2):197-208. doi: 10.2217/epi.15.98.

70. Yang J, Shen MH. Polyethylene glycol-mediated cell fusion. Methods Mol Biol. 2006;325:59-66. doi: 10.1385/1-59745-005-7:59. PMID: 16761719.

71. Li Y, Kröger M, Liu WK. Endocytosis of PEGylated nanoparticles accompanied by structural and free energy changes of the grafted polyethylene glycol. Biomaterials. 2014 Oct;35(30):8467-78. doi: 10.1016/j.biomaterials.2014.06.032

72. Fang Y, Xue J, Gao S, Lu A, Yang D, Jiang H, He Y, Shi K. Cleavable PEGylation: a strategy for overcoming the "PEG dilemma" in efficient drug delivery. Drug Deliv. 2017 Dec;24(sup1):22-32. doi: 10.1080/10717544.2017.1388451.

73. Park S, Choi YK, Kim S, Lee J, Im W. CHARMM-GUI Membrane Builder for Lipid Nanoparticles with Ionizable Cationic Lipids and PEGylated Lipids. J Chem Inf Model. 2021 Oct 25;61(10):5192-5202. doi: 10.1021/acs.jcim.1c00770.

74. Lee J, Patel DS, Ståhle J, Park SJ, Kern NR, Kim S, Lee J, et al. CHARMM-GUI Membrane Builder for Complex Biological Membrane Simulations with Glycolipids and Lipoglycans. J Chem Theory Comput. 2019 Jan 8;15(1):775-786. doi: 10.1021/acs.jctc.8b01066.

75. Kovtun O, Dickson VK, Kelly BT, Owen DJ, Briggs JAG. Architecture of the AP2/clathrin coat on the membranes of clathrin-coated vesicles. Sci Adv. 2020 Jul 22;6(30):eaba8381. doi: 10.1126/sciadv.aba8381.

76. Inoue Y, Tanaka N, Tanaka Y, Inoue S, Morita K, Zhuang M, Hattori T, Sugamura K. Clathrin-dependent entry of severe acute respiratory syndrome coronavirus into target cells expressing ACE2 with the cytoplasmic tail deleted. J Virol. 2007 Aug;81(16):8722-9. doi: 10.1128/JVI.00253-07.

77. Chang CC, Wu M, Yuan F. Role of specific endocytic pathways in electrotransfection of cells. Mol Ther Methods Clin Dev. 2014 Dec 17;1:14058. doi: 10.1038/mtm.2014.58.

78. Wang LH, Rothberg KG, Anderson RG. Mis-assembly of clathrin lattices on endosomes reveals a regulatory switch for coated pit formation. J Cell Biol. 1993;123:1107–1117.

79. Canfrán-Duque A, Barrio LC, Lerma M, de la Peña G, Serna J, Pastor O,. First-Generation Antipsychotic Haloperidol Alters the Functionality of the Late Endosomal/Lysosomal Compartment in Vitro. Int J Mol Sci. 2016 Mar 18;17(3):404. doi: 10.3390/ijms17030404.

80. Daniel WA. Mechanisms of cellular distribution of psychotropic drugs. Significance for drug action and interactions. Prog Neuropsychopharmacol Biol Psychiatry. 2003 Feb;27(1):65-73. doi: 10.1016/s0278-5846(02)00317-2. PMID: 12551728.

81. Popova, N.V.; Deyev, I.E.; Petrenko, A.G. Clathrin-mediated endocytosis and adaptor proteins. Acta Nat. 2013, 5, 62–73.

82. Meyer N, Henkel L, Linder B, Zielke S, Tascher G, Trautmann S, et al. Autophagy activation, lipotoxicity and lysosomal membrane permeabilization synergize to promote pimozide- and loperamide-induced glioma cell death. Autophagy. 2021 Nov;17(11):3424-3443. doi: 10.1080/15548627.2021.1874208.

83. Su Y, Liu M, Liang K, Liu X, Song Y, Deng Y. Evaluating the Accelerated Blood Clearance Phenomenon of PEGylated Nanoemulsions in Rats by Intraperitoneal Administration. AAPS PharmSciTech. 2018 Oct;19(7):3210-3218. doi: 10.1208/s12249-018-1120-2

84. Liu M, Chu Y, Liu H, Su Y, Zhang Q, Jiao J, et al. Accelerated Blood Clearance of Nanoemulsions Modified with PEG-Cholesterol and PEG-Phospholipid Derivatives in Rats: The Effect of PEG-Lipid Linkages and PEG Molecular Weights. Mol Pharm. 2020 Apr 6;17(4):1059-1070. doi: 10.1021/acs.molpharmaceut.9b00770.

85. Chaurio RA, Janko C, Muñoz LE, Frey B, Herrmann M, Gaipl US. Phospholipids: key players in apoptosis and immune regulation.

Molecules. 2009 Nov 30;14(12):4892-914. doi: 10.3390/molecules14124892

86. Zhang H, Han X, Alameh MG, Shepherd SJ, Padilla MS, Xue L, et al. Rational design of anti-inflammatory lipid nanoparticles for mRNA delivery. J Biomed Mater Res A. 2022 May;110(5):1101-1108. doi: 10.1002/jbm.a.37356.

87. Lin WC, Blanchette CD, Ratto TV, Longo ML. Lipid asymmetry in DLPC/DSPC-supported lipid bilayers: a combined AFM and fluorescence microscopy study. Biophys J. 2006 Jan 1;90(1):228-37. doi: 10.1529/biophysj.105.067066.

88. Benne N, Leboux RJT, Glandrup M, van Duijn J, Lozano Vigario F, Neustrup MA, Romeijn S, Galli F, Kuiper J, Jiskoot W, Slütter B. Atomic force microscopy measurements of anionic liposomes reveal the effect of liposomal rigidity on antigen-specific regulatory T cell responses. J Control Release. 2020 Feb;318:246-255. doi: 10.1016/j.jconrel.2019.12.003.

89. Batista-Duharte A, Pera A, Aliño SF, Solana R. Regulatory T cells and vaccine effectiveness in older adults. Challenges and prospects. Int Immunopharmacol. 2021 Jul;96:107761. doi: 10.1016/j.intimp.2021.107761

90. Galván-Peña S, Leon J, Chowdhary K, Michelson DA, Vijaykumar B, Yang L, et al. MGH COVID-19 Collection & Processing Team, Mathis D, Benoist C. Profound Treg perturbations correlate with COVID-19 severity. Proc Natl Acad Sci U S A. 2021 Sep 14;118(37):e2111315118. doi: 10.1073/pnas.2111315118.

91. Stapel B, Sieve I, Falk CS, Bleich S, Hilfiker-Kleiner D, Kahl KG. Second generation atypical antipsychotics olanzapine and aripiprazole reduce expression and secretion of inflammatory

cytokines in human immune cells. J Psychiatr Res. 2018 Oct;105:95-102. doi: 10.1016/j.jpsychires.2018.08.017.

92. Ponsford MJ, Pecoraro A, Jolles S. Clozapine-associated secondary antibody deficiency. Curr Opin Allergy Clin Immunol. 2019 Dec;19(6):553-562. doi: 10.1097/ACI.0000000000000592. PMID: 31567398.

93. Leykin I, Mayer R, Shinitzky M. Short and long-term immunosuppressive effects of clozapine and haloperidol. Immunopharmacology. 1997 Aug;37(1):75-86. doi: 10.1016/s0162-3109(97)00037-4. PMID: 9285246.

94. May M, Beauchemin M, Vary C, Barlow D, Houseknecht KL. The antipsychotic medication, risperidone, causes global immunosuppression in healthy mice. PLoS One. 2019 Jun 26;14(6):e0218937. doi: 10.1371/journal.pone.0218937.

95. Jutila A, Söderlund T, Pakkanen AL, Huttunen M, Kinnunen PK. Comparison of the effects of clozapine, chlorpromazine, and haloperidol on membrane lateral heterogeneity. Chem Phys Lipids. 2001 Aug;112(2):151-63. doi: 10.1016/s0009-3084(01)00175-x.

96. Pandurangi AK, Buckley PF. Inflammation, Antipsychotic Drugs, and Evidence for Effectiveness of Anti-inflammatory Agents in Schizophrenia. Curr Top Behav Neurosci. 2020;44:227-244. doi: 10.1007/7854_2019_91.

97. May M, Beauchemin M, Vary C, Barlow D, Houseknecht KL. The antipsychotic medication, risperidone, causes global immunosuppression in healthy mice. PLoS One. 2019 Jun 26;14(6):e0218937. doi: 10.1371/journal.pone.0218937.

98. Al-Amin MM, Nasir Uddin MM, Mahmud Reza H. Effects of antipsychotics on the inflammatory response system of patients with schizophrenia in peripheral blood mononuclear cell cultures. Clin

Psychopharmacol Neurosci. 2013 Dec;11(3):144-51. doi: 10.9758/cpn.2013.11.3.144. Epub 2013 Dec 24. PMID: 24465251

99. Sherman MA, Linthicum DS, Bolger MB. Haloperidol binding to monoclonal antibodies: conformational analysis and relationships to D-2 receptor binding. Mol Pharmacol. 1986 Jun;29(6):589-98. PMID: 2423865.

100. Goldsmith SK. Haloperidol reduces IgG immunoreactivity in the rat brain. Int J Neuropsychopharmacol. 2002 Dec;5(4):309-13. doi: 10.1017/s146114570200305x. PMID: 14710722.

101. Lozano R, Marin R, Santacruz MJ, Pascual A. Selective Immunoglobulin M Deficiency Among Clozapine-Treated Patients: A Nested Case-Control Study. Prim Care Companion CNS Disord. 2015 Jul 2;17(4):10.4088/PCC.15m01782. doi: 10.4088/PCC.15m01782.

102. Schleuning MJ, Duggan A, Reem GH. Inhibition by chlorpromazine of lymphokine-specific mRNA expression in human thymocytes. Eur J Immunol. 1989 Aug;19(8):1491-5. doi: 10.1002/eji.1830190822. PMID: 2550248.

103. Ficarra S, Russo A, Barreca D, Giunta E, Galtieri A, Tellone E. Short-Term Effects of Chlorpromazine on Oxidative Stress in Erythrocyte Functionality: Activation of Metabolism and Membrane Perturbation. Oxid Med Cell Longev. 2016;2016:2394130. doi: 10.1155/2016/2394130.

104. Kelly DL, Li X, Kilday C, Feldman S, Clark S, Liu F, Buchanan RW, Tonelli LH. Increased circulating regulatory T cells in medicated people with schizophrenia. Psychiatry Res. 2018 Nov;269:517-523. doi: 10.1016/j.psychres.2018.09.006.

105. Himmerich H, Milenović S, Fulda S, Plümäkers B, Sheldrick AJ, Michel TM, Kircher T, Rink L. Regulatory T cells increased while

IL-1β decreased during antidepressant therapy. J Psychiatr Res. 2010 Nov;44(15):1052-7. doi: 10.1016/j.jpsychires.2010.03.005

106. Paloncýová M, Čechová P, Šrejber M, Kührová P, Otyepka M. Role of Ionizable Lipids in SARS-CoV-2 Vaccines As Revealed by Molecular Dynamics Simulations: From Membrane Structure to Interaction with mRNA Fragments. J Phys Chem Lett. 2021 Nov 18;12(45):11199-11205. doi: 10.1021/acs.jpclett.1c03109.

107. Gao X, Huang L. Potentiation of cationic liposome-mediated gene delivery by polycations. Biochemistry. 1996 Jan 23;35(3):1027-36. doi: 10.1021/bi952436a. PMID: 8547238.

108. Han, X., Zhang, H., Butowska, K. et al. An ionizable lipid toolbox for RNA delivery. Nat Commun 12, 7233 (2021). https://doi.org/10.1038/s41467-021-27493-0

109. Soulet D, Gagnon B, Rivest S, Audette M, Poulin R. A fluorescent probe of polyamine transport accumulates into intracellular acidic vesicles via a two-step mechanism. J Biol Chem. 2004 Nov 19;279(47):49355-66. doi: 10.1074/jbc.M401287200.

110. Jiang Y, Lu Q, Wang Y, Xu E, Ho A, Singh P, et al. Quantitating Endosomal Escape of a Library of Polymers for mRNA Delivery. Nano Lett. 2020 Feb 12;20(2):1117-1123. doi: 10.1021/acs.nanolett.9b04426

111. Goldman SD, Funk RS, Rajewski RA, Krise JP. Mechanisms of amine accumulation in, and egress from, lysosomes. Bioanalysis. 2009 Nov;1(8):1445-59. doi: 10.4155/bio.09.128.

112. Li J, He Y, Wang W, Wu C, Hong C, Hammond PT. Polyamine-Mediated Stoichiometric Assembly of Ribonucleoproteins for Enhanced mRNA Delivery. Angew Chem Int Ed Engl. 2017 Oct 23;56(44):13709-13712. doi: 10.1002/anie.201707466.

113. Ding F, Zhang H, Cui J, Li Q, Yang C. Boosting ionizable lipid nanoparticle-mediated in vivo mRNA delivery through optimization of lipid amine-head groups. Biomater Sci. 2021 Nov 9;9(22):7534-7546. doi: 10.1039/d1bm00866h. PMID: 34647548.

114. Merkley SD, Chock CJ, Yang XO, Harris J, Castillo EF. Modulating T Cell Responses via Autophagy: The Intrinsic Influence Controlling the Function of Both Antigen-Presenting Cells and T Cells. Front Immunol. 2018 Dec 14;9:2914. doi: 10.3389/fimmu.2018.02914

115. Alsaleh G, Panse I, Swadling L, Zhang H, Richter FC, Meyer A, Lord J, Barnes E, Klenerman P, Green C, Simon AK. Autophagy in T cells from aged donors is maintained by spermidine and correlates with function and vaccine responses. Elife. 2020 Dec 15;9:e57950. doi: 10.7554/eLife.57950.

116. Squassina A, Manchia M, Chillotti C, Deiana V, Congiu D, Paribello F, et al. Differential effect of lithium on spermidine/spermine N1-acetyltransferase expression in suicidal behaviour. Int J Neuropsychopharmacol. 2013 Nov;16(10):2209-18. doi: 10.1017/S1461145713000655.

117. Yadav M, Parle M, Jindal DK, Sharma N. Potential effect of spermidine on GABA, dopamine, acetylcholinesterase, oxidative stress and proinflammatory cytokines to diminish ketamine-induced psychotic symptoms in rats. Biomed Pharmacother. 2018 Feb;98:207-213. doi: 10.1016/j.biopha.2017.12.016.

118. Lefèvre PL, Palin MF, Murphy BD. Polyamines on the reproductive landscape. Endocr Rev. 2011 Oct;32(5):694-712. doi: 10.1210/er.2011-0012. Epub 2011 Jul 26. PMID: 21791568.

119. Aassve A, Cavalli N, Mencarini L, Plach S, Sanders S. Early assessment of the relationship between the COVID-19 pandemic and

births in high-income countries. Proc Natl Acad Sci U S A. 2021 Sep 7;118(36):e2105709118. doi: 10.1073/pnas.2105709118.

120. McLaren RA Jr, Trejo FE, Blitz MJ, Bianco A, Limaye M, Brustman L, et al. COVID-related "lockdowns" and birth rates in New York. Am J Obstet Gynecol MFM. 2021 Nov;3(6):100476. doi: 10.1016/j.ajogmf.2021.100476

121. Firpo MR, Mastrodomenico V, Hawkins GM, Prot M, Levillayer L, Gallagher T, Simon-Loriere E, Mounce BC. Targeting Polyamines Inhibits Coronavirus Infection by Reducing Cellular Attachment and Entry. ACS Infect Dis. 2021 Jun 11;7(6):1423-1432. doi: 10.1021/acsinfecdis.0c00491.

122. Bourgin M, Derosa L, Silva CAC, Goubet AG, Dubuisson A, et al. Circulating acetylated polyamines correlate with Covid-19 severity in cancer patients. Aging (Albany NY). 2021 Sep 13;13(17):20860-20885. doi: 10.18632/aging.203525

123. Fiori LM, Turecki G. Implication of the polyamine system in mental disorders. J Psychiatry Neurosci. 2008 Mar;33(2):102-10. PMID: 18330456; PMCID: PMC2265312.

124. Gross JA, Turecki G. Suicide and the polyamine system. CNS Neurol Disord Drug Targets. 2013 Nov;12(7):980-8. doi: 10.2174/18715273113129990095.

125. Zhao YC, Chi YJ, Yu YS, Liu JL, Su RW, Ma XH, Shan CH, Yang ZM. Polyamines are essential in embryo implantation: expression and function of polyamine-related genes in mouse uterus during peri-implantation period. Endocrinology. 2008 May;149(5):2325-32. doi: 10.1210/en.2007-1420.

126. Heiczman A, Tóth M. Effect of chlorpromazine on the synthesis of neutral lipids and phospholipids from [3H]glycerol in the primordial

human placenta. Placenta. 1995 Jun;16(4):347-58. doi: 10.1016/0143-4004(95)90092-6. PMID: 7567797.

127. Tang H, Mourad S, Zhai SD, Hart RJ. Dopamine agonists for preventing ovarian hyperstimulation syndrome. Cochrane Database Syst Rev. 2016 Nov 30;11(11):CD008605. doi: 10.1002/14651858.CD008605.pub3. Update in: Cochrane Database Syst Rev. 2021 Apr 14;4:CD008605.

128. Eygeris Y, Patel S, Jozic A, Sahay G. Deconvoluting Lipid Nanoparticle Structure for Messenger RNA Delivery. Nano Lett. 2020 Jun 10;20(6):4543-4549. doi: 10.1021/acs.nanolett.0c01386.

129. Sebastiani F, Yanez Arteta M, Lerche M, Porcar L, Lang C, Bragg RA, et al. Apolipoprotein E Binding Drives Structural and Compositional Rearrangement of mRNA-Containing Lipid Nanoparticles. ACS Nano. 2021 Apr 27;15(4):6709-6722. doi: 10.1021/acsnano.0c10064.

130. Guo SJ, Ma CG, Hu YY, Bai G, Song ZJ, Cao XQ. Solid lipid nanoparticles for phytosterols delivery: The acyl chain number of the glyceride matrix affects the arrangement, stability, and release. Food Chem. 2022 Jun 7;394:133412. doi: 10.1016/j.foodchem.2022.133412.

131. Yuan L, Zhang F, Shen M, Jia S, Xie J. Phytosterols Suppress Phagocytosis and Inhibit Inflammatory Mediators via ERK Pathway on LPS-Triggered Inflammatory Responses in RAW264.7 Macrophages and the Correlation with Their Structure. Foods. 2019 Nov 16;8(11):582. doi: 10.3390/foods8110582.

132. Sharma N, Tan MA, An SSA. Phytosterols: Potential Metabolic Modulators in Neurodegenerative Diseases. Int J Mol Sci. 2021 Nov 12;22(22):12255. doi: 10.3390/ijms222212255. PMID: 34830148; PMCID: PMC8618769.

133. Gamba P, Testa G, Gargiulo S, Staurenghi E, Poli G, Leonarduzzi G. Oxidized cholesterol as the driving force behind the development of Alzheimer's disease. Front Aging Neurosci. 2015 Jun 19;7:119. doi: 10.3389/fnagi.2015.00119.

134. Cenik B, Cenik C, Snyder MP, Brown ES. Plasma sterols and depressive symptom severity in a population-based cohort. PLoS One. 2017 Sep 8;12(9):e0184382. doi: 10.1371/journal.pone.0184382. PMID: 28886149; PMCID: PMC5590924.

135. Balasubramanian I, Faheem A, Padhy SK, Menon V. Psychiatric adverse reactions to COVID-19 vaccines: A rapid review of published case reports. Asian J Psychiatr. 2022 May;71:103129. doi: 10.1016/j.ajp.2022.103129.

136. Chen S, Aruldass AR, Cardinal RN. Mental health outcomes after SARS-CoV-2 vaccination in the United States: A national cross-sectional study. J Affect Disord. 2022 Feb 1;298(Pt A):396-399. doi: 10.1016/j.jad.2021.10.134.

137. Jones KT, Zhen J, Reith ME. Importance of cholesterol in dopamine transporter function. J Neurochem. 2012 Dec;123(5):700-15. doi: 10.1111/jnc.12007.

138. Erro R, Buonomo AR, Barone P, Pellecchia MT. Severe Dyskinesia After Administration of SARS-CoV2 mRNA Vaccine in Parkinson's Disease. Mov Disord. 2021 Oct;36(10):2219. doi: 10.1002/mds.28772.

139. Digney A, Keriakous D, Scarr E, Thomas E, Dean B. Differential changes in apolipoprotein E in schizophrenia and bipolar I disorder. Biol Psychiatry. 2005 Apr 1;57(7):711-5. doi: 10.1016/j.biopsych.2004.12.028. PMID: 15820227.

140. Vik-Mo AO, Fernø J, Skrede S, Steen VM. Psychotropic drugs up-regulate the expression of cholesterol transport proteins including ApoE in cultured human CNS- and liver cells. BMC Pharmacol. 2009 Aug 29;9:10. doi: 10.1186/1471-2210-9-10.

141. Dean B, Laws SM, Hone E, Taddei K, Scarr E, Thomas EA, et al. Increased levels of apolipoprotein E in the frontal cortex of subjects with schizophrenia. Biol Psychiatry. 2003 Sep 15;54(6):616-22. doi: 10.1016/s0006-3223(03)00075-1

142. Luquain-Costaz C, Kockx M, Anastasius M, Chow V, Kontush A, Jessup W, Kritharides L. Increased ABCA1 (ATP-Binding Cassette Transporter A1)-Specific Cholesterol Efflux Capacity in Schizophrenia. Arterioscler Thromb Vasc Biol. 2020 Nov;40(11):2728-2737. Doi: 10.1161/ATVBAHA.120.314847.

143. Korade Ž, Liu W, Warren EB, Armstrong K, Porter NA, Konradi C. Effect of psychotropic drug treatment on sterol metabolism. Schizophr Res. 2017 Sep;187:74-81. doi: 10.1016/j.schres.2017.02.001. Epub 2017 Feb 12. PMID: 28202290; PMCID: PMC555446

Chapter 11
COVID-19 mRNA Therapeutics and Schizophrenia

Chapter 10 examines the interaction between COVID-19 mRNA vaccine and psychotropic drugs, while chapter 11 takes a closer look at the role of schizophrenia in the efficacy of these vaccines.

It is now established that the SARS-CoV-2 virus usurps the endocytic pathway (EP) to infect human cells. Since several psychotropic drugs ingress host cells via the EP, these agents may deny viral entry through this portal. Indeed, other antivirals, hydroxychloroquine or ivermectin block viral endocytosis, protecting against infection.

The second modality SARS-CoV-2 virus infects human cells is by fusing with the plasma membrane.This prompts fusion of host cells with each other, forming syncytial structures. Therefore, infection progresses from one infected cell to all fused cells through the shared cytosol. Fused cells trigger cellular senescence and resistance to apoptosis (cell death).

SARS-CoV-2 and RNA therapeutics have reopened the research on cell-cell fusion or syncytia formation. This is significant as fused cells can occur in the absence of viral infection, such as in normal aging and neuropathology.

Pfizer and Moderna COVID-19 vaccines are composed of LNP containing a modified messenger RNA (mRNA) that encodes for the Spike S protein (1) (2) (3). The LNP transfection likely involves particle engulfment by the host immune cells due to their resemblance to apoptotic bodies, vesicles with externalized phosphatidylserine (ePS). As the LNPs are decorated with PS-like ionizable phospholipids, including 1,2-distearoyl-sn-glycero-3-

phosphocholine (DSPCs) that "encourage" human phagocytes to internalize the LNP (4) (5) (6).

The LNP technology mimics viral envelopes with ePS, a universal "eat me" signal that directs immune cells to engulf the particle (7) (8). However, as ePS is also a "fuse me" signal, LNPs may inadvertently facilitate the formation of pathological syncytia (9) (10). Moreover, ePS may activate a disintegrin and metalloprotease 10 and 17 (ADAM 10) (ADAM 17), master regulators of syncytia formation, contributing further to this process (11) (12).

LNP-incorporated mRNA comprises a technological success which goes beyond vaccines, opening new avenues for developing "smart" therapeutics that can be delivered with pinpoint precision to specific subcellular structures (13). The development of such therapeutics is anticipated to redefine clinical pathways, for communicable and non-communicable diseases. However, these therapies may not be ready for worldwide application in their present molecular form.

The question has been asked before, about the potential toxicity of lipid formulations, especially those delivering cancer therapeutics (14). Pathological cell-cell fusion may be the root cause of vaccine adverse effects, including giant cell myocarditis, heart failure, and infertility. Indeed, cardiomyocyte fusion is a newly discovered mechanism contributing to pathological cardiac hypertrophy (15). Fusion is probably induced by the LNP components DSPC and polyethylene glycol (PEG), and not by the mRNA itself.

Messenger RNA vaccines, an overview

To elicit the formation of neutralizing antibodies, exogenously administered mRNA must avoid the obstacles described in the previous chapter (16) (17). This is accomplished by hiding the nucleic acid backbone in LNPs, and adding N1-methyl pseudouridine (m1Ψ) to the mRNA (18) (19) (Fig. 1). The coding region of mRNA is flanked by two untranslated regions (UTRs) followed by a polyadenylated (polyA) tail at 3' and a cap at 5' for further structural stabilization and protection (Fig. 1) (17) (19) (20).

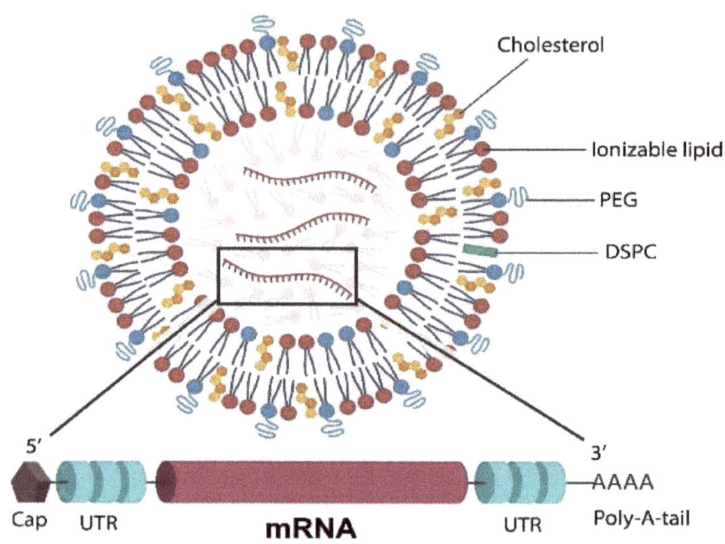

Fig. 11.1 N1-methylpseudouridine (m1Ψ)-modified mRNA (in the rectangle) is surrounded by a lipid nanoparticle (LNP) comprised of 1,2-distearoyl-sn-glycero-3-phosphocholine (DSPC), cholesterol, and an ionizable lipid. Polyethylene glycol (PEG) is conjugated with the lipid molecules to increase the mRNA duration of action. The mRNA encodes for the full-length S antigen and is flanked by two untranslated regions (UTRs) and a polyadenylated (polyA) tail at the 3' end for stabilization. A cap at the 5' end offers further protection from exonuclease recognition.

As mRNA vaccines are based primarily on pre-fusion epitopes, cell-cell fusion may continue among host cells, allowing viral infection to continue by syncytia formation (3) (16). This is significant, as it could account for the recurrence of COVID-19 symptoms in fully vaccinated individuals (3) (21) (22). In addition, this may explain the post-vaccination events associated with cell-cell fusion, including giant cell myocarditis, giant cell arteritis, and Creutzfeldt-Jakob Disease, recorded in the Vaccine Adverse Event Reporting System (VAERS) database (23) (24) (25) (26) (27).

What is cell-cell fusion?

Cell-cell fusion is a physiological or pathological process in which one or more adjacent cells merge their plasma membranes, cytoplasm, nuclei, and intracellular organelles, generating multinucleated syncytia, often with novel, emerging properties (28). Under normal circumstances, cell-cell fusion occurs during fertilization and placentation as well as during the formation of myoblasts, including the cardiac myoblasts (29). Likewise, in the CNS, astrocytes engender physiological syncytia via connexins (30) (31).

Several viruses, including SARS-CoV-2, exploit host physiological fusion drivers (fusogenic) as these molecules induce premature cellular senescence and immunosuppression, phenotypes hospitable for viral replication and immune evasion (32) (33). Indeed, cell-cell fusion is triggered by ePS, a marker of low immunogenicity, exploited by the SARS-CoV-2 virus to enter host cells undetected (9) (34) (35) (36). Virus-upregulated intracellular calcium (Ca^{2+}) activates transmembrane protein 16F (TMEM16F), which in turn flips PS from the inner to the outer layer of cell membranes, promoting fusion (9).

Viruses, including SARS-CoV-2, can enter host cells via endocytosis or cell-cell fusion, suggesting that endocytosis inhibition may not always prevent the infection (37) (38) (39). Endocytosis requires viral protein attachment to a cell surface receptor and internalization of the virus/receptor complex into the host cell. For example, SARS-CoV-2 binds to host angiotensin-converting enzyme-2 (ACE-2) via its S1 protein, followed by endocytosis. On the other hand, ePS activates ADAM17, inducing cell-cell fusion via furin cleaving site (FCS) located within the S2 protein, a pathway independent of S1/ACE-2 (40) (41) (42) (43).

Vaccine core: the synthetic mRNA

In contrast to traditional vaccines that present a plethora of viral proteins to the host immune cells, COVID-19 mRNA-based therapeutics are limited to the antigen of interest (AOI) and elicit antibodies only against the receptor binding site (RBS) (1) (12) (44). For the complete success of the above method, it must be assumed that the SARS-CoV-2 virus cannot ingress host cells by an alternative pathway. However, several studies have highlighted other potential routes of viral ingress, including metalloprotease, integrins, glucose-regulating protein 78 (GRP78), antibody-dependent enhancement, cell-penetrating peptides, and HERVs (45) (46) (47).

LNPs

Although transfection data is proprietary primarily, interrogation of LNP components can provide clues about the mRNA ingress into human cells (6). For example, LNPs contain ionizable lipids, phospholipid 1,2-distearoyl-sn-glycero-3-phosphocholine (DSPC), and cholesterol that can attract host phagocytes to internalize the particle (48) (49) (50). Ionizable lipids and DSPC resemble ePS and communicate readiness for engulfment (51). Aside from comprising an established "eat me" signal, ePS can also convey "fuse me" cues to host phagocytes, initiating pathological syncytia (10). The LNP component, cholesterol, is also a promoter of pathological cell-cell fusion as it can alter the asymmetry of cell membranes (50). Moreover, as cell-cell fusion leads to premature cellular senescence and immunosuppression, it may partly explain the immune dysfunction documented in some vaccinated individuals (52) (53) (54).

Formation of multiple nuclei

PEG was added to the LNP to stabilize and prolong the mRNA duration of action (Fig. 1). The extensive utilization of PEG over the past few decades suggests that preexisting antibodies could trigger hypersensitivity to vaccines containing this molecule (55) (56). Aside from allergy, PEG is also an established chemical fusogen that can generate pathology by promoting multinucleation, aneuploidy, and genomic instability (57) (58) (59) (60). In addition, PEG upregulates intracellular $Ca^{2=}$, activating the transmembrane protein 16F (TMEM16F), a lipid scramblase that flips PS on the cell surface, triggering fusion, premature cellular senescence, and immunosuppression (61) (62) (63). As these phenotypes are virus-friendly, PEG-induced cell-cell fusion may inadvertently facilitate not only SARS-CoV-2 but also other viral infections (61) (65) (66) (67). Furthermore, ePS-activated ADAM 10 and 17 promote syncytia formation via the has never been used in an approved vaccine previously; therefore, its presence in Pfizer-BioNTech and Moderna -1273 therapeutics, raised concerns, especially regarding anaphylactic and fusogenic adverse effects (53) (68) (69). Moreover, PEG promotes temporary permeabilization of the BBB, a property exploited by the pharmaceutical industry for CNS delivery systems (70) (71) (72). This may account, at least in part, for the VAERS-reported neuropsychiatric symptoms, from "brain fog" to neurodegeneration (73) (74) (75). Furthermore, earlier studies have demonstrated that PEG may interfere with the conformational stability of proteins, indicating that syncytia, cellular senescence, and impaired protein folding are highly intertwined (76) (77) (78). While the attention to PEG and the need to further study its relation to the potential vaccine adverse reactions is logical and appropriate, it must be noted that excipients other than PEG might also be involved in such reported adverse events (79).

DSPC and ionizable lipids

To deliver the liposome cargo to human immune cells, mRNA therapeutics must trick host phagocytes into internalizing LNPs, as discussed in Chapter 10 (80) (81). This is accomplished by decorating the liposomal particles with ionizable lipids and DSPC, an anionic phospholipid that mimics ePS and conveys readiness for phagocytosis (82) (83).

Pfizer and Moderna vaccines were designed to "imitate" dying cells or apoptotic bodies by utilizing ionizable lipids and DSPC, which delivers mRNA directly to the immune cells' translation machinery (5). However, DSPC's resemblance to PS may inadvertently activate ADAM 10 and 17, promoting cell-cell fusion and subsequent pathology (40).

Together, LNPs mimicking ePS are engulfed by host immune cells and generate anti-S antibodies by delivering the mRNA cargo to host ribosomes. However, in some cases, the disruption of the plasma cell membrane may inadvertently engender iatrogenic syncytia by activating the metalloprotease pathway.

The autophagy–lysosomal pathway in SMI

Virus-induced first-episode psychosis (FEP) is critical to elucidating the link between SARS-CoV-2 and SMI. In other words, establishing how COVID-19 induces psychosis may help clarify the underlying pathophysiology of SMI.

Approximately 4% of people exposed to any viral outbreak develop psychosis. This is significantly higher than 015%, the median incidence for psychosis in the general population, highlighting viral infection as an independent risk factor for SMI (41).

The autophagy–lysosomal pathway has emerged as the common denominator of COVID-19 and psychosis, suggesting that a better understanding of virus-human protein-protein interaction (interactome) could elucidate the etiopathogenesis of SMI (42).

Autophagy refers to an intracellular system of vesicles that degrade defective proteins, dysfunctional mitochondria, and lysosomes. These molecules are recycled via autophagosomes that fuse with lysosomes. Autophagosomes fuse with lysosomes to form phagolysosomes in which the cargo is digested.

The EP is the second intracellular system comprised of vesicles that remove the surface receptors by sinking them into the cytoplasm to be recycled. These vesicles, early and late endosomes, merge with the lysosomes, where recycling occurs. The lysosome joins autophagy and endocytosis by fusing autophagosomes and lysosomes. Interestingly, antipsychotic drugs and the SARS-CoV-2 virus disrupt the autophagosome-lysosome fusion, disconnecting the two systems.

The first SARS-CoV-2 interactome study has identified that viral antigen open reading frame 3 (ORF 3) interaction with human Rab 7 protein disrupts the fusion of the autophagosome with the lysosome, thus preventing the removal of damaged proteins and defective mitochondria or lysosomes (autophagy). These findings align with previous studies, which emphasized the role of autophagy in the pathogenesis of SCZ (43). Indeed, others found that olanzapine, a widely used antipsychotic drug, acts at the level of the autophagy and lysosomal pathway (44).

Taken together, the SARS-CoV-2 virus, COVID-19 mRNA vaccine, and many psychotropic drugs enter human cells via the EP. Therefore, understanding this route is imperative for clarifying the pathogenesis of SMI,

Another common denominator between the virus and neuropsychiatric disorders is fusion. Fusion of SARS-CoV-2 with human cell membrane, fusion of host cells to each other, and fusion of autophagosome and lysosome are disrupted because the virus hijacks human fusogens to control cell-cell fusion.

Conclusions

The mRNA virus and vaccines shifted the attention of researchers and clinicians to the EP, a standard route for viruses, SMI, and cancer.

The mRNA vaccines represent the first large-scale administration of LNPs and represent the avant-garde of novel delivery systems for therapeutics. The pandemic and vaccines also highlighted a rarely studied phenomenon: syncytia formation documented in SCZ, dementias, and aging in general.

On a positive note, the COVID-19 pandemic has clarified many unknown pathophysiological mechanisms of SMI, including autophagy, microbial translocation, and cellular senescence.

Chapter 11 References:

1. Rijkers GT, Weterings N, Obregon-Henao A, Lepolder M, Dutt TS, van Overveld FJ, Henao-Tamayo M. Antigen Presentation of mRNA-Based and Virus-Vectored SARS-CoV-2 Vaccines. Vaccines (Basel). 2021 Aug 3;9(8):848. doi: 10.3390/vaccines9080848.

2. Bergwerk M, Gonen T, Lustig Y, Amit S, Lipsitch M, Cohen C, et al. Covid-19 Breakthrough Infections in Vaccinated Health Care Workers. N Engl J Med. 2021 Oct 14;385(16):1474-1484. doi: 10.1056/NEJMoa2109072.

3. Hein S, Benz NI, Eisert J, Herrlein ML, Oberle D, Dreher M, Stingl JC, Hildt C, Hildt E. Comirnaty-Elicited and Convalescent Sera Recognize Different Spike Epitopes. Vaccines (Basel). 2021 Dec 1;9(12):1419. doi: 10.3390/vaccines9121419.

4. Sakai-Kato K, Yoshida K, Takechi-Haraya Y, Izutsu KI. Physicochemical Characterization of Liposomes That Mimic the Lipid Composition of Exosomes for Effective Intracellular Trafficking. Langmuir. 2020 Oct 27;36(42):12735-12744. doi: 10.1021/acs.langmuir.0c02491.

5. Lotter C, Alter CL, Bolten JS, Detampel P, Palivan CG, Einfalt T, Huwyler J. Incorporation of phosphatidylserine improves the efficiency of lipid lipid-based gene delivery systems. Eur J Pharm Biopharm. 2022 Mar;172:134-143. doi: 10.1016/j.ejpb.2022.02.007.

6. Cao Y, Gao GF. mRNA vaccines: A matter of delivery. EClinicalMedicine. 2021 Feb 3;32:100746. doi 10.1016/j.eclinm.2021.100746. PMID: 33644722

7. Liu J, Conboy JC. Phase Behavior of Planar Supported Lipid Membranes Composed of Cholesterol and 1,2-Distearoyl-sn-Glycerol-3-Phosphocholine Examined by Sum-Frequency

Vibrational Spectroscopy. Vib Spectrosc. 2009 May 26;50(1):106-115. doi: 10.1016/j.vibspec.2008.09.004

8.   Bohan D, Ert HV, Ruggio N, Rogers KJ, Badreddine M, Aguilar Briseño JA, et al. Phosphatidylserine Receptors Enhance SARS-CoV-2 Infection: AXL as a Therapeutic Target for COVID-19. bioRxiv [Preprint]. 2021 Jun 24:2021.06.15.448419. doi: 10.1101/2021.06.15.448419. Update in: PLoS Pathog. 2021 Nov 19;17(11):e1009743. PMID: 34159331; PMCID: PMC8219095.

9.   Whitlock JM, Chernomordik LV. Flagging fusion: Phosphatidylserine signaling in cell-cell fusion. J Biol Chem. 2021;296:100411. doi:10.1016/j.jbc.2021.100411

10.   Kim GW, Park SY, Kim IS. Novel function of stabilin-2 in myoblast fusion: the recognition of extracellular phosphatidylserine as a "fuse-me" signal. BMB Rep. 2016 Jun;49(6):303-4. doi: 10.5483/bmbrep.2016.49.6.078.

11.   Yamamoto M, Gohda J, Kobayashi A, Tomita K, Hirayama Y, Naohiko Koshikawa, et al. Metalloproteinase-Dependent and TMPRSS2-Independent Cell Surface Entry Pathway of SARS-CoV-2 Requires the Furin Cleavage Site and the S2 Domain of Spike Protein. ASM Journal (2022). DOI: https://doi.org/10.1128/mbio.00519-22

12.   Theuerkauf SA, Michels A, Riechert V, Maier TJ, Flory E, Cichutek K, Buchholz CJ. Quantitative assays reveal cell fusion at minimal levels of SARS-CoV-2 spike protein and fusion from without. iScience. 2021 Mar 19;24(3):102170. doi: 10.1016/j.isci.2021.102170.

13.   Pardi N., Hogan M.J., Porter F.W., Weissman D. mRNA vaccines - a new era in vaccinology. Nat Rev Drug Discov. 2018;17:261–279. doi: 10.1038/nrd.2017.243

14. Kulkarni JA, Cullis PR, van der Meel R. Lipid Nanoparticles Enabling Gene Therapies: From Concepts to Clinical Utility. Nucleic Acid Ther. 2018 Jun;28(3):146-157. doi: 10.1089/nat.2018.0721

15. A Colliva, S Vodret, W Bongiovanni, S Zacchigna, Cardiomyocyte fusion as a new mechanism contributing to pathological cardiac hypertrophy, Cardiovascular Research, Volume 118, Issue Supplement_1, June 2022, cvac066.092, https://doi.org/10.1093/cvr/cvac066.092

16. Andries O, Mc Cafferty S, De Smedt SC, Weiss R, Sanders NN, Kitada T. N(1)-methyl pseudouridine-incorporated mRNA outperforms pseudouridine-incorporated mRNA by providing enhanced protein expression and reduced immunogenicity in mammalian cell lines and mice. J Control Release. 2015 Nov 10;217:337-44. doi: 10.1016/j.jconrel.2015.08.051.

17. Schoenmaker L, Witzigmann D, Kulkarni JA, et al. mRNA-lipid nanoparticle COVID-19 vaccines: Structure and stability. Int J Pharm. 2021;601:120586. doi:10.1016/j.ijpharm.2021.120586

18. Nance KD, Meier JL. Modifications in an Emergency: The Role of N1-Methylpseudouridine in COVID-19 Vaccines. ACS Cent Sci. 2021 May 26;7(5):748-756. doi: 10.1021/acscentsci.1c00197.

19. Gebre, M.S., Rauch, S., Roth, N. et al. Optimization of non-coding regions for a non-modified mRNA COVID-19 vaccine. Nature 601, 410–414 (2022). https://doi.org/10.1038/s41586-021-04231-6

20. Jeeva S, Kim KH, Shin CH, Wang BZ, Kang SM. An Update on mRNA-Based Viral Vaccines. Vaccines (Basel). 2021;9(9):965. Published 2021 Aug 29. doi:10.3390/vaccines9090965

21. Hu, J., Chen, X., Lu, X. et al. A spike protein S2 antibody efficiently neutralizes the Omicron variant. Cell Mol Immunol 19, 644–646 (2022). https://doi.org/10.1038/s41423-022-00847-4

22. Ren, F., Zhang, N., Zhang, L. et al. Alternative Polyadenylation: a new frontier in post post-transcriptional regulation. Biomark Res 8, 67 (2020). https://doi.org/10.1186/s40364-020-00249-6

23. Sung K, McCain J, King KR, Hong K, Aisagbonhi O, Adler ED, Urey MA. Biopsy-Proven Giant Cell Myocarditis Following the COVID-19 Vaccine. Circ Heart Fail. 2022 Apr;15(4):e009321. doi: 10.1161/CIRCHEARTFAILURE.121.009321.

24. Lazebnik Y. Cell fusion as a link between the SARS-CoV-2 spike protein, COVID-19 complications, and vaccine side effects. Oncotarget. 2021;12(25):2476-2488. Published 2021 Dec 7. doi:10.18632/oncotarget.28088

25. Anzola AM, Trives L, Martínez-Barrio J, Pinilla B, Álvaro-Gracia JM, Molina-Collada J. New-onset giant cell arteritis following COVID-19 mRNA (BioNTech/Pfizer) vaccine: a double-edged sword?. Clin Rheumatol. 2022;41(5):1623-1625. doi:10.1007/s10067-021-06041-7

26. Kidson C, Moreau MC, Asher DM, et al. Cell fusion induced by scrapie and Creutzfeldt-Jakob virus-infected brain preparations. Proc Natl Acad Sci U S A. 1978;75(6):2969-2971. doi:10.1073/pnas.75.6.2969

27. Perez JC, Moret-Chalmin C, Montagnier L. Towards the emergence of a new neurodegenerative Creutzfeldt-Jakob disease: Twenty-six cases of CJD were declared a few days after a COVID-19 "vaccine" Jab. Preprint May 2022 DOI: 10.13140/RG.2.2.14427.03366

28. Lin, L., Li, Q., Wang, Y. et al. Syncytia formation during SARS-CoV-2 lung infection: a disastrous unity to eliminate lymphocytes. Cell Death Differ 28, 2019–2021 (2021). https://doi.org/10.1038/s41418-021-00795-y

29. Kar M, Ghosh D, Sengupta J. Molecular correlates of syncytialization in muscle and placenta. Indian J Physiol Pharmacol. 2007 Oct-Dec;51(4):311-25. PMID: 18476385.

30. Refaeli R, Doron A, Benmelech-Chovav A, Groysman M, Kreisel T, Loewenstein Y, Goshen I. Features of hippocampal astrocytic domains and their spatial relation to excitatory and inhibitory neurons. Glia. 2021 Oct;69(10):2378-2390. doi: 10.1002/glia.24044.

31. Katoozi S, Skauli N, Zahl S, Deshpande T, Ezan P, Palazzo C, Steinhäuser C, Frigeri A, Cohen-Salmon M, Ottersen OP, Amiry-Moghaddam M. Uncoupling of the Astrocyte Syncytium Differentially Affects AQP4 Isoforms. Cells. 2020 Feb 7;9(2):382. doi: 10.3390/cells9020382.

32. de De Souza Cardoso R, Viana RMM, Vitti BC, Coelho ACL, de Jesus BLS, de Paula Souza J, Pontelli MC, Murakami T, Ventura AM, Ono A, Arruda E. Human Respiratory Syncytial Virus Infection in a Human T Cell Line Is Hampered at Multiple Steps. Viruses. 2021 Feb 2;13(2):231. doi: 10.3390/v13020231

33. Vance TDR, Lee JE. Virus and eukaryote fusogen superfamilies. Curr Biol. 2020 Jul 6;30(13):R750-R754. doi: 10.1016/j.cub.2020.05.029. PMID: 32634411; PMCID: PMC7336913.

34. Hörnich BF, Großkopf AK, Schlagowski S, Tenbusch M, Kleine-Weber H, Neipel F, et al. SARS-CoV-2 and SARS-CoV Spike-Mediated Cell-Cell Fusion Differ in Their Requirements for Receptor Expression and Proteolytic Activation. J Virol. 2021 Apr 12;95(9):e00002-21. doi: 10.1128/JVI.00002-21.

35. Birge, R., Boeltz, S., Kumar, S. et al. Phosphatidylserine is a global immunosuppressive signal in efferocytosis, infectious disease, and

cancer. Cell Death Differ 23, 962–978 (2016).
https://doi.org/10.1038/cdd.2016.11

36. Gal H, Krizhanovsky V. Cell fusion induced senescence. Aging (Albany, NY). 2014;6(5):353-354. doi:10.18632/aging.100670

37. Chou T. Stochastic entry of enveloped viruses: fusion versus endocytosis. Biophys J. 2007;93(4):1116-1123. doi:10.1529/biophysj.107.106708

38. Kumar CS, Dey D, Ghosh S, Banerjee M. Breach: Host Membrane Penetration and Entry by Nonenveloped Viruses. Trends Microbiol. 2018 Jun;26(6):525-537. doi: 10.1016/j.tim.2017.09.010. Epub 2017 Oct 25. PMID: 29079499.

39. Yamauchi Y, Greber UF. Principles of Virus Uncoating: Cues and the Snooker Ball. Traffic. 2016 Jun;17(6):569-92. doi: 10.1111/tra.12387.

40. Sommer A, Kordowski F, Büch J, Maretzky T, Evers A, Andrä J, et al. Phosphatidylserine exposure is required for ADAM17 sheddase function. Nat Commun. 2016 May 10;7:11523. doi: 10.1038/ncomms11523

41. Nirisha PL, Bhaskaran AS, Yedavally NA, Suchandra HH, Manjunatha N, Kumar CN, Math SB. First episode psychosis and COVID-19: A case series and mini review. Asian J Psychiatr. 2022 Jul;73:103123. doi: 10.1016/j.ajp.2022.103123.

42. Liang H, Luo D, Liao H, Li S. Coronavirus Usurps the Autophagy-Lysosome Pathway and Induces Membranes Rearrangement for Infection and Pathogenesis. Front Microbiol. 2022 Mar 2;13:846543. doi: 10.3389/fmicb.2022.846543.

43. Merenlender-Wagner A, Malishkevich A, Shemer Z, Udawela M, Gibbons A, Scarr E, Dean B, Levine J, Agam G, Gozes I. Autophagy

has a key role in the pathophysiology of schizophrenia. Mol Psychiatry. 2015 Feb;20(1):126-32. doi: 10.1038/mp.2013.174.

44. Chen, Xi, Wang, Z., Zheng, P., Dongol, A., Xie, Y., Ge, X., Zheng, M., Dang, X., Seyhan, Z. B., Nagaratnam, N., Yu, Y., & Huang, X.-F. (2023). Impaired mitophagosome–lysosome fusion mediates olanzapine-induced aging. Aging Cell, 22, e14003. https://doi.org/10.1111/acel.14003

Chapter 12
Ancestral Malaria and COVID-19 Critical Illness

When cells, including neurons and red blood cells, are ready to die (a process called apoptosis), they externalize phosphatidylserine on the outer leaflet of cell membrane, signaling to the immune system readiness for engulfment by phagocytes.

When Plasmodium falciparum, the etiological agent of malaria infects red blood cells, they externalize phosphatidylserine, a hallmark of injured and dying cells.

Phosphatidylserine is negatively charged, therefore, attracts positively charged phenothiazines, such as chlorpromazine. These antipsychotics attach to the dying cell, accelerating its elimination. As infected red blood cells are cleared, a process called eryptosis, the clinical course of malaria improves. Positively charged antimalarial drugs, chloroquine, and hydroxychloroquine, clear damaged, infected or cancer cells in a similar manner.

Cancer cells are negatively charged due to externalized phosphatidylserine and are directly targeted by CPZ, chloroquine, and hydroxychloroquine, indicating that malaria, cancer, and mental illness meet at the endocytic pathway. Indeed, chloroquine inhibits the proliferation of several malignancies, including colon, breast, glioblastoma, head, and neck, suggesting that treatment should focus on the EP.

> COVID-19 has shed light on the similarity between cancer, neuropsychiatric disorders, and viruses, especially on the fact that antipsychotic and antiparasitic drugs eliminate malignancies without the adverse effects of conventional chemotherapy. Chloroquine, and hydroxychloroquine are also classified as senolytic drugs, suggesting that other agents from this category may kill cancer cells.

The long arm of malaria

Malaria is an old enemy of mankind that, throughout the past centuries, exacted a heavy toll on the population of Africa and the surrounding regions. To protect against malaria, residents of these areas have gradually developed plasmodium-resistant phenotypes of red blood cells (RBCs), marked by glucose 6 phosphate dehydrogenase (G6PD) deficiency, thalassemia, and hemoglobin C. Although these modified RBCs may block plasmodium entry, individuals with these changes are more susceptible to hemolysis and iron-mediated oxidative stress. This, in turn, promotes infections, hypertension, cancer, and neuropsychiatric disorders (1).

Several studies have reported that *Plasmodium falciparum*-infected red blood cells externalize phosphatidylserine (ePS), a phenomenon observed in severe COVID-19 illness (2). As ePS is negatively charged, it repels the negatively charged SARS-CoV-2 virus, suggesting that PS externalization may be a compensatory phenomenon (3).

<u>Antipsychotic drugs</u>

Antipsychotic drugs are zwitterionic (ionized) amphiphiles that are both hydrophilic (water soluble) and hydrophobic (insoluble in water). Phenothiazines, such as chlorpromazine (CPZ), are positively charged and attach to negatively charged ePS, facilitating the elimination of infected red blood cells and the subsequent amelioration of malaria symptoms (4). Like CPZ, positively charged antimalarial drugs, chloroquine, and hydroxychloroquine, clear damaged, infected, or cancer cells. Indeed, chloroquine inhibits the proliferation of colon, breast, glioblastoma, head and neck cancers (5). For this reason, several of these drugs are being repurposed for cancer.

Neuropsychiatric manifestations of malaria

Neuropsychiatric manifestations of malaria have been known since the ancient era. However, they were more thoroughly studied only in World War I when French Army physicians encountered malaria during a campaign in Northern Greece. More recent studies demonstrated that ROS play a major role in the pathogenesis of malaria and the CNS manifestations of this infection. For example, excessive ROS was shown to directly activate the inflammasomes, molecular structures involved in inflammatory processes, including neuroinflammation. Interestingly, some antipsychotic drugs, including clozapine, inhibit the inflammasomes, indicating antiinflammatory properties. In addition, the SARS-CoV-2 viral protein open reading frame 3a (OPR3a) appears to activate the inflammasomes, highlighting a pathway for virus-induced neuroinflammation.

Does COVID-19 target people with impaired redox systems?

Different ethnic groups exhibit various degrees of SARS-CoV-2 binding affinity, indicating that ethnic bioweapons could be developed based on this property. Another characteristic found primarily in African Americans and people from the Mediterranean Basin is increased levels of ROS and lower glutathione due to ancestral exposure to malaria. For example, COVID-19 prognosis depends on the premorbid redox reserves of antioxidant enzymes glucose 6 phosphate dehydrogenase (G6PD) and glutathione peroxidase (GPX). SARS-CoV-2 virus lowers G6PD via elevated ANG II, aldosterone, and NADPH oxidase, a major oxidant axis (Figure 1). In addition, SARS-CoV-2 lowers GPX directly, predisposing to more oxidation. When this occurs in individuals with hereditary G6PD deficiency (observed in populations with ancestral exposure to malaria), the resultant redox failure may trigger COVID-19 critical illness (Figure 12.1).

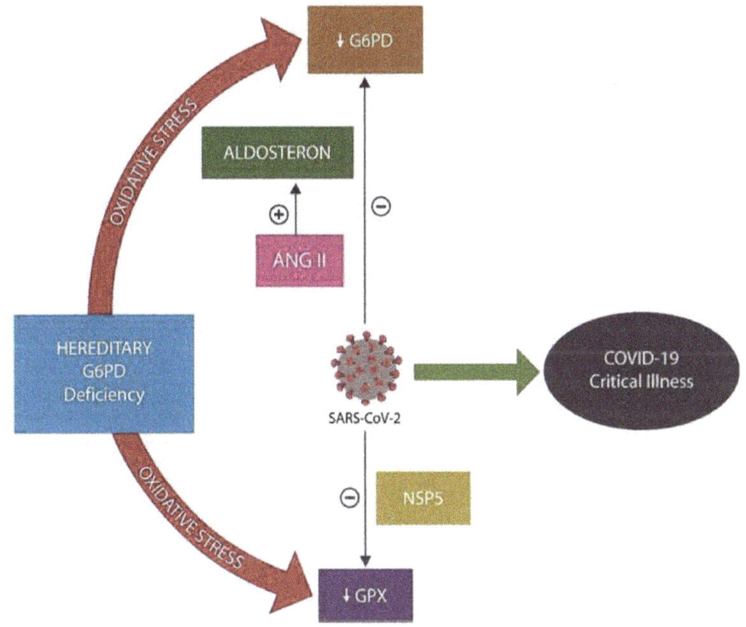

Figure 12.1. The SARS-CoV-2 virus causes oxidative stress by inhibiting both GPX (directly) and G6PD (indirectly via ANG II and aldosterone-upregulated NADPH oxidase). Individuals with hereditary G6PD deficiency are at higher mortality risk as the loss of antioxidant enzymes is more profound and oxidative stress higher.

The SARS-CoV-2 virus causes oxidative stress by inhibiting both GPX (directly) and G6PD (indirectly via ANG II and aldosterone-upregulated NADPH oxidase). Individuals with hereditary G6PD deficiency are at higher mortality risk as the loss of antioxidant enzymes is more profound and oxidative stress higher. Since some ethnic groups are more deficient in G6PD than others, COVID-19 can be considered an ethnic bioweapon.

Several recent studies have supported this model, establishing that G6PD-deficient individuals, including many African Americans, are more likely to have an unfavorable COVID-19 prognosis (6). Moreover, G6PD deficiency was associated with cardiovascular disease, hypertension, liver fibrosis, and iron dyshomeostasis, highlighting the importance of redox balance in this pathology.

Mental illness gone viral.

The virus's connection with neuropsychiatric disorders has been around for many centuries. In ancient times, Thucydides reported "total and immediate loss of memory" in the survivors of the "plague of Athens," a disease suggestive of viral encephalitis. Fast-forwarding to our time, recent MRI studies have found specific neuroimaging markers in herpes simplex encephalitis, a condition marked by neuropsychiatric pathology, including amnesia and psychosis. In addition, novel genetic studies have demonstrated that the HK2 retrovirus, frequently detected in the genome of drug addicts, was an ancestral pathogen incorporated into human DNA, further linking viruses to neuropathology.

Over the past century, numerous studies have associated in-utero or early postnatal viral infections with the development of SCZ and ASD later in life (7). For example, women pregnant during the 1964 rubella epidemic in the United States gave birth to offspring that frequently developed ASD or SCZ later in life, suggesting that other viruses, probably including COVID-19, may be succeeded by similar sequelae (8) (9). In addition, obsessive-compulsive disorder (OCD), SCZ, attention deficit hyperactivity disorder (ADHD), and Tourette syndrome were traced to prenatal viral infections (10). Moreover, neurodegenerative disorders, especially Parkinson's disease (PD), were documented to surge after prior pandemics, including the 1918 influenza, suggesting that COVID-19 may also promote neurodegeneration. On the positive side, the SARS-CoV-2 virus may prompt the development of novel PD therapies, including angiotensin receptor blockers (ARBs) and angiotensin-converting enzyme inhibitors (ACEi) that have demonstrated efficacy in animal models of this disorder.

Aside from prenatal viral exposure, several new studies reported that dormant CNS viruses could also engender SMI (11). For example, a recent report found that compared to controls, patients with SCZ demonstrated higher titers of Borna disease virus (BDV) immune complexes (12). Others have connected influenza A, varicella-zoster, herpes simplex, hepatitis C, and human immunodeficiency virus with the development of severe psychiatric disorders (13).

Autoantibodies against N-methyl-D-aspartate (NMDA) receptor (NMDARs), demonstrated in suicide and SCZ, were recently found to be the result of molecular mimicry between the M2 protein of influenza A virus and NMDARs (14). Moreover, the molecular resemblance between an H1N1 influenza antigen and a human hypocretin molecule triggers narcolepsy as virus-induced hypocretin modification may elicit autoantibodies (15).

Untreated patients with SCZ were reported to be at high risk of COVID-19 complications, probably due to SARS-CoV-2-associated neuroinflammation, an established risk factor for many psychiatric disorders. On the other hand, psychotropic drugs possess anti-inflammatory properties that may lower SARS-CoV-2-mediated neuroinflammation, accounting for the neuroprotective effects of these agents (16). In addition, as shown above, antipsychotics from the phenothiazine group block the EP, preventing viral endocytosis.

<u>The gulag syndrome</u>

Anxiety, depression, and PTSD have been demonstrated during the COVID-19 pandemic, suggesting that the draconic measures some governments took to isolate people led to a higher prevalence of neuropsychiatric illness, forming together a constellation of symptoms that can go by "the Gulag syndrome." Indeed, in some areas of Australia and China, people were confined to home gulags for many months in a row. As mentioned in the section on prosopagnosia, mask mandates may have led to defects in facial recognition during childhood development.

Conclusion

The COVID-19 pandemic has exacerbated the disease course in many psychiatric patients as mandatory social isolation and decreased frequency of therapeutic meetings promoted fear and uncertainty in this fragile population. The restrictive measures associated with the pandemic have often led to d medication nonadherence, increased depression, anxiety, and substance use disorders, frequently contributing to unfavorable outcomes.

On a positive note, the SARS-CoV-2 virus may be a catalyst for a better understanding of viruses' role in the pathogenesis of psychiatric illness. As SARS-CoV-2 (and probably other viruses) utilize the same molecular machinery as neuropsychiatric illnesses, a better understanding of these mechanisms will lead to better therapies. Indeed, the EP and antioxidant enzymes may become new psychiatric targets, expanding the current dopamine and serotonin models to include viruses and microbes.

Chapter 12 References:

1. Bocchetta A. Psychotic mania in glucose-6-phosphate-dehydrogenase-deficient subjects. Ann Gen Hosp Psychiatry. 2003;2(1):6. Published 2003 Jun 13. doi:10.1186/1475-2832-2-6

2. N'Guessan, K.F., Patel, P.H. & Qi, X. SapC-DOPS – a Phosphatidylserine-targeted Nanovesicle for selective Cancer therapy. Cell Commun Signal 18, 6 (2020). https://doi.org/10.1186/s12964-019-0476-6

3. Luisetto M, Tarro G, Edbey K, Khan FA, Ilman A, et al. Coronavirus COVID-19 surface properties: Electrical charges status. Int J Clin Microbiol Biochem Technol. 2021; 4: 016-027.

4. Olivier JL, Chachaty C, Wolf C, Daveloose D, Bereziat G. Binding of two spin-labelled derivatives of chlorpromazine to human erythrocytes. Biochem J. 1989 Dec 15;264(3):633-41. doi: 10.1042/bj2640633.

5. Ovejero-Sánchez M, Rubio-Heras J, Vicente de la Peña MDC, San-Segundo L, Pérez-Losada J, González-Sarmiento R, Herrero AB. Chloroquine-Induced DNA Damage Synergizes with Nonhomologous End Joining Inhibition to Cause Ovarian Cancer Cell Cytotoxicity. Int J Mol Sci. 2022 Jul 7;23(14):7518. doi: 10.3390/ijms23147518.

6. Youssef JG, Zahiruddin F, Youssef G, et al. G6PD deficiency and severity of COVID-19 pneumonia and acute respiratory distress syndrome: the tip of the iceberg? Ann Hematol. 2021;100(3):667-673. doi:10.1007/s00277-021-04395-1

7. McGrath JJ, Pemberton MR, Welham JL, Murray RM. Schizophrenia and the influenza epidemics of 1954, 1957 and 1959: a southern hemisphere study. Schizophr Res. 1994 Dec;14(1):1-8. doi: 10.1016/0920-9964(94)90002-7. PMID: 7893616.

8. Hutton J. Does Rubella Cause Autism: A 2015 Reappraisal? Front Hum Neurosci. 2016;10:25. Published 2016 Feb 1. doi:10.3389/fnhum.2016.00025

9. Brown AS, Begg MD, Gravenstein S, Schaefer CA, Wyatt RJ, Bresnahan M, Babulas VP, Susser ES. Serologic evidence of prenatal influenza in the etiology of schizophrenia. Arch Gen Psychiatry. 2004 Aug;61(8):774-780. doi: 10.1001/archpsyc.61.8.774. PMID: 15289276.

10. Dickerson F, Jones-Brando L, Ford G, Genovese G, Stallings C, Origoni A, O'Dushlaine C, Katsafanas E, Sweeney K, Khushalani S, Yolken R. Schizophrenia is Associated With an Aberrant Immune Response to Epstein-Barr Virus. Schizophr Bull. 2019 Sep 11;45(5):1112-1119. doi: 10.1093/schbul/sby164.

11. Breier A. 39. VIRUSES AND SCHIZOPHRENIA: IMPLICATIONS FOR PATHOPHYSIOLOGY AND TREATMENT. Schizophr Bull. 2018;44(Suppl 1):S61-S62. doi:10.1093/schbul/sby014.158

12. Zaliunaite V, Steibliene V, Bode L, Podlipskyte A, Bunevicius R, Ludwig H. Primary psychosis and Borna disease virus infection in Lithuania: a case-control study. BMC Psychiatry. 2016;16(1):369. Published 2016 Nov 3. doi:10.1186/s12888-016-1087-z.

13. Coughlin SS. Anxiety and Depression: Linkages with Viral Diseases. Public Health Rev. 2012;34(2):7. doi:10.1007/BF03391675

14. Kępińska AP, Iyegbe CO, Vernon AC, Yolken R, Murray RM, Pollak TA. Schizophrenia and Influenza at the Centenary of the 1918-1919 Spanish Influenza Pandemic: Mechanisms of Psychosis Risk. Front Psychiatry. 2020;11:72. Published 2020 Feb 26. doi:10.3389/fpsyt.2020.00072

15. Luo G, Ambati A, Lin L, Bonvalet M, Partinen M, Ji X, Maecker HT, Mignot EJ. Autoimmunity to hypocretin and molecular mimicry to flu in type 1 narcolepsy. Proc Natl Acad Sci USA. 2018 Dec 26;115(52): E12323-E12332. doi: 10.1073/pnas.1818150116. Epub 2018 Dec 12. PMID: 30541895; PMCID: PMC6310865.

16. Kozloff N, Mulsant BH, Stergiopoulos V, Voineskos AN. The COVID-19 Global Pandemic: Implications for People With Schizophrenia and Related Disorders. Schizophr Bull. 2020 Jul 8;46(4):752-757. doi: 10.1093/schbul/sbaa051. PMID: 32343342; PMCID: PMC7197583

Part II Therapies

Chapter 13
Biophysical Medicine: Music of the Spheres

> Biophysical interventions, such as oscillations, electrical stimulation, magnetic fields, and music, have been used as forms of treatment from antiquity to the present time. For example, Pythagoras and Aristotle proposed that the celestial bodies were driven by the Music of the Spheres, mediated by a frequency permeating the entire universe. Others, including Nikola Tesla, have stated that specific frequences bring synchrony between Man and God. It is believed that a frequency of 528Hz possesses transformative powers and may be the frequency Tesla talked about.
>
> In the brain, frequences in the gamma range are known to synchronize distant networks, likely engendering a communication platform. Patients with schizophrenia, depression and other significant mental illnesses cannot generate gamma band frequences, but can they be induced?

Eighty years ago, in 1944, Erwin Schrödinger wrote a famous book called "What is Life," in which he applied the laws of physics to biology. This was one of the most influential books of the 20th century that inspired many researchers, ultimately leading to the discovery of the genetic code and the epigenome. During this endeavor, Schrödinger encountered difficulties applying entropy to the living matter as the latter did not seem to bend easily to the second law of thermodynamics. In physics, entropy drives disorder and reflects the system's randomness. To revert the system to order, an outside energy source is required. In other words, the cosmos can only be generated from chaos with energy from elsewhere. However, living organisms produce energy, limiting or reversing entropy without an external energy source.

Schrödinger attempted to solve this dilemma, stating that living matter had inbuilt mechanisms, such as mitochondria, which generate energy, bringing the system back to order. To reverse entropy, the mitochondrion requires a host capable of providing nutrients for energy.

Schrödinger concluded that applying physics to biology is imperfect, as living matter may be driven by laws that have yet to be discovered but will eventually become part of science. For example, to validate Schrödinger's hypothesis, life must contain "order inside the chaos," something conceivable in quantum but not in Newtonian physics.

Entropy in neuropsychiatry was initially obtained to study consciousness. There are views that SCZ and MDD are disorders of consciousness; thus, their entropy can be measured (1) (2). Entropy provides an essential tool for quantifying the brain's work, such as information processing. Indeed, the ability to measure functional interactivity between various brain regions that drive consciousness is a strength of entropy. For example, a recent entropy study has identified early warning signals (EWSs) of depression and patient's transition between stable and unstable states (3). Another study examined the EEG entropy and found it abnormal in SCZ patients (4).

In 1621, Robert Burton wrote "The Anatomy of Melancholy," one of the first books on depression and one of the most influential in the 17th century. In this book, Burton hinted at entropy when discussing melancholy and the role of equilibrium among blood, phlegm, yellow bile, and black bile. Today, we would call this equilibrium maximal entropy, which is not very different from the name Burton used.

Conceptualization of neuropsychiatric pathology in terms of entropy has opened the door for alternative treatments, including therapeutic medicine, acupuncture, energy, yoga, and vibrational therapy, as well as rediscovering the value of introspection and its more modern avatar interoception.

Oscillations and vibrations in nature have been studied since antiquity, but their application in medicine has taken centuries. Nikola Tesla envisioned a universe driven by frequencies, while in our time, two separate groups have detected acoustic oscillations emitted by the Universe (5). Moreover, a recent Italian study found that, compared to other frequencies, music tuned at 432 Hz can optimize the heart rate, blood pressure, and respiration, linking select frequencies to human well-being (6). Another study analyzed music by its entropy and found that it captured unique characteristics, including the type, artist, style, and genre, suggesting that entropy can provide researchers with more information than neuroimaging (6). Moreover, coherent musical vibration was found to optimize hemodynamics, neurological, and musculoskeletal parameters, emphasizing the role of music as therapy (7).

Together, this data shows that the Newtonian model of medical thinking may be limited as the human body is more than the sum of its components. The new paradigm sees humans as complex energy fields with unique oscillations intertwined with the physical and cellular systems (8). Physiological brain oscillations in the gamma range were demonstrated to increase empathy, suggesting the involvement of IC and ACC (9). In addition, specific vibrational frequencies were presented even without music to improve overall health (7). Along this line, a study on depressed college students utilizing a whole-body vibration platform showed improved mood, emphasizing the beneficial effects of vibration (10).

At the cellular level, neuronal oscillations can spread and synchronize with neuronal cells at distant brain areas, likely engender consciousness (11).

Neuronal membranes play a key role in the generation and transmission of action potentials and synchronization. Cellular and mitochondrial membranes are composed of lipid bilayers containing phospholipids, cholesterol, and sphingolipids, such as ceramide. The lipid bilayer, which is susceptible to peroxidation, promotes premature cellular senescence (12). Lipid peroxidation disrupts neuronal cells by altering the biophysical properties of plasma membranes, disrupting neurotransmission.

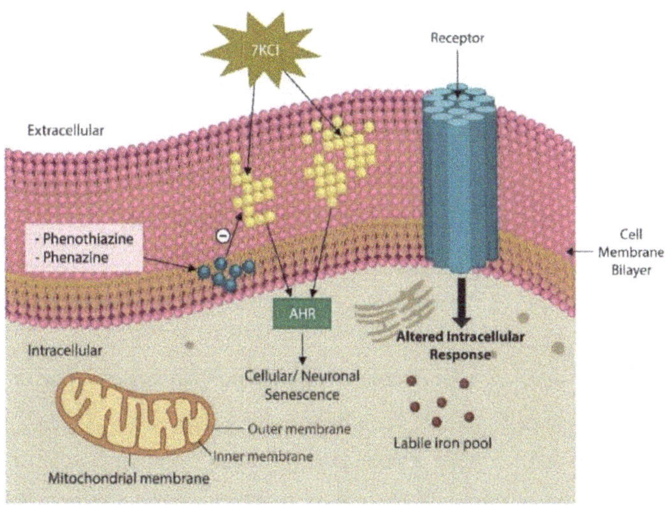

When intracellular iron is upregulated, the lipid bilayer of the neuronal membrane is easily oxidated. Oxysterols, including 7-ketocholesterol (a toxic oxide), and oxidated phospholipids alter the biophysical properties of cell membranes, disrupting neurotransmission. In addition, oxidized lipids activate AhR, triggering

premature neuronal senescence. Phenazines, Phenothiazines, and their derivatives intercalate themselves into the lipid bilayer, repairing the lipids. The mitochondrial membrane is also oxidated, especially by upregulated intracellular iron.

Biophysical interventions

The future of medicine will likely involve more biophysical modalities and fewer drugs. Natural compounds are likely to be preferred by the general public (see the section on AhR inhibitors)

1. Auricular vagal nerve stimmulation (aVNS)

Electrical stimulation of the auricular transcutaneous vagal nerve is a modality that can alter the work of the neural cells, bringing therapeutic benefits. The Vagus nerve links the brain directly to several visceral organs, including the GI tract.

Vagus nerve stimulation (VNS) is an invasive procedure that requires the implantation of a pulse generator and electrodes. As the auricular nerve travels superficially and projects to the nucleus of the solitary tract (NTS) where vagal branches also reach, aVNS could yield results comparable to those of the VNS without the risks of invasive surgery (13).

Aside from its central role of increasing norepinephrine, endorphins, and 5-HT, VNS was shown to optimize the permeability of the gut barrier, averting microbial translocation (14). This is significant as migration of commensal flora (or its components) outside the GI tract is a hallmark of SMI. For this reason, VNS should be used as an adjunct to other treatments.

2. Gamma band entrainment

Gamma oscillations on EEG are rapid brain waves (30-100 Hz) implicated in higher neural functions, including working memory, attention, and probably consciousness (17). It is believed that gamma waves are generated by the GABA interneurons that secrete somatostatin (SST). Gamma oscillations are absent in SCZ and MDD, suggesting a defect of interneurons and/or SST (15). Other studies have associated loss of gamma rhythm with aggressive behaviors in forensic psychiatric patients (see the section on iron, and ferroptosis).

The question asked more and more often has been "Can gamma waves be induced in schizophrenic brains to ameliorate the symptoms?" Most researchers and clinicians believe that the gamma band can be elicited by exposing the patient to this rhythm. This can be accomplished by various brain stimulation techniques described below (16).

3. Pulsed electromagnetic field therapy (PEMF)

Magnetotherapy can be static or pulsed and is generated by the electric current flowing through a coil, producing an electromagnetic field. Exposure to magnets is an old therapy that has been revisited as we have learned more about the biophysical impact on human biological processes.

A recent large study, based on 8-week PEMF treatment for patients with treatment-resistant depression found a beneficial role of this modality, indicating that PEMF can be used as an augmentation strategy with other treatments.

PEMF has been used in many conditions, including chronic pain, wound healing, postoperative pain, and depression. In psychiatry, larger studies are needed to confirm these findings and to compare efficacy with other modalities and/or treatments.

4. Electroconvulsive therapy (ECT)

ECT is the most effective treatment for severe depression and treatment-resistant depression. This biophysical intervention is believed to lower GSK3β and upregulate adult neurogenesis in the hippocampus.

Another ECT target is the microbiome as one study found a decreased abundance of *Clostridium* spp. after ECT, suggesting that this modality may combat depression by altering the composition of gut microorganisms (18). This may be significant as some *Clostridium spp.* produce butyrate, a short-chain fatty acid (SCFA), with antidepressant properties (19). In addition, GMV increase after ECT was documented, suggesting that this modality likely protects the GABA interneurons, upregulating the production of SST by these cells. Furthermore, another study found that ECT can upregulate SST, an anxiolytic and antidepressant hormone generated both in the CNS and locally (20) (21).

5. Vibration therapy

Whole Body Vibration is a modality known to physical therapists but novel to neuropsychiatry. There is a growing body of evidence that whole-body vibration may improve cognition in humans (22).

Oscillatory activity may be a fundamental rule of nature. In the human body, cytoskeletal proteins crosstalk with the intracellular and extracellular molecules, engendering global molecular networks as described by Agnati LF, et al (23). Along this line, it was hypothesized that inside the cytoskeletal protein tubulin, memories can be preserved in a quantum manner, especially in Ca2+/calmodulin-dependent protein kinase II (CaMKII) (24). Interestingly, a preclinical study found that vibration (produced by the Tibetan singing bowls) decreased CaMKII in the prefrontal cortex, lowering anxiety (25).

Taken together, whole-body vibration may benefit SCZ patients as it lowers CaMKII, a molecule linked to pathology.

6. Photobiomodulation (PBM)

Is a light-based biophysical intervention, consisting of near-infrared light obtained from a laser or light-emitting diodes (LEDs) that modulate the homeostasis of various body processes, including mood and sleep (26). Transcranial-applied light is absorbed by the mitochondrion of neuronal or glial cells, ameliorating organelle function (27).

PBN has obtained FDA approval for chronic pain, while an indication for neuromodulation is currently being considered. More studies are needed to identify the optimal dose and the likely responders to this modality.

Light-emitting diodes (LEDs) rely on semiconductors, which convert electrical currents into incoherent narrow-spectrum light. LEDs have gained popularity lately, especially for SCZ, as several studies found a positive correlation. Light from white light-emitting diodes is detected by melanopsin-expressing photosensitive retinal ganglion cells. These cells participate in the circadian rhythm, melatonin secretion, alertness, and sleep regulation. Blue light-emitting diodes were demonstrated to increase alertness, suggesting beneficial effects in SCZ with negative symptoms as well as depression.

Chapter 13: References:

1. Venkatasubramanian G. Understanding schizophrenia as a disorder of consciousness: biological correlates and translational implications from quantum theory perspectives. Clin Psychopharmacol Neurosci. 2015 Apr 30;13(1):36-47. doi: 10.9758/cpn.2015.13.1.36.

2. Whiteley, C.M. (2021). Depression as a Disorder of Consciousness. The British Journal for the Philosophy of Science.

3. Pham TD. Identifying critical transitions in major depression with fuzzy recurrence entropy. ALL LIFE2022, VOL. 15, NO. 1, 1086–1100https://doi.org/10.1080/26895293.2022.2132017

4. Xiang J, Tian C, Niu Y, Yan T, Li D, Cao R, Guo H, Cui X, Cui H, Tan S, Wang B. Abnormal Entropy Modulation of the EEG Signal in Patients With Schizophrenia During the Auditory Paired-Stimulus Paradigm. Front Neuroinform. 2019 Feb 19;13:4. doi: 10.3389/fninf.2019.00004. PMID: 30837859; PMCID: PMC6390065.

5. Miller CJ, Nichol RC, Batuski DJ. Acoustic oscillations in the early universe and today. Science. 2001 Jun 22;292(5525):2302-3. doi: 10.1126/science.1060440. Epub 2001 May 24. PMID: 11375481.

6. Calamassi D, Pomponi GP. Music Tuned to 440 Hz Versus 432 Hz and the Health Effects: A Double-blind Cross-over Pilot Study. Explore (NY). 2019 Jul-Aug;15(4):283-290. doi: 10.1016/j.explore.2019.04.001. Epub 2019 Apr 6. Erratum in: Explore (NY). 2020 Jan - Feb;16(1):8. PMID: 31031095.

7. Bartel L, Mosabbir A. Possible Mechanisms for the Effects of Sound Vibration on Human Health. Healthcare (Basel). 2021 May 18;9(5):597. doi: 10.3390/healthcare9050597. PMID: 34069792; PMCID: PMC8157227.

8. Beri K. A future perspective for regenerative medicine: understanding the concept of vibrational medicine. Future Sci OA. 2018 Jan 5;4(3):FSO274. doi: 10.4155/fsoa-2017-0097. PMID: 29568563; PMCID: PMC5859346.

9. Miu AC, Balteş FR. Empathy manipulation impacts music-induced emotions: a psychophysiological study on opera. PLoS One. 2012;7(1):e30618. doi: 10.1371/journal.pone.0030618. Epub 2012 Jan 24. PMID: 22292000; PMCID: PMC3265492.

10. Chawla G, Azharuddin M, Ahmad I, Hussain ME. Effect of Whole-body Vibration on Depression, Anxiety, Stress, and Quality of Life in College Students: A Randomized Controlled Trial. Oman Med J. 2022 Jul 31;37(4):e408. doi: 10.5001/omj.2022.72.

11. Myrov, V., Siebenhühner, F., Juvonen, J.J. et al. The rhythmicity of neuronal oscillations delineates their cortical and spectral architecture. Commun Biol 7, 405 (2024). https://doi.org/10.1038/s42003-024-06083-y

12. Suda, K., et al. (2024). Plasma membrane damage limits replicative lifespan in yeast and induces premature senescence in human fibroblasts. Nature Aging. doi.org/10.1038/s43587-024-00575-6.

13. Verma N, Mudge JD, Kasole M, Chen RC, Blanz SL, Trevathan JK, Lovett EG, Williams JC, Ludwig KA. Auricular Vagus Neuromodulation Systematic Review on Quality of Evidence and Clinical Effects. Front Neurosci. 2021 Apr 30;15:664740. doi: 10.3389/fnins.2021.664740. PMID: 33994937; PMCID: PMC8120162.

14. Mogilevski T, Rosella S, Aziz Q, Gibson PR. Transcutaneous vagal nerve stimulation protects against stress-induced intestinal barrier dysfunction in healthy adults. Neurogastroenterol Motil. 2022 Apr 28:e14382. doi: 10.1111/nmo.14382

15. Fitzgerald PJ, Watson BO. Gamma oscillations as a biomarker for major depression: an emerging topic. Transl Psychiatry. 2018 Sep 4;8(1):177. doi: 10.1038/s41398-018-0239-y. PMID: 30181587; PMCID: PMC6123432.

16. Blanco-Duque C, Chan D, Kahn MC, Murdock MH, Tsai L-H. Audiovisual gamma stimulation for the treatment of neurodegeneration. J Intern Med. 2024; 295: 146–170.

17. Panagiotaropoulos TI, Deco G, Kapoor V, Logothetis NK. Neuronal discharges and gamma oscillations explicitly reflect visual consciousness in the lateral prefrontal cortex. Neuron. 2012 Jun;74(5):924-935. DOI: 10.1016/j.neuron.2012.04.013. PMID: 22681695.

18. Kanayama M, Hayashida M, Hashioka S, Miyaoka T, Inagaki M. Decreased Clostridium Abundance after Electroconvulsive Therapy in the Gut Microbiota of a Patient with Schizophrenia. Case Rep Psychiatry. 2019 Feb 25;2019:4576842. doi: 10.1155/2019/4576842.

19. Stoeva MK, Garcia-So J, Justice N, Myers J, Tyagi S, Nemchek M, McMurdie PJ, Kolterman O, Eid J. Butyrate-producing human gut symbiont, Clostridium butyricum, and its role in health and disease. Gut Microbes. 2021 Jan-Dec;13(1):1-28. doi: 10.1080/19490976.2021.1907272.

20. Mikkelsen JD, Woldbye DP. Accumulated increase in neuropeptide Y and somatostatin gene expression of the rat in response to repeated electroconvulsive stimulation. J Psychiatr Res. 2006 Mar;40(2):153-9. doi: 10.1016/j.jpsychires.2005.02.005.

21. Engin E, Treit D. Anxiolytic and antidepressant actions of somatostatin: the role of sst2 and sst3 receptors. Psychopharmacology (Berl). 2009 Oct;206(2):281-9. doi: 10.1007/s00213-009-1605-5.

22. Shantakumari N, Ahmed M. Whole body vibration therapy and cognitive functions: a systematic review. AIMS Neurosci. 2023 May 18;10(2):130-143. doi: 10.3934/Neuroscience.2023010.

23. Agnati LF, Zunarelli E, Genedani S, Fuxe K. On the existence of a global molecular network enmeshing the whole central nervous system: physiological and pathological implications. Curr Protein Pept Sci. 2006 Feb;7(1):3-15. doi: 10.2174/138920306775474086.

24. Craddock TJ, Tuszynski JA, Hameroff S. Cytoskeletal signaling: is memory encoded in microtubule lattices by CaMKII phosphorylation? PLoS Comput Biol. 2012;8(3):e1002421. doi: 10.1371/journal.pcbi.1002421. Epub 2012 Mar 8. PMID: 22412364; PMCID: PMC3297561

25. Misrani A, Tabassum S, Wang T, Huang H, Jiang J, Diao H, Zhao Y, Huang Z, Tan S, Long C, Yang L. Vibration-reduced anxiety-like behavior relies on ameliorating abnormalities of the somatosensory cortex and medial prefrontal cortex. Neural Regen Res. 2024 Jun 1;19(6):1351-1359. doi: 10.4103/1673-5374.385840.

26. Gonzalez-Lima, F, and Barrett, DW. Augmentation of cognitive brain functions with transcranial lasers. Front Syst Neurosci. (2014) 8:36. doi: 10.3389/fnsys.2014.00036

27. Mochizuki-Oda, N, Kataoka, Y, Cui, Y, Yamada, H, Heya, M, and Awazu, K. Effects of near-infra-red laser irradiation on adenosine triphosphate and adenosine diphosphate contents of rat brain tissue. Neurosci Lett. (2002) 323:207–10. doi: 10.1016/s0304-3940(02)00159-3

Chapter 14
Mitochondrial Transfer and Transplantation

Mitochondria are intracellular organelles that were once bacteria and became "domesticated." They currently function in symbiosis with human cells. Mitochondria generate energy in the form of ATP and play a major role in averting depression, a pathology marked by low energy-related symptoms (1).

However, mitochondria's role does not end here. Mitochondria also regulate human life span and health span (2). Studies of people from Blue Zones, areas of the world with the highest number of centenarians, have identified socialization and interconnectedness as the main pillars of longevity. Here comes the mitochondrion.

It has been shown that mitochondrial variation modulates individual differences in sociability. In addition, cell-free mitochondrial DNA (cf-mtDNA) is a marker of inflammatory disease that is upregulated by psychological stress and social isolation (3). Cf-mtDNA is a measure of psychosocial stress and is considered a PTSD biomarker (4). For example, it is now known that loneliness and insufficient socialization activate cf-mtDNA/toll-like receptor 9 (TLR9) signaling while reducing cf-mtDNA attenuates social stress (5).

Isolation-upregulated cf-mtDNA acts as a damage-associated molecular pattern (DAMP), triggering "sterile" inflammation by activating the inflammasomes (6). Elevated levels of cf-mtDNA may be a marker of stress vulnerability, explaining why some individuals develop PTSD in response to stress, but others do not. A recent study looked at this aspect in veterans with PTSD and demonstrated that cf-mtDNA mirrors glucocorticoid sensitivity, a measure of vulnerability to stress-related disorders (7). Indeed, mitochondria can leave the cell and function in the extracellular compartment where it regulates the metabolism and immunity, processes marked by upregulation of cf-mDNA.

Taken together, the mitochondrion is more than an energy-producing battery. This organelle, found at the interface of biological and psychological stress, unifies the sterile and non-sterile inflammation into a single pathology.

A former bacterium, the mitochondrion has retained the ability to communicate with intestinal microbes, contributing to the gut-brain axis. For example, metabolites produced by the gut microbes interact directly with brain mitochondria, regulating neuronal function. For example, the short-chain fatty acid (SCFA) butyrate generated by gut microbiota crosses the BBB and ameliorates depression by interacting with neuronal mitochondria (8).

Mitochondria are implicated in innate immunity via mitochondrial antiviral signaling protein (MAVS), a pathway frequently hijacked by viruses that disrupts host defenses.

Mitochondria are composed of an inner and outer membrane, the latter being in close contact with mitochondria-associated membranes (MAMs), which connect the organelle to the "lipid factory of the cell," the endoplasmic reticulum (ER).

The mitochondrion contains its AhR (mitoAhR), which binds oxidized lipids, including cholesterol. While inhibitors are therapeutic, overactivated AhR may lead to neuropathology, including SCZ. Ceramide is a sphingolipid that, when excessive, may become toxic and activates GSK-3β, a kinase implicated in SCZ. Conversely, Lithium, several antipsychotics, Kaempferol, and Berberine inhibit GSK-3β, lowering ROS and deactivating mitoAhR (Fig.1). This is significant as Berberine and Kaempferol are natural products that exert antipsychotic actions without the adverse effects of conventional psychotropic agents.

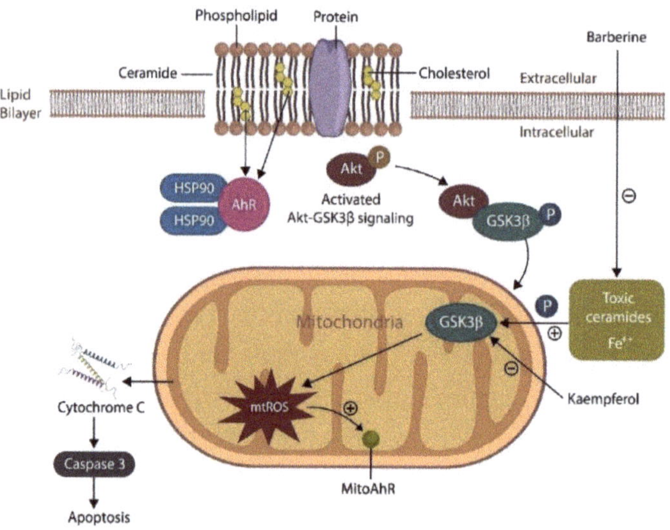

Fig. 14.1 shows AhR represented in the cytosol and mitochondria (mitoAhR). Akt negatively phosphorylates GSK-3β, inhibiting its function. Toxic ceramides and iron activate GSK-3β, resulting in excessive mitochondrial ROS (mtROS), which activates mitoAhR, triggering organelle death. mtROS can also cause mitochondrial demise by activating cytochrome C and caspase 3. Natural compounds, berberine and kaempferol inhibit GSK-3β, averting organelle death.

Antipsychotic drugs and mitochondria

Novel studies examining the relationship between the mitochondrion and antipsychotic drugs revealed that typical and atypical antipsychotics disrupt mitochondrial function in neurons and other tissues, decreasing ATP production and disrupting the membrane potential (9) (10). It appears that SCZ itself, as well as treatment with antipsychotic drugs, disrupts mitochondria, a phenomenon like GMV reduction that both SCZ and its treatment can trigger.

Mitochondria, the powerhouses of the cell, play a crucial role in energy production, iron homeostasis, and biosynthesis of essential cellular components like lipids, amino acids, and nucleic acids. This central role also means that mitochondrial dysfunction can lead to lipid peroxidation and increased intracellular iron, predisposing to ferroptosis, a nonapoptotic cell death marked by low glutathione peroxidase 4 (GPX 4).

Impaired mitochondrial function in SCZ may be caused by the loss of superoxide dismutase 2 (SOD2), a mitochondrial enzyme known as Manganese Superoxide Dismutase, which lowers mtROS by eliminating the toxic superoxide (11). Earlier studies found that loss of SOD2 can result in several pathological phenotypes, including SCZ (12). Moreover, GMV reduction can occur in primary mitochondrial disorders, suggesting that impaired mitochondria and brain atrophy go hand in hand (13).

Mitochondrial transplantation

The history of mitochondrial transplantation is a testament to its potential. Starting in the 1980s, experiments with various cell types and mitochondrial sources have shown that this technique, when performed for 1-2 hours, can successfully supply organelles to mitochondria-depleted cells. The successful transplantation in cardiomyocytes, confirmed by the presence of mitochondrial DNA in the heart tissue, is a promising step forward (18) (19).

Mitochondrial transplantation to rescue neurons from ferroptosis is currently possible and was performed successfully in animals and humans; however, to my knowledge, it has not been attempted in MDD or SCZ (20).

Rescuing the mitochondrion with MLR, Kaempferol, and Berberine is a strategy for averting GSK-3β overactivation by toxic ceramides, oxysterols, or oxidized phospholipids. In addition, SSRIs were demonstrated to facilitate mitochondrial transfer, emphasizing a potential strategy for restoring the neurometabolic balance in SMI and neurodegeneration.

Mitochondrial transfer

Intercellular mitochondrial transfer can occur in physiological or pathological circumstances via TNTs or EVs.

Noncanonical mitochondrial transfer can occur via cell-cell fusion, synaptosomes, or dendritic networks. Cell-cell fusion can occur in senescent neurons that re-enter the cell cycle and remain indefinitely fused.

Aside from their role in the intracellular compartment, a growing body of evidence indicates that mitochondria are secreted into the extracellular space under physiological or pathological circumstances, where they play a crucial role in regulating metabolism and immunity (21).

Preclinical studies have shown that mitochondrial transplantation decreases LPS-induced depression, emphasizing it as a potential therapy for MDD (22). Indeed, as mentioned above, SSRIs were demonstrated to enhance mitochondrial transfer from astrocytes to neurons, suggesting a non-synaptic mechanism.

Mitochondrial transfer or transplantation for premature cellular senescence

Exogenous mitochondrial transplantation can improve mitochondrial dysfunction and alleviate cellular senescence, reducing senescent markers. These include senescence-associated β-galactosidase, upregulated nuclear factor NF-κB, increased inflammatory cytokines, and cyclin-dependent kinase inhibitors p21 and p16 (23). This is significant as mitochondrial dysfunction is rarely studied as a hallmark of cellular senescence, SASP, or resistance to apoptosis. Moreover, recent studies found that rapid brain oscillations require intact mitochondria (24).

Premature cellular senescence, a characteristic of SMI, has been associated with dysfunctional mitochondrion and excessive SASP (25). For example, deleting mitochondria in senescent cells lowers inflammation, and the cell cycle is not reactivated, suggesting that SASP may drive the senescent phenotype.

In neuronal cells, mitochondria move in the axon via the actin cytoskeleton when the distance is short and microtubules for longer distances. More giant cells, such as VENS, require long transport, suggesting higher chances of mitochondrial damage and loss. Frontotemporal lobar degeneration likely targets VENS preferentially due to a higher percentage of damaged mitochondria. Indeed, impaired mitochondrial/ER signaling was documented in bvFTD, suggesting that mitochondrial transplantation could benefit this disorder (26).

Putting it all together, mitochondria play a crucial role in SMI by controlling sterile inflammation, stress, neuronal senescence, and rapid brain waves. Mitochondrial transplantation or transfer could replace the damaged organelles with exogenous, healthy mitochondria, likely improving the outcome in SCZ and MDD.

Chapter 14 References:

1. Khan, M.; Baussan, Y.; Hebert-Chatelain, E. Connecting Dots between Mitochondrial Dysfunction and Depression. Biomolecules 2023, 13, 695. https://doi.org/10.3390/biom13040695

2. Akbari M, Kirkwood TBL, Bohr VA. Mitochondria are the signaling pathways that control longevity and health span. Ageing Res Rev. 2019 Sep;54:100940. doi: 10.1016/j.arr.2019.100940. Epub 2019 Aug 12. PMID: 31415807; PMCID: PMC7479635.

3. Möller M, Du Preez JL, Viljoen FP, Berk M, Emsley R, Harvey BH. Social isolation rearing induces mitochondrial, immunological, neurochemical, and behavioral deficits in rats and is reversed by clozapine or N-acetyl cysteine. Brain Behav Immun. 2013 May;30:156-67. doi: 10.1016/j.bbi.2012.12.011.

4. Trumpff C, Marsland AL, Basualto-Alarcón C, Martin JL, Carroll JE, Sturm G, Vincent AE, Mosharov EV, Gu Z, Kaufman BA, Picard M. Acute psychological stress increases serum circulating cell-free mitochondrial DNA. Psychoneuroendocrinology. 2019 Aug;106:268-276. doi: 10.1016/j.psyneuen.2019.03.026.

5. Tripathi, A., Bartosh, A., Whitehead, C. et al. Activation of cell-free mtDNA-TLR9 signaling mediates chronic stress-induced social behavior deficits. Mol Psychiatry 28, 3806–3815 (2023). https://doi.org/10.1038/s41380-023-02189-76.

6. Fleshner M, Crane CR. Exosomes, DAMPs, and miRNA: Stress Physiology and Immune Homeostasis Features. Trends Immunol. 2017 Oct;38(10):768-776. doi: 10.1016/j.it.2017.08.002.

7. Blalock, Z.N., Wu, G.W.Y., Lindqvist, D. et al. Circulating cell-free mitochondrial DNA levels and glucocorticoid sensitivity in a cohort of male veterans with and without combat-related PTSD. Transl

Psychiatry 14, 22 (2024). https://doi.org/10.1038/s41398-023-02721-x

8. Luu, M., and Visekruna, A. (2019). Short-chain fatty acids: bacterial messengers modulating the immunometabolism of T cells. Eur. J. Immunol. 49, 842–848. doi: 10.1002/eji.201848009

9. Chan ST, McCarthy MJ, Vawter MP. Psychiatric drugs impact mitochondrial function in the brain and other tissues. Schizophr Res. 2020 Mar;217:136-147. doi: 10.1016/j.schres.2019.09.007

10. Burkhardt, C., Kelly, J. P., Lim, Y. H., Filley, C. M. & Parker, W. D. Jr. Neuroleptic medications inhibit complex I of the electron transport chain. Ann. Neurol. 33, 512–517 (1993).

11. Srivastava, V., Buzas, B., Momenan, R. et al. Association of SOD2, a Mitochondrial Antioxidant Enzyme, with Gray Matter Volume Shrinkage in Alcoholics. Neuropsychopharmacol 35, 1120–1128 (2010). https://doi.org/10.1038/npp.2009.217

12. Wang DF, Cao B, Xu MY, Liu YQ, Yan LL, Liu R, Wang JY, Lu QB. Meta-Analyses of Manganese Superoxide Dismutase Activity, Gene Ala-9Val Polymorphism, and the Risk of Schizophrenia. Medicine (Baltimore). 2015 Sep;94(36):e1507. doi: 10.1097/MD.0000000000001507.

13. Gropman AL. Neuroimaging in mitochondrial disorders. Neurotherapeutics. 2013 Apr;10(2):273-85. doi: 10.1007/s13311-012-0161-6. PMID: 23208728; PMCID: PMC3625392.

14. Engwa G.A., Ayuk E.L., Igbojekwe B.U., Unaegbu M. Potential Antioxidant Activity of New Tetracyclic and Pentacyclic Nonlinear Phenothiazine Derivatives. Biochem. Res. Int. 2016;2016:9896575. Doi: 10.1155/2016/9896575.

15. Clark MA, Shay JW. Mitochondrial transformation of mammalian cells. Nature. (1982) 295:605–7. doi: 10.1038/295605a0

16. Katrangi E, D'Souza G, Boddapati SV, Kulawiec M, Singh KK, Bigger B, et al. Xenogenic transfer of isolated murine mitochondria into human rho0 cells can improve respiratory function. Rejuvenation Res. (2007) 10:561–70. doi: 10.1089/rej.2007.0575

17. Pacak AP, Preble JM, Kondo H, Seibel P, Levitsky S, del Nido PJ, et al. Actin-dependent mitochondrial internalization in cardiomyocytes: evidence for rescue of mitochondrial function. Biol Open. (2015) 4:622–6. doi: 10.1242/bio.20151147818.

18. Hayakawa K, Esposito E, Wang X, Terasaki Y, Liu Y, Xing C, et al. Transfer of mitochondria from astrocytes to neurons after stroke. Nature. (2016) 535:551–5. doi: 10.1038/nature18928

19. Ali Pour P, Hosseinian S, Kheradvar A. Mitochondrial transplantation in cardiomyocytes: foundation, methods, and outcomes. Am J Physiol Cell Physiol. (2021) 321:C489–503. doi: 10.1152/ajpcell.00152.2021

20. Sasaki, D., Abe, J., Takeda, A. et al. Transplantation of MITO cells, mitochondria-activated cardiac progenitor cells, to the ischemic myocardium of mice enhances the therapeutic effect. Sci Rep 12, 4344 (2022). https://doi.org/10.1038/s41598-022-08583-521.

21. Suh, J., Lee, YS. Mitochondria are secretory organelles and therapeutic cargos. Exp Mol Med 56, 66–85 (2024). https://doi.org/10.1038/s12276-023-01141-722.

22. Wang Y, Ni J, Gao C, Xie L, Zhai L, Cui G, Yin X. Mitochondrial transplantation attenuates lipopolysaccharide-induced depression-

like behaviors. Prog Neuropsychopharmacol Biol Psychiatry. 2019 Jul 13;93:240-249. doi: 10.1016/j.pnpbp.2019.04.010.

23. Noh SE, Lee SJ, Lee TG, Park KS, Kim JH. Inhibition of cellular senescence hallmarks by mitochondrial transplantation in senescence-induced ARPE-19 cells. Neurobiol Aging. 2023 Jan;121:157-165. doi: 10.1016/j.neurobiolaging.2022.11.003.

24. Zhao, J., Zhu, H., Duan, K. et al. Dysbindin-1 regulates mitochondrial fission and gamma oscillations. Mol Psychiatry 26, 4633–4651 (2021). https://doi.org/10.1038/s41380-021-01038-9

25. Correia-Melo C, Marques FDM, Anderson R, Hewitt G, Hewitt R, Cole J, Carroll BM, Miwa S, Birch J, Merz A, Rushton MD, Charles M, Jurk D, Tait SWG, Czapiewski R, Greaves L, Nelson G, Bohlooly-Y M, Rodriguez-Cuenca S, Vidal-Puig A, Mann D, Saretzki G, Quarato G, Green DR, Adams PD, von Zglinicki T, Korolchuk VI & Passos JF (2016) Mitochondria are required for pro-ageing features of the senescent phenotype. EMBO J 35, 724–42

26. Lau, D.H.W., Hartopp, N., Welsh, N.J. et al. Disruption of ER–mitochondria signaling in frontotemporal dementia and related amyotrophic lateral sclerosis. Cell Death Dis 9, 327 (2018). https://doi.org/10.1038/s41419-017-0022-7

Chapter 15
IL-22 – The "Guardian" of Gut Barrier, A New Schizophrenia Therapy

Emil Kraepelin believed that dementia praecox, the disorder we now call SCZ, was caused by brain poisoning with toxins generated in other parts of the body, especially the mouth, intestine, or genitals (1). In this regard, Kraepelin hinted at the microbiome and believed that microbial molecules could drive the pathogenesis of SMI. However, the infectious model of SCZ drew limited attention until the launching of the Human Microbiome Project and the discovery of innate lymphoid cells (ILCs).

The gut and schizophrenia

Several recent studies have connected SCZ with microbial translocation from the GI tract into the host systemic circulation, eventually reaching the brain (2) (3) (4) (5). Microbial translocation refers to migrating intestinal microorganisms or their components into host tissues by passing through the intestinal barrier to reach mesenteric lymph nodes and systemic circulation. In the CNS, bacteria or their components can trigger psychosis by several mechanisms, including inflammation, impaired autophagy, premature cellular senescence, and aberrant microglial activation (6) (7) (8) (9).

The evidence of microbial translocation in schizophrenia

1. Patients with SCZ have a high prevalence of IBD, such as ulcerative colitis and Chron's disease, conditions associated with increased gut barrier permeability and microbial migration outside the GI tract (10-12).

2. Patients with SCZ present with elevated bacterial translocation markers, including soluble CD14 (sCD14), lipopolysaccharide lipopolysaccharide-binding protein (LBP), and cf-mDNA, emphasizing microbial migration from the immune-tolerant GI tract into the bacteria-intolerant systemic circulation (13-15).

3. Patients with SCZ exhibit increased BBB permeability, enabling bacteria and toxins to ingress the CNS (16) (17) (18) (19).

4. The 2011 outbreak of *Escherichia coli (E. coli)* in Germany has been associated with sporadic cases of new onset of psychosis, connecting this pathogen to neuropsychiatric illnesses (20-21). In addition, *E. coli* has been implicated in urinary tract infection (UTI), conditions often associated with new-onset psychosis or SCZ exacerbation, linking this bacterium to psychopathology (22-23).

Hypothesis

I have hypothesized earlier that recombinant human interleukin-22 (IL-22) can alleviate psychotic symptoms by blocking microbial translocation. In addition, IL-22 shares several properties with antipsychotic drugs, as summarized in Table 15.1.

Antipsychotic drugs	IL-22	References
JAK-STAT activation	JAK-STAT activation	33; 91
Neuroprotective	Neuroprotective	37; 92
IFN-γ inhibitor	IFN-γ inhibitor	60; 64; 93
Activate autophagy	Activate autophagy	86; 88; 94
Antibacterial/antiviral	Antibacterial/antiviral	83; 84; 95; 96

Table 15.1. Recombinant human IL-22 comparison with antipsychotic drugs

Interleukin-22, the "guardian" of gut barrier.

During the human immunodeficiency virus (HIV) epidemic in the 1980s, microbial translocation drew the attention of researchers and clinicians as this virus depleted IL-22, enabling lipopolysaccharide (LPS) migration into host tissues (22) (23) (Fig. 15.1). Indeed, patients with HIV are more likely to develop new new-onset psychosis compared to the general population, suggesting that dysfunctional gut barrier may play a role in this pathology (24-29).

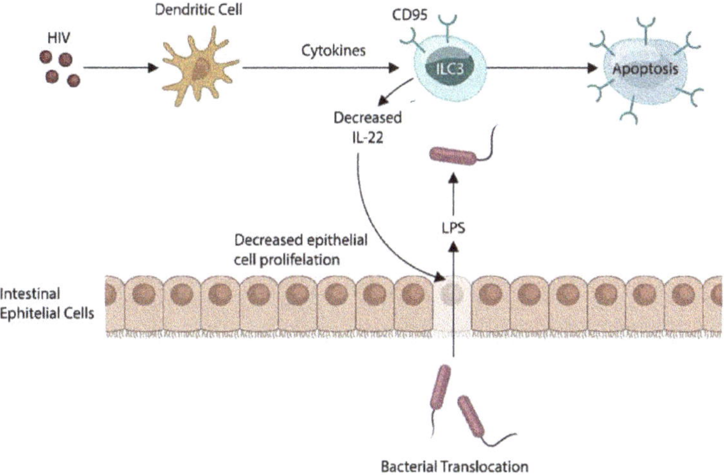

Fig. 15.1 HIV induces apoptotic loss of innate lymphoid cells, type 3 (ILC3), lowering IL22, the guardian of the gut barrier. This, in turn, promotes microbial translocation into the systemic circulation. Activated host immunity maintains a state of low-grade inflammation, a pathology found in schizophrenia.

Discovered in 2000, IL-22 is a member of the IL-10 family generated by several lymphocyte types, including T helper (Th) 17 cells, γδ T cells, NKCs, and innate lymphoid cells (ILCs) (30). IL-22 controls several IEC functions, including mucus formation, permeability, and synthesis of complement and antimicrobial peptides (AMPs), indicating that this cytokine functions as the master regulator of gut barrier permeability (31). AhR regulates IL-22 in its tissue remodeling action.

The crosstalk between IL-22 and its receptor (IL-22R), a dimeric protein comprised of IL-22R1 and IL-10R2, activates the JAK/STAT pathway, a critical antibacterial and antiviral system, protecting against infections (32-33). As IL22R contains IL-10R2, it can be cross-activated by IL-10, a cytokine previously connected to SCZ (34-36). In addition, several studies have shown that IL-22 possesses neuroprotective properties, and its disruption has been associated with SCZ (37-39). Moreover, aside from safeguarding neuronal cells, IL-22 protects against COVID-19, influenza, and IBD, indicating that supplementation with this cytokine may ameliorate or alleviate these pathologies (39-42).

IL-22 and innate lymphoid cells (ILCs)

Novel studies have reported that a subgroup of natural killer cells (NKCs) produce IL-22, enhancing the gut barrier and thus averting translocation (43) (44) (45). Indeed, research over the past two decades has connected defective NKCs with both IBD and SCZ (46) (47) (48) (49). Moreover, in the CNS, NKCs participate in adult neurogenesis, cognition, and cellular senescence, suggesting that under pathological circumstances, these processes may be disrupted (50) (53).

NKCs belong to innate lymphoid cells (ILCs), mucosa-anchored non-T, non-B lymphocytes, which also include ILC-1, ILC-2, and ILC-3 (52) (Fig.2). These systems play a pivotal role in gut barrier homeostasis, nutrient transport, and immune tolerance of both food proteins and gut commensals (52) (53). The ILCs in CNS have been implicated in neuropathology, including SCZ, MDD, and neurodegeneration (55) (56) (57).

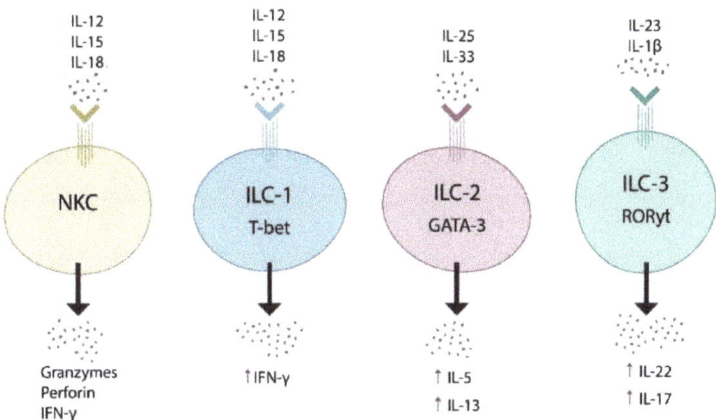

Fig. 15.2 Innate lymphoid cells comprise NKCs and innate lymphoid cells type 1, 2, and 3 (ILC-1, ILC-2, and ILC-3). These cells are activated by various cytokines (top), release other cytokines (bottom), and express transcription factors, including T-bet, GATA-3, and RORγt. Under pathological circumstances, these lymphoid systems may lead to IBD and microbial translocation, contributing to schizophrenia. A subgroup of gut NKCs produces IL-22, maintaining the gut barrier homeostasis (not shown).

For example, aberrant activation of NKCs by IL-12, IL-15, and IL-18 was reported in IBD and SCZ, linking ILCs to both conditions (58) (59). In addition, NKCs-generated interferon-γ (IFN-γ) has been linked to SCZ, emphasizing the critical role of ILCs in neuropathology. On the other hand, conventional antipsychotic drugs have been shown to suppress IFN-γ, suggesting that, at least in part, IL-22 may contribute to the pathogenesis of SCZ (60) (61) (62). Indeed, dysfunctional IFN-γ was associated with losing dopaminergic neurons in PD, connecting ILCs to DA pathology (63). Like antipsychotic agents, IL-22 is an IFN-γ inhibitor, suggesting a mechanism through which IL-22 may alleviate the symptoms of SCZ (64).

Taken together, dysfunctional ILCs, including NKCs, connect IBD with SCZ. In contrast, IL-22 likely exhibits antipsychotic properties by lowering microbial translocation, restoring intestinal barrier integrity, and suppressing IFN-γ. Moreover, IL-22 promotes protective autophagy and facilitates iron storage in ferritin, reducing the risk of lipid peroxidation, a pathology linked with SCZ.

Psychosis and gut microbes

The BBB, comprised of specialized endothelial cells (ECs) kept together by TJs, regulates the CNS entry of peripheral molecules, including gut microbes and toxins. Interestingly, experimental colitis has been shown to increase BBB permeability, indicating a crosstalk between the gut barrier and BBB that, under pathological circumstances, may enable intestinal microbes to reach the brain (65).

The link between gut bacteria and SCZ has been documented for several decades. For example, antibodies against various *E. coli* proteins were detected in patients with SCZ but not healthy controls (66). In addition, SCZ and colibactin, an *E. coli* toxin, were demonstrated to trigger premature cellular senescence and thymic dysfunction (67-70). On the other hand, IL-22 drives the regeneration of the thymus, restoring the homeostasis of senescent cells and, according to one study, induces rejuvenation (71-73).

Several gut and urinary tract microbes, including *E. coli*, were associated with SCZ, while IL-22 was shown to neutralize this pathogen (74-78). Other gut microbes, including *Hafnei alvei, Pseudomonas aeruginosa, Pseudomonas putida, and Klebsiella pneumoniae*, have been associated with SCZ, further enhancing the infectious paradigm (79-80).

Taken together, intestinal inflammation can alter the BBB, enabling microbes, including *E. coli*, to enter the CNS. Antibodies against microbial antigens (which often mimic human proteins) trigger pathology in distant organs, including the brain. IL-22 opposes translocation by lowering gut barrier permeability and enhancing thymic function to strengthen host immune defenses.

Human recombinant IL-22 is currently in Phase II clinical trials for the treatment of COVID-19, COVID-19 pneumonia, acute pancreatitis, chronic, acute liver failure, alcoholic hepatitis, and graft versus host disease (GVHD) (NCT02406651). Several studies have evaluated the safety, pharmacokinetics, pharmacodynamics, and tolerability of human recombinant IL-22, demonstrating that this is a safe compound with favorable pharmacological parameters (81) (82).

Aside from functioning as the guardian of the intestinal barrier, IL-22 possesses antibacterial and antiviral properties, probably by enhancing autophagy (83) (84) (85). Impaired autophagy has been documented in both SCZ and IBD, while enhanced autophagy is a property of many antipsychotic drugs, including clozapine (85) (86) (87) (88) (89). Moreover, like antipsychotics, recombinant IL-22 lowers INF-γ and protects the intestinal barrier against IBD and microbial translocation (60) (64) (89) (90)

Conclusions

Recombinant human IL-22 is an antibacterial and antiviral molecule that promotes tissue repair and autophagy. Like antipsychotic drugs, IL-22 suppresses INF-γ, promoting neuroprotection. In addition, it drives thymic regeneration, opposing premature cellular and immune senescence. In clinical trials, IL-22 decreased serum triglycerides, correcting dyslipidemia (often found in SCZ patients), and presented with anti-inflammatory properties, warranting further evaluation for SCZ.

Chapter 15 References:

1. Noll R. Kraepelin's 'lost biological psychiatry'? Autointoxication, organotherapy, and surgery for dementia praecox. Hist Psychiatry. 2007 Sep;18(71 Pt 3):301-20. doi: 10.1177/0957154X07078705.

2. Wang C, Zhang T, He L, Fu JY, Deng HX, Xue XL, Chen BT. Bacterial Translocation Associates With Aggression in Schizophrenia Inpatients. Front Syst Neurosci. 2021 Sep 29;15:704069. doi: 10.3389/fnsys.2021.704069.

3. Severance EG, Gressitt KL, Stallings CR, Origoni AE, Khushalani S, Leweke FM, Dickerson FB, Yolken RH. Discordant patterns of bacterial translocation markers and implications for innate immune imbalances in schizophrenia. Schizophr Res. 2013 Aug;148(1-3):130-7. doi: 10.1016/j.schres.2013.05.018.

4. Zhu, F., Ju, Y., Wang, W. et al. Metagenome-wide association of gut microbiome features for schizophrenia. Nat Commun 11, 1612 (2020). https://doi.org/10.1038/s41467-020-15457-9

5. Dickerson F, Severance E, Yolken R. The microbiome, immunity, and schizophrenia and bipolar disorder. Brain Behav Immun. 2017 May;62:46-52. doi: 10.1016/j.bbi.2016.12.010.6.

6. Sibony M, Abdullah M, Greenfield L, Raju D, Wu T, Rodrigues DM, Galindo-Mata E, Mascarenhas H, Philpott DJ, Silverberg MS, Jones NL. Microbial Disruption of Autophagy Alters Expression of the RISC Component AGO2, a Critical Regulator of the miRNA Silencing Pathway. Inflamm Bowel Dis. 2015 Dec;21(12):2778-86. doi: 10.1097/MIB.0000000000000553.

7. Secher T, Samba-Louaka A, Oswald E, Nougayrède JP. Escherichia coli-producing colibactin triggers premature and transmissible senescence in mammalian cells. PLoS One. 2013 Oct 8;8(10):e77157. doi: 10.1371/journal.pone.0077157.

8. Franchi L, Muñoz-Planillo R, Núñez G. Sensing and reacting to microbes through the inflammasomes. Nat Immunol. 2012 Mar 19;13(4):325-32. doi: 10.1038/ni.2231.

9. Fernández-Arjona MDM, Grondona JM, Fernández-Llebrez P, López-Ávalos MD. Microglial activation by microbial neuraminidase through TLR2 and TLR4 receptors. J Neuroinflammation. 2019 Dec 2;16(1):245. doi: 10.1186/s12974-019-1643-9. PMID: 31791382

10. Sung KY, Zhang B, Wang HE, Bai YM, Tsai SJ, Su TP, Chen TJ, Hou MC, Lu CL, Wang YP, Chen MH. Schizophrenia and risk of new-onset inflammatory bowel disease: a nationwide longitudinal study. Aliment Pharmacol Ther. 2022 May;55(9):1192-1201. doi: 10.1111/apt.16856.

11. Bernstein CN, Hitchon CA, Walld R, Bolton JM, Sareen J, Walker JR, Graff LA, Patten SB, Singer A, Lix LM, El-Gabalawy R, Katz A, Fisk JD, Marrie RA; CIHR Team in Defining the Burden and Managing the Effects of Psychiatric Comorbidity in Chronic Immunoinflammatory Disease. Increased Burden of Psychiatric Disorders in Inflammatory Bowel Disease. Inflamm Bowel Dis. 2019 Jan 10;25(2):360-368. doi: 10.1093/ibd/izy235.

12. Marrie RA, Walld R, Bolton JM, Sareen J, Walker JR, Patten SB, Singer A, Lix LM, Hitchon CA, El-Gabalawy R, Katz A, Fisk JD, Bernstein CN; CIHR Team in Defining the Burden and Managing the Effects of Psychiatric Comorbidity in Chronic Immunoinflammatory Disease. Increased incidence of psychiatric disorders in immune-mediated inflammatory disease. J Psychosom Res. 2017 Oct;101:17-23. doi: 10.1016/j.jpsychores.2017.07.015

13. Wang C, Zhang T, He L, Fu JY, Deng HX, Xue XL, Chen BT. Bacterial Translocation Associates With Aggression in

Schizophrenia Inpatients. Front Syst Neurosci. 2021 Sep 29;15:704069. doi: 10.3389/fnsys.2021.704069.

14. Severance EG, Gressitt KL, Stallings CR, Origoni AE, Khushalani S, Leweke FM, Dickerson FB, Yolken RH. Discordant patterns of bacterial translocation markers and implications for innate immune imbalances in schizophrenia. Schizophr Res. 2013 Aug;148(1-3):130-7. doi: 10.1016/j.schres.2013.05.018.

15. Szeligowski T, Yun AL, Lennox BR, Burnet PWJ. The Gut Microbiome and Schizophrenia: The Current State of the Field and Clinical Applications. Front Psychiatry. 2020 Mar 12;11:156. doi: 10.3389/fpsyt.2020.00156.

16. Najjar S, Pahlajani S, De Sanctis V, Stern JNH, Najjar A, Chong D. Neurovascular Unit Dysfunction and Blood-Brain Barrier Hyperpermeability Contribute to Schizophrenia Neurobiology: A Theoretical Integration of Clinical and Experimental Evidence. Front Psychiatry. 2017 May 23;8:83. doi: 10.3389/fpsyt.2017.00083.

17. Puvogel, S., Alsema, A., Kracht, L. et al. Single-nucleus RNA sequencing of midbrain blood-brain barrier cells in schizophrenia reveals subtle transcriptional changes with overall preservation of cellular proportions and phenotypes. Mol Psychiatry 27, 4731–4740 (2022). https://doi.org/10.1038/s41380-022-01796-0

18. Greene C, Hanley N, Campbell M. Blood-brain barrier associated tight junction disruption is a hallmark feature of major psychiatric disorders. Transl Psychiatry. 2020 Nov 2;10(1):373. doi: 10.1038/s41398-020-01054-3.

19. Cheng Y, Wang T, Zhang T, Yi S, Zhao S, Li N, Yang Y, Zhang F, Xu L, Shan B, Xu X, Xu J. Increased Blood-Brain Barrier Permeability of the Thalamus Correlated With Symptom Severity and Brain Volume Alterations in Patients With Schizophrenia. Biol

Psychiatry Cogn Neurosci Neuroimaging. 2022 Oct;7(10):1025-1034. doi: 10.1016/j.bpsc.2022.06.006.

20. Kleimann A, Toto S, Eberlein CK, Kielstein JT, Bleich S, Frieling H, Sieberer M. Psychiatric symptoms in patients with Shiga toxin-producing E. coli O104:H4 induced haemolytic-uraemic syndrome. PLoS One. 2014 Jul 9;9(7):e101839. doi: 10.1371/journal.pone.0101839.

21. Wiwanitkit V. Psychosis and E. coli Infection: A Forgotten Issue. Indian J Psychol Med. 2012 Oct;34(4):407-8. doi: 10.4103/0253-7176.108241.

22. Graham KL, Carson CM, Ezeoke A, Buckley PF, Miller BJ. Urinary tract infections in acute psychosis. J Clin Psychiatry. 2014 Apr;75(4):379-85. doi: 10.4088/JCP.13m08469

23. Buchholz U, Bernard H, Werber D, Böhmer MM, Remschmidt C, Wilking H, Deleré Y, an der Heiden M, Adlhoch C, Dreesman J, Ehlers J, Ethelberg S, Faber M, Frank C, Fricke G, Greiner M, Höhle M, Ivarsson S, Jark U, Kirchner M, Koch J, Krause G, Luber P, Rosner B, Stark K, Kühne M. German outbreak of Escherichia coli O104:H4 associated with sprouts. N Engl J Med. 2011 Nov 10;365(19):1763-70. doi: 10.1056/NEJMoa1106482.

24. Sandler NG, Douek DC. Microbial translocation in HIV infection: causes, consequences and treatment opportunities. Nat Rev Microbiol. 2012 Sep;10(9):655-66. doi: 10.1038/nrmicro2848.

25. Kim CJ, Nazli A, Rojas OL, Chege D, Alidina Z, Huibner S, Mujib S, Benko E, Kovacs C, Shin LY, Grin A, Kandel G, Loutfy M, Ostrowski M, Gommerman JL, Kaushic C, Kaul R. A role for mucosal IL-22 production and Th22 cells in HIV-associated mucosal immunopathogenesis. Mucosal Immunol. 2012 Nov;5(6):670-80. doi: 10.1038/mi.2012.72.

26. Harris MJ, Jeste DV, Gleghorn A, Sewell DD. New-onset psychosis in HIV-infected patients. J Clin Psychiatry. 1991 Sep;52(9):369-76. PMID: 1894589.

27. de Ronchi D, Faranca I, Forti P, Ravaglia G, Borderi M, Manfredi R, Volterra V. Development of acute psychotic disorders and HIV-1 infection. Int J Psychiatry Med. 2000;30(2):173-83. doi: 10.2190/PLGX-N48F-RBHJ-UF8K. PMID: 11001280.

28. Alciati A, Fusi A, D'Arminio Monforte A, Coen M, Ferri A, Mellado C. New-onset delusions and hallucinations in patients infected with HIV. J Psychiatry Neurosci. 2001 May;26(3):229-34. PMID: 11394192; PMCID: PMC1408305.

29. Sewell DD. Schizophrenia and HIV. Schizophr Bull. 1996;22(3):465-73. doi: 10.1093/schbul/22.3.465. PMID: 8873297.

30. Dudakov JA, Hanash AM, Jenq RR, Young LF, Ghosh A, Singer NV, West ML, Smith OM, Holland AM, Tsai JJ, Boyd RL, van den Brink MR. Interleukin-22 drives endogenous thymic regeneration in mice. Science. 2012 Apr 6;336(6077):91-5. doi: 10.1126/science.1218004. Epub 2012 Mar 1. PMID: 22383805

31. Keir M, Yi Y, Lu T, Ghilardi N. The role of IL-22 in intestinal health and disease. J Exp Med. 2020 Feb 13;217(3):e20192195. doi: 10.1084/jem.20192195.

32. Arshad T, Mansur F, Palek R, Manzoor S, Liska V. A Double Edged Sword Role of Interleukin-22 in Wound Healing and Tissue Regeneration. Front Immunol. 2020 Sep 17;11:2148. doi: 10.3389/fimmu.2020.02148.

33. Ezeonwumelu IJ, Garcia-Vidal E, Ballana E. JAK-STAT Pathway: A Novel Target to Tackle Viral Infections. Viruses. 2021 Nov 27;13(12):2379. doi: 10.3390/v13122379. PMID: 34960648; PMCID: PMC8704679.

34. Perusina Lanfranca M, Lin Y, Fang J, Zou W, Frankel T. Biological and pathological activities of interleukin-22. J Mol Med (Berl). 2016 May;94(5):523-34. doi: 10.1007/s00109-016-1391-6.

35. Fu G, Zhang W, Dai J, Liu J, Li F, Wu D, Xiao Y, Shah C, Sweeney JA, Wu M, Lui S. Increased Peripheral Interleukin 10 Relate to White Matter Integrity in Schizophrenia. Front Neurosci. 2019 Feb 7;13:52. doi: 10.3389/fnins.2019.00052.

36. Kapelski P, Skibinska M, Maciukiewicz M, Pawlak J, Zaremba D, Twarowska-Hauser J. Family-based association study of interleukin 10 (IL10) and interleukin 10 receptor alpha (IL10RA) functional polymorphisms in schizophrenia in Polish population. J Neuroimmunol. 2016 Aug 15;297:92-7. doi: 10.1016/j.jneuroim.2016.05.010.

37. Mattapallil MJ, Kielczewski JL, Zárate-Bladés CR, St Leger AJ, Raychaudhuri K, Silver PB, Jittayasothorn Y, Chan CC, Caspi RR. Interleukin 22 ameliorates neuropathology and protects from central nervous system autoimmunity. J Autoimmun. 2019 Aug;102:65-76. doi: 10.1016/j.jaut.2019.04.017. Epub 2019 May 9. PMID: 31080013; PMCID: PMC6667188

38. Rachel Caspi, Mary Mattapallil, Rachael Rigden, Carlos Zarate-Blades, Phyllis Silver, Dror Luger, Chi Chao Chan; Neuroprotective effects of IL-22 during CNS inflammation (CCR4P.203). J Immunol 1 May 2015; 194 (1_Supplement): 118.3.

39. Subbanna M, Shivakumar V, Talukdar PM, Narayanaswamy JC, Venugopal D, Berk M, Varambally S, Venkatasubramanian G, Debnath M. Role of IL-6/RORC/IL-22 axis in driving Th17 pathway mediated immunopathogenesis of schizophrenia. Cytokine. 2018 Nov;111:112-118. doi: 10.1016/j.cyto.2018.08.016.

40. Barthelemy A, Sencio V, Soulard D, Deruyter L, Faveeuw C, Le Goffic R, Trottein F. Interleukin-22 Immunotherapy during Severe Influenza Enhances Lung Tissue Integrity and Reduces Secondary Bacterial Systemic Invasion. Infect Immun. 2018 Jun 21;86(7):e00706-17. doi: 10.1128/IAI.00706-17.

41. Albayrak N, Orte Cano C, Karimi S, Dogahe D, Van Praet A, Godefroid A, Del Marmol V, Grimaldi D, Bondue B, Van Vooren JP, Mascart F, Corbière V. Distinct Expression Patterns of Interleukin-22 Receptor 1 on Blood Hematopoietic Cells in SARS-CoV-2 Infection. Front Immunol. 2022 Mar 29;13:769839. doi: 10.3389/fimmu.2022.769839.

42. Li LJ, Gong C, Zhao MH, Feng BS. Role of interleukin-22 in inflammatory bowel disease. World J Gastroenterol. 2014 Dec 28;20(48):18177-88. doi: 10.3748/wjg.v20.i48.18177

43. Cella M, Fuchs A, Vermi W, Facchetti F, Otero K, Lennerz JK, Doherty JM, Mills JC, Colonna M. A human natural killer cell subset provides an innate source of IL-22 for mucosal immunity. Colonna M. Interleukin-22-producing natural killer cells and lymphoid tissue inducer-like cells in mucosal immunity. Immunity. 2009 Jul 17;31(1):15-23. doi: 10.1016/j.immuni.2009.06.008. Nature. 2009 Feb 5;457(7230):722-5. doi: 10.1038/nature07537. Epub 2008 Nov 2.

44. Colonna M. Interleukin-22-producing natural killer cells and lymphoid tissue inducer-like cells in mucosal immunity. Immunity. 2009 Jul 17;31(1):15-23. doi: 10.1016/j.immuni.2009.06.008. PMID: 19604490.

45. Kumar P, Thakar MS, Ouyang W, Malarkannan S. IL-22 from conventional NK cells are epithelial regenerative and inflammation protective during influenza infection. Mucosal Immunol. 2013 Jan;6(1):69-82. doi: 10.1038/mi.2012.49.

46. Zaiatz Bittencourt V, Jones F, Tosetto M, Doherty GA, Ryan EJ. Dysregulation of Metabolic Pathways in Circulating Natural Killer Cells Isolated from Inflammatory Bowel Disease Patients. J Crohns Colitis. 2021 Aug 2;15(8):1316-1325. doi: 10.1093/ecco-jcc/jjab014. PMID: 33460436;

47. Fernandez-Egea E, Vértes PE, Flint SM, Turner L, Mustafa S, Hatton A, Smith KG, Lyons PA, Bullmore ET. Peripheral Immune Cell Populations Associated with Cognitive Deficits and Negative Symptoms of Treatment-Resistant Schizophrenia. PLoS One. 2016 May 31;11(5):e0155631. doi: 10.1371/journal.pone.0155631.

48. Tarantino N, Leboyer M, Bouleau A, Hamdani N, Richard JR, Boukouaci W, Ching-Lien W, Godin O, Bengoufa D, Le Corvoisier P, Barau C, Ledudal K, Debré P, Tamouza R, Vieillard V. Natural killer cells in first-episode psychosis: an innate immune signature? Mol Psychiatry. 2021 Sep;26(9):5297-5306. doi: 10.1038/s41380-020-01008-7.

49. Steel AW, Mela CM, Lindsay JO, Gazzard BG, Goodier MR. Increased proportion of CD16(+) NK cells in the colonic lamina propria of inflammatory bowel disease patients, but not after azathioprine treatment. Aliment Pharmacol Ther. 2011 Jan;33(1):115-26. doi: 10.1111/j.1365-2036.2010.04499.x.

50. Sedgwick AJ, Ghazanfari N, Constantinescu P, Mantamadiotis T, Barrow AD. The Role of NK Cells and Innate Lymphoid Cells in Brain Cancer. Front Immunol. 2020 Jul 31;11:1549. doi: 10.3389/fimmu.2020.01549.

51. Jin WN, Shi K, He W, Sun JH, Van Kaer L, Shi FD, Liu Q. Neuroblast senescence in the aged brain augments natural killer cell cytotoxicity leading to impaired neurogenesis and cognition. Nat Neurosci. 2021 Jan;24(1):61-73. doi: 10.1038/s41593-020-00745-w.

52. Vivier E, Artis D, Colonna M, Diefenbach A, Di Santo JP, Eberl G, et al. Innate Lymphoid Cells: 10 Years On. Cell. 2018 Aug 23;174(5):1054-1066. doi: 10.1016/j.cell.2018.07.017.

53. Artis, D., Spits, H. The biology of innate lymphoid cells. Nature 517, 293–301 (2015). https://doi.org/10.1038/nature14189

54. Fan H, Wang A, Wang Y, Sun Y, Han J, Chen W, Wang S, Wu Y, Lu Y. Innate Lymphoid Cells: Regulators of Gut Barrier Function and Immune Homeostasis. J Immunol Res. 2019 Dec 20;2019:2525984. doi: 10.1155/2019/2525984.

55. Borovcanin MM, Minic Janicijevic S, Jovanovic IP, Gajovic NM, Jurisevic MM, Arsenijevic NN. Type 17 Immune Response Facilitates Progression of Inflammation and Correlates with Cognition in Stable Schizophrenia. Diagnostics (Basel). 2020 Nov 10;10(11):926. doi: 10.3390/diagnostics10110926.

56. Barichello T. The role of innate lymphoid cells (ILCs) in mental health. Discov Ment Health. 2022;2(1):2. doi: 10.1007/s44192-022-00006-1. Epub 2022 Feb 7. PMID: 35224555; PMCID: PMC8855986.

57. Yeung, S.SH., Ho, YS. & Chang, R.CC. The role of meningeal populations of type II innate lymphoid cells in modulating neuroinflammation in neurodegenerative diseases. Exp Mol Med 53, 1251–1267 (2021). https://doi.org/10.1038/s12276-021-00660-5

58. Uchiyama, K., Takagi, T., Mizushima, K. et al. Increased mucosal IL-12 expression is associated with relapse of ulcerative colitis. BMC Gastroenterol 21, 122 (2021). https://doi.org/10.1186/s12876-021-01709-5

59. Langer V, Vivi E, Regensburger D, Winkler TH, Waldner MJ, Rath T, Schmid B, Skottke L, Lee S, Jeon NL, Wohlfahrt T, Kramer V, Tripal P, Schumann M, Kersting S, Handtrack C, Geppert CI,

Suchowski K, Adams RH, Becker C, Ramming A, Naschberger E, Britzen-Laurent N, Stürzl M. IFN-γ drives inflammatory bowel disease pathogenesis through VE-cadherin-directed vascular barrier disruption. J Clin Invest. 2019 Nov 1;129(11):4691-4707. doi: 10.1172/JCI124884.

60. Kato T, Monji A, Hashioka S, Kanba S. Risperidone significantly inhibits interferon-gamma-induced microglial activation in vitro. Schizophr Res. 2007 May;92(1-3):108-15. doi: 10.1016/j.schres.2007.01.019.

61. Wilson KE, Demyanovich H, Rubin LH, Wehring HJ, Kilday C, Kelly DL. Relationship of Interferon-γ to Cognitive Function in Midlife Women with Schizophrenia. Psychiatr Q. 2018 Dec;89(4):937-946. doi: 10.1007/s11126-018-9591-6

62. Arolt V, Weitzsch C, Wilke I, Nolte A, Pinnow M, Rothermundt M, Kirchner H. Production of interferon-gamma in families with multiple occurrence of schizophrenia. Psychiatry Res. 1997 Feb 7;66(2-3):145-52. doi: 10.1016/s0165-1781(96)03023-5

63. Mount MP, Lira A, Grimes D, Smith PD, Faucher S, Slack R, Anisman H, Hayley S, Park DS. Involvement of interferon-gamma in microglial-mediated loss of dopaminergic neurons. J Neurosci. 2007 Mar 21;27(12):3328-37. doi: 10.1523/JNEUROSCI.5321-06.2007.

64. Pennino D, Bhavsar PK, Effner R, Avitabile S, Venn P, Quaranta M, Marzaioli V, Cifuentes L, Durham SR, Cavani A, Eyerich K, Chung KF, Schmidt-Weber CB, Eyerich S. IL-22 suppresses IFN-γ-mediated lung inflammation in asthmatic patients. J Allergy Clin Immunol. 2013 Feb;131(2):562-70. doi: 10.1016/j.jaci.2012.09.036.

65. Natah SS, Mouihate A, Pittman QJ, Sharkey KA. Disruption of the blood-brain barrier during TNBS colitis. Neurogastroenterol Motil.

2005 Jun;17(3):433-46. doi: 10.1111/j.1365-2982.2005.00654.x. PMID: 15916631.

66. Chen BY, Hsu CC, Chen YZ, Lin JJ, Tseng HH, Jang FL, Chen PS, Chen WN, Chen CS, Lin SH. Profiling antibody signature of schizophrenia by Escherichia coli proteome microarrays. Brain Behav Immun. 2022 Nov;106:11-20. doi: 10.1016/j.bbi.2022.07.162.

67. Secher T, Samba-Louaka A, Oswald E, Nougayrède JP. Escherichia coli-producing colibactin triggers premature and transmissible senescence in mammalian cells. PLoS One. 2013 Oct 8;8(10):e77157. doi: 10.1371/journal.pone.0077157.

68. Papanastasiou E, Gaughran F, Smith S. Schizophrenia as segmental progeria. J R Soc Med. 2011 Nov;104(11):475-84. doi: 10.1258/jrsm.2011.110051.

69. Mizuno Y, Muraoka M, Shimabukuro K, Toda K, Miyagawa K, Yoshimatsu H, Tsuchiya M. Inflammatory bowel diseases and thymus disorder: reactivity of thymocytes with monoclonal antibodies. Bull Tokyo Dent Coll. 1990 May;31(2):137-41. PMID: 2131166

70. Watanabe M, Funahashi T, Suzuki T, Nomura S, Nakazawa T, Noguchi T, Tsukada Y. Antithymic antibodies in schizophrenic sera. Biol Psychiatry. 1982 Jun;17(6):699-710. PMID: 6125218.

71. Pan B, Wang D, Li L, Shang L, Xia F, Zhang F, Zhang Y, Gale RP, Xu M, Li Z, Xu K. IL-22 Accelerates Thymus Regeneration via Stat3/Mcl-1 and Decreases Chronic Graft-versus-Host Disease in Mice after Allotransplants. Biol Blood Marrow Transplant. 2019 Oct;25(10):1911-1919. doi: 10.1016/j.bbmt.2019.06.002.

72. Falk W. A ticket to the gut for thymic T cells. Gut. 2006 Jul;55(7):910-2. doi: 10.1136/gut.2005.087288. PMID: 16766746; PMCID: PMC1856347.

73. Shang L, Duah M, Xu Y, Liang Y, Wang D, Xia F, Li L, Sun Z, Yan Z, Xu K, Pan B. Dynamic of plasma IL-22 level is an indicator of thymic output after allogeneic hematopoietic cell transplantation. Life Sci. 2021 Jan 15;265:118849. doi: 10.1016/j.lfs.2020.118849.

74. Li Y, Wang J, Li Y, Wu H, Zhao S, Yu Q. Protecting intestinal epithelial cells against deoxynivalenol and E. coli damage by recombinant porcine IL-22. Vet Microbiol. 2019 Apr;231:154-159. doi: 10.1016/j.vetmic.2019.02.027.

75. Aujla SJ, Chan YR, Zheng M, Fei M, Askew DJ, Pociask DA, Reinhart TA, McAllister F, Edeal J, Gaus K, Husain S, Kreindler JL, Dubin PJ, Pilewski JM, Myerburg MM, Mason CA, Iwakura Y, Kolls JK. IL-22 mediates mucosal host defense against Gram-negative bacterial pneumonia. Nat Med. 2008 Mar;14(3):275-81. doi: 10.1038/nm1710.

76. Le PT, Pearce MM, Zhang S, Campbell EM, Fok CS, Mueller ER, Brincat CA, Wolfe AJ, Brubaker L. IL22 regulates human urothelial cell sensory and innate functions through modulation of the acetylcholine response, immunoregulatory cytokines and antimicrobial peptides: assessment of an in vitro model. PLoS One. 2014 Oct 29;9(10):e111375. doi: 10.1371/journal.pone.0111375.

77. Ingersoll MA, Starkey MR. Interleukin-22 in urinary tract disease - new experimental directions. Clin Transl Immunology. 2020 Jun 7;9(6):e1143. doi: 10.1002/cti2.1143.

78. Ronald A. The etiology of urinary tract infection: traditional and emerging pathogens. Am J Med. 2002 Jul 8;113 Suppl 1A:14S-19S. doi: 10.1016/s0002-9343(02)01055-0

79. Rudzki L, Szulc A. "Immune Gate" of Psychopathology-The Role of Gut Derived Immune Activation in Major Psychiatric Disorders.

Front Psychiatry. 2018 May 29;9:205. doi:
10.3389/fpsyt.2018.00205

80. Maes M, Vojdani A, Geffard M, Moreira EG, Barbosa DS, Michelin
AP, Semeão LO, Sirivichayakul S, Kanchanatawan B. Schizophrenia
phenomenology comprises a bifactorial general severity and a single-
group factor, which are differently associated with neurotoxic
immune and immune-regulatory pathways. Biomol Concepts. 2019
Nov 17;10(1):209-225. doi: 10.1515/bmc-2019-0023.

81. Tang KY, Lickliter J, Huang ZH, Xian ZS, Chen HY, Huang C, Xiao
C, Wang YP, Tan Y, Xu LF, Huang YL, Yan XQ. Safety,
pharmacokinetics, and biomarkers of F-652, a recombinant human
interleukin-22 dimer, in healthy subjects. Cell Mol Immunol. 2019
May;16(5):473-482. doi: 10.1038/s41423-018-0029-8.

82. Arab JP, Sehrawat TS, Simonetto DA, Verma VK, Feng D, Tang T,
Dreyer K, Yan X, Daley WL, Sanyal A, Chalasani N, Radaeva S,
Yang L, Vargas H, Ibacache M, Gao B, Gores GJ, Malhi H, Kamath
PS, Shah VH. An Open-Label, Dose-Escalation Study to Assess the
Safety and Efficacy of IL-22 Agonist F-652 in Patients With
Alcohol-associated Hepatitis. Hepatology. 2020 Aug;72(2):441-453.
doi: 10.1002/hep.31046.

83. Dempsey, L. Antimicrobial IL-22. Nat Immunol 18, 373 (2017).
https://doi.org/10.1038/ni.3722

84. Das S, St Croix C, Good M, Chen J, Zhao J, Hu S, Ross M,
Myerburg MM, Pilewski JM, Williams J, Wenzel SE, Kolls JK, Ray
A, Ray P. Interleukin-22 Inhibits Respiratory Syncytial Virus
Production by Blocking Virus-Mediated Subversion of Cellular
Autophagy. iScience. 2020 Jul 24;23(7):101256. doi:
10.1016/j.isci.2020.101256.

85. Shao, L., Xiong, X., Zhang, Y. et al. IL-22 ameliorates LPS-induced acute liver injury by autophagy activation through ATF4-ATG7 signaling. Cell Death Dis 11, 970 (2020). https://doi.org/10.1038/s41419-020-03176-4

86. Merenlender-Wagner, A., Malishkevich, A., Shemer, Z. et al. Autophagy has a key role in the pathophysiology of schizophrenia. Mol Psychiatry 20, 126–132 (2015). https://doi.org/10.1038/mp.2013.174

87. Iida T, Onodera K, Nakase H. Role of autophagy in the pathogenesis of inflammatory bowel disease. World J Gastroenterol. 2017 Mar 21;23(11):1944-1953. doi: 10.3748/wjg.v23.i11.1944.

88. Mo R, Lai R, Lu J, Zhuang Y, Zhou T, Jiang S, Ren P, Li Z, Cao Z, Liu Y, Chen L, Xiong L, Wang P, Wang H, Cai W, Xiang X, Bao S, Xie Q. Enhanced autophagy contributes to protective effects of IL-22 against acetaminophen-induced liver injury. Theranostics. 2018 Jul 30;8(15):4170-4180. doi: 10.7150/thno.25798.

89. Kim SH, Park S, Yu HS, Ko KH, Park HG, Kim YS. The antipsychotic agent clozapine induces autophagy via the AMPK-ULK1-Beclin1 signaling pathway in the rat frontal cortex. Prog Neuropsychopharmacol Biol Psychiatry. 2018 Feb 2;81:96-104. doi: 10.1016/j.pnpbp.2017.10.012.

90. Kim YK, Suh IB, Kim H, Han CS, Lim CS, Choi SH, Licinio J. The plasma levels of interleukin-12 in schizophrenia, major depression, and bipolar mania: effects of psychotropic drugs. Mol Psychiatry. 2002;7(10):1107-14. doi: 10.1038/sj.mp.4001084. PMID: 12476326.

91. Singh RK, Dai Y, Staudinger JL, Muma NA. Activation of the JAK-STAT pathway is necessary for desensitization of 5-HT2A receptor-stimulated phospholipase C signaling by olanzapine, clozapine, and

MDL 100907. Int J Neuropsychopharmacol. 2009 Jun;12(5):651-65. doi: 10.1017/S1461145708009590.

92. He J, Kong J, Tan QR, Li XM. Neuroprotective effect of atypical antipsychotics in cognitive and non-cognitive behavioral impairment in animal models. Cell Adh Migr. 2009 Jan-Mar;3(1):129-37. doi: 10.4161/cam.3.1.7401. Epub 2009 Jan 13. PMID: 19372744; PMCID: PMC2675159.

93. Kato T, Mizoguchi Y, Monji A, Horikawa H, Suzuki SO, Seki Y, Iwaki T, Hashioka S, Kanba S. Inhibitory effects of aripiprazole on interferon-gamma-induced microglial activation via intracellular Ca2+ regulation in vitro. J Neurochem. 2008 Jul;106(2):815-25. doi: 10.1111/j.1471-4159.2008.05435.x

94. Vucicevic L, Misirkic-Marjanovic M, Harhaji-Trajkovic L, Maric N, Trajkovic V. Mechanisms and therapeutic significance of autophagy modulation by antipsychotic drugs. Cell Stress. 2018 Oct 25;2(11):282-291. doi: 10.15698/cst2018.11.161. PMID: 31225453; PMCID: PMC6551804

95. Girgis RR, Lieberman JA. Anti-viral properties of antipsychotic medications in the time of COVID-19. Psychiatry Res. 2021 Jan;295:113626. doi: 10.1016/j.psychres.2020.113626.

96. Nehme H, Saulnier P, Ramadan AA, Cassisa V, Guillet C, Eveillard M, Umerska A. Antibacterial activity of antipsychotic agents, their association with lipid nanocapsules and its impact on the properties of the nanocarriers and antibacterial activity. PLoS One. 2018 Jan 3;13(1):e0189950. doi: 10.1371/journal.pone.0189950

Chapter 16
Lessons from COVID-19: The FURIN Gene and Mental Illness

> COVID-19 usurps human furin, a protein implicated in PTSD and other mental illnesses. Furin also plays a key role in pathogen weaponization, increased virulence by gain of function. The exploitation of furin by the SARS-CoV-2 virus is one out of many indicators that this pathogen may have been intended as a biological weapon.

Posttraumatic stress disorder (PTSD) is a severe neuropsychiatric illness triggered by psychological stress, which, like SCZ, is marked by premature cellular senescence. Direct molecular aging due to psychosocial stress was documented recently by the detection of senescent markers, including p16INK4a, in PTSD patients (1) (2). Endothelial cells (ECs), due to their vascular architecture and turnover rate, are the first to be affected by the aging process and generate the most significant burden of senescent cells in the body (3) (4) (5) (6). Therefore, the vessels age first, and this explains the high comorbidity of cardiovascular disease (CVD) with PTSD (7).

The FURIN gene, a new player in neuropsychiatric illness, is highly expressed in ECs and regulates cellular senescence via brain-derived neurotrophic factor (BDNF) (8) (9) (10) (11). Furin is a proprotein convertase that converts precursor proteins into their biologically active forms, such as pro-BDNF to BDNF. BDNF is elevated in PTSD, implicating overactive ECs furin (12). The ability to activate toxins or pathogens, such as anthrax, by proteolytic cleavage brought FURIN to the forefront of the bioweapon manufacturing programs, where it remained up to the present day (13) (14).

Psychological stress and vascular aging

Stress-induced aging has been known for centuries; however, the molecular underpinning of this process remains unclear. Cellular senescence, the building block of organismal aging, is a default program of replicative arrest in which the cell permanently exits the cell cycle, rewires its metabolism, and attempts to repair the genome (15). Senescence affects ECs first, increasing the levels of BDNF, an angiogenesis-promoting neurotrophin that facilitates the sprouting of new vessels to replace the damaged ones (5) (16) (17). Indeed, senescent cells upregulate BDNF because it is a component of SASP (11). In PTSD, BDNF levels are elevated, probably due to furin-induced cellular senesce (12) (18) (19).

BDNF is derived from pro-BDNF, an inactive precursor protein that requires proteolytic cleavage by furin or plasmin to be converted into the biologically active form. Furin protein, encoded by the FURIN gene, is a calcium (Ca^{2+}) dependent serine protease that plays a key role in activating numerous endogenous and exogenous proteins into functional molecules. Furin and plasmin activate BDNF, while plasminogen activator inhibitor 1 (PAI-1) does the opposite, inhibiting plasmin and furin and suppressing their proteolytic activity (20).

Over the past decades, furin drew the attention of researchers and clinicians for two reasons: the 1950s and 1960s weaponization of anthrax by the Soviet Union and its vital role in COVID-19 virulence. The former triggered an intensive biological arms race, which stopped only after the "Sverdlovsk anthrax outbreak of 1979" that killed 64 people (21). The collective memories of anthrax weaponization programs and the discovery of the FURIN gene in 1990 raised the question of whether other pathogens, especially viruses, could be manipulated to gain extra functions, such as increased infectivity.

Despite the pandemic and worldwide concerns about weaponizing this virus, the study of COVID-19 led to a better understanding of furin. The virus hijacks human furin to cleave the S (spike) protein into S1 and S2, increasing infectivity. This takes place via an arginine-rich sequence in the S antigen. This sequence, PRRAR (proline-arginine-arginine-alanine-arginine), hijacks human furin, interfering with the conversion of pre-BDNF into BDNF.

Furin, previously implicated in SMI, is decreased in SCZ, dementias, and PTSD and increased in epilepsy, suggesting a new target (8) (22) (23) (24). In addition, furin is intertwined with the serotonergic system, possibly interfering with the mechanism of action of SSRIs (25). Moreover, several cancers upregulate BDNF, probably due to its angiogenetic properties, to facilitate metastatic dissemination (26). As ECs release large amounts of BDNF, exploitation of endothelia leads to SARS-CoV-2 control over this growth factor (27) (28) (29).

The fearmongering hormone, plasmin activator inhibitor-1 (PAI-1)

Psychosocial stress-induced EC senescence disrupts fibrin breakdown by plasmin activator inhibitor-1 (PAI-1) and tissue plasminogen activator (tPA). PAI-1 is a serine protease inhibitor that blocks the proteolytic activity of furin and plasmin, disrupting the conversion of pro-BDNF into BDNF (30). For example, elevated PAI-1/BDNF ratio was documented in PTSD and dementias, while low furin, PAI-1, and BDNF characterize SCZ (20) (31) (32) (33).

Furin inhibition by PAI-1 leads to the accumulation of pro-BDNF, a negative regulator of synaptic plasticity, predisposing to PTSD. Moreover, AhR upregulates pro-BDNF, highlighting the therapeutic role of AhR inhibitors in PTSD (34). In contrast, glycogen synthase kinase three beta (GSK-3β) has a detrimental effect on PTSD via AhR inhibition by phosphorylation (23) (35).

Premature EC senescence in SCZ and bvFTD is well-established, indicating increased intestinal permeability due to the senescent endothelial barrier (36) (37). This promotes microbial migration into host tissues, contributing further to the development of PTSD symptoms by neuroinflammation. For example, as gut commensal flora expresses adrenergic receptors, it may elicit antibodies against these proteins upon translocation. Anti-adrenergic antibodies cross-react with the host adrenergic system, resulting in anxiety and fear (38) (39). For this reason, PAI-1 has been associated with stress, stress-related disorders, MDD, and SCZ (40) (41) (42) (43) (44) (45)

Microtubules-Encoded Traumatic Memories

Under physiological circumstances, tau protein is a microtubular stabilizer believed to participate in tubulin memory storage and retrieval. Microtubules are cytoskeletal components formed by tubulin polymerization and held together by tau protein. It was hypothesized that microtubular lattices encode memories in a quantum manner via calcium-calmodulin-dependent protein kinase II (CaMKII) (46).

A recent preclinical study found that social stress disrupts memory by impairing tubulin polymerization, suggesting that PTSD-related traumatic amnesia and hypermnesia may reflect microtubular pathology (47) (48). The microtubules' connection to memory is further substantiated by organ transplantation studies, which have demonstrated the acquisition of donor personality traits in the recipients of heart transplants (49). This phenomenon, reported in about 36.2% of transplants, highlights the role of microtubules in storing and retrieving memories (50) (51) (52).

Under physiological circumstances, GSK-3β phosphorylates tau protein, stabilizing microtubular conformation. However, excessive tau phosphorylation destabilizes microtubules, altering recall (53) (54). Indeed, microtubule-destabilizing agents, including chemotherapy, colchicine, and fluoride (added to drinking water), were associated with defective recall as well as behavioral disturbances (55) (56). Since the same agents activate microglia, it is not surprising that they may induce neurotoxicity and neuronal loss (57).

Recent studies have shown that tau protein engages in brain oscillatory activity, contributing to the rapid gamma waves implicated in higher cognitive functions (58).

Taken together, under pathological circumstances, GSK-3β may engage in hyperphosphorylation of tau protein, maintaining traumatic memories and promoting fear-induced aggressive behavior.

Therapeutic strategies

In two previous articles, we have discussed potential novel therapies for PTSD (59) (60). Here, we present a unique membrane lipid replacement (MLR) strategy augmented with kaempferol and berberine. This combination of natural compounds suppresses GSK-3β by three distinct mechanisms, producing a cumulative effect.

Membrane Lipid Replacement

MLR is a technique that utilizes healthy, natural glycerophospholipids to substitute the oxidized components of the plasma membranes lipid bilayer, thus restoring the physiological fluidity of cell and mitochondrial membranes. The membrane lipid bilayer comprises phospholipids, cholesterol, and ceramide, which disrupt neurotransmission when oxidized. Oxidized lipids, including oxysterols, phospholipids, and toxic ceramide, are gradually replaced with natural glycerophospholipids, restoring membrane homeostasis.

This approach, based on the oral supplementation with natural phospholipids and antioxidants, was demonstrated to halt the dissemination of cellular senescence to the neighboring, healthy cells, probably by inhibiting SASP (61) (62) (63). Moreover, MLR was shown to facilitate cell membranes and the damaged mitochondrial inner and outer membranes with natural lipid species. Indeed, loss of lyso-phosphatidylethanolamine (LPE), phosphatidylglycerol (PG), and phosphatidylinositol (PI) in senescent mitochondria was shown to cause organelle demise. Conversely, replacement with healthy lipids promotes mitochondrial homeostasis (64).

Phosphoinositide-Dependent Kinase 1 (PDK-1) Inhibitors

It has been hypothesized that cellular senescence and proliferation arrest are permanent and irreversible. However, novel data have shown that inhibitors of phosphoinositide-dependent kinase 1 (PDK-1), such as kaempferol (also an AhR antagonist), may reverse the senescent phenotype (65). On the other hand, PDK1 activation of protein kinase B (Akt) and GSK-3β contributes to the pathogenesis of SCZ (66). In contrast, PDK-1 inhibitors combined with MLR and berberine may exert antipsychotic properties by inhibiting GSK-3β while avoiding the typical adverse effects of conventional antipsychotics.

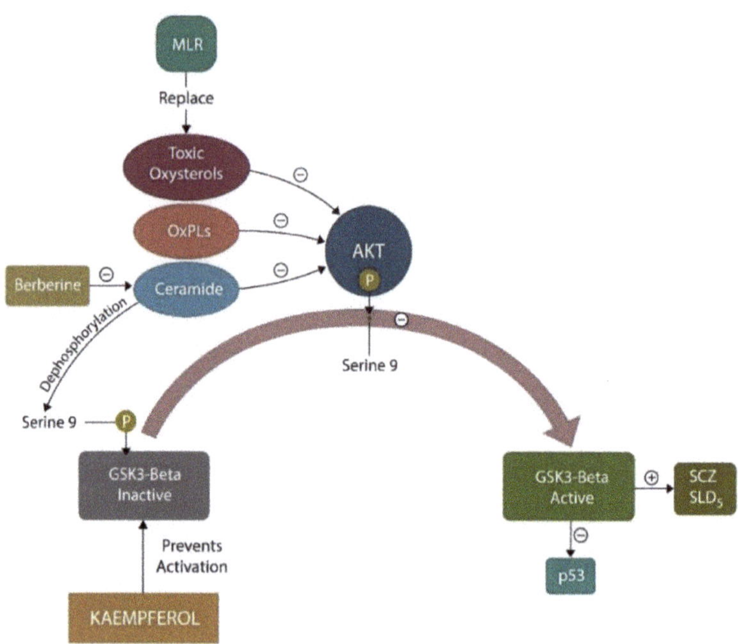

Fig. 16.2 MLR supplies natural glycerophospholipids to replace the oxidized phospholipids (OxPL), cholesterol, and ceramide. Under normal circumstances, lipids from the membrane bilayer activate Akt, inhibiting GSK-3β by phosphorylation at serine 9. Without lipidomic input, GSK-3β suppresses p53, disrupting genomic repair. Kaempferol prevents GSK-3β activation, while Berberine opposes GSK-3β by inhibiting ceramide and preventing serine 9 phosphorylation.

Berberine

Berberine is a plant alkaloid extracted from Hydrastis canadensis, Phellodendron Chinese, Coptis chinensis, and Berberis aquifolium, which has been used in Asia for centuries due to its antimicrobial and anthelminthic properties. Berberine is used in CVD, hyperlipidemia, diabetes, and hypertension as it reduces toxic ceramide, lowering insulin resistance caused by this toxin (67) (68). Moreover, berberine recently received attention as a potential anticancer agent, a property related to altering the cell cycle dynamics, autophagy, and cellular senescence (69). Indeed, berberine ameliorates cellular senescence by inhibiting cyclins and p16 (70). Furthermore, berberine alleviates anxiety, suggesting beneficial effects in PTSD (71). In ECs, berberine inhibits proliferation (72). Table 1 summarizes the natural inhibitors of PDK-1, some of which are also AhR inhibitors.

PDK1 Inhibitor	Plant	References
Kaempferol	Fruits, vegetables, and herbs	[73]
Quercetin	Onions, kale, broccoli	[74]
Myricetin	Oranges, berries, tomatoes, nuts, tea	[75]
Epigallocatechin-3 gallate	Green tea	[76]
Lupiwighteone isoflavone	Glycyrrhiza glabra; Lotus pedunculatus	[77]
Delphinidin	Citrus fruits	[78]
Honokiol	Cherries, berries, grapes	[79]
Delphinidin	Cranberries, concord grapes, pomegranates	[80]

Table. 16.1

Natural PDK-1 inhibitors

In conclusion, like other neuropsychiatric conditions, PTSD is associated with premature ECs senescence, increased permeability of gut barrier and BBB, altered fibrinolysis, and upregulated BDNF that often leads to comorbidities.

Chapter 16 References:

1. Rentscher KE, Carroll JE, Repetti RL, Cole SW, Reynolds BM, Robles TF. Chronic stress exposure and daily stress appraisals relate to biological aging marker p16 INK4a. Psychoneuroendocrinology. 2019;102:139–148. doi: 10.1016/j.psyneuen.2018.12.006

2. Razzoli M, Nyuyki-Dufe K, Gurney A, et al. Social stress shortens lifespan in mice. Aging Cell. 2018;17(4):e12778. doi: 10.1111/acel.12778

3. Yousefzadeh MJ et al. Tissue specificity of senescent cell accumulation during physiologic and accelerated aging of mice. Aging Cell 19, e13094 (2020). 10.1111/acel.13094

4. Grosse L et al. Defined p16(High) Senescent Cell Types Are Indispensable for Mouse Healthspan. Cell Metab 32, 87–99.e86 (2020). 10.1016/j.cmet.2020.05.002

5. Piao L, Zhao G, Zhu E, Inoue A, Shibata R, Lei Y, Hu L, Yu C, Yang G, Wu H, Xu W, Okumura K, Ouchi N, Murohara T, Kuzuya M, Cheng XW. Chronic Psychological Stress Accelerates Vascular Senescence and Impairs Ischemia-Induced Neovascularization: The Role of Dipeptidyl Peptidase-4/Glucagon-Like Peptide-1-Adiponectin Axis. J Am Heart Assoc. 2017 Sep 28;6(10):e006421. doi: 10.1161/JAHA.117.006421.

6. Lehmann ML, Poffenberger CN, Elkahloun AG, Herkenham M. Analysis of cerebrovascular dysfunction caused by chronic social defeat in mice. Brain Behav Immun. 2020 Aug;88:735-747. doi: 10.1016/j.bbi.2020.05.030.

7. Beristianos MH, Yaffe K, Cohen B, Byers AL. PTSD and Risk of Incident Cardiovascular Disease in Aging Veterans. Am J Geriatr Psychiatry. 2016 Mar;24(3):192-200. doi: 10.1016/j.jagp.2014.12.003. Epub 2014 Dec 9. PMID: 25555625.

8. Zhang Y, Gao X, Bai X, Yao S, Chang YZ, Gao G. The emerging role of furin in neurodegenerative and neuropsychiatric diseases. Transl Neurodegener. 2022 Aug 23;11(1):39. doi: 10.1186/s40035-022-00313-1.

9. Yang X, Yang W, McVey DG, Zhao G, Hu J, Poston RN, Ren M, Willeit K, Coassin S, Willeit J, Webb TR, Samani NJ, Mayr M, Kiechl S, Ye S. FURIN Expression in Vascular Endothelial Cells Is Modulated by a Coronary Artery Disease-Associated Genetic Variant and Influences Monocyte Transendothelial Migration. J Am Heart Assoc. 2020 Feb 18;9(4):e014333. doi: 10.1161/JAHA.119.014333.

10. AbdelMassih AF, Ye J, Kamel A, Mishriky F, Ismail HA, Ragab HA, El Qadi L, Malak L, Abdu M, El-Husseiny M, Ashraf M, Hafez N, AlShehry N, El-Husseiny N, AbdelRaouf N, Shebl N, Hafez N, Youssef N, Afdal P, Hozaien R, Menshawey R, Saeed R, Fouda R. A multicenter consensus: A role of furin in the endothelial tropism in obese patients with COVID-19 infection. Obes Med. 2020 Sep;19:100281. doi: 10.1016/j.obmed.2020.100281.

11. Anerillas C, Herman AB, Munk R, Garrido A, Lam KG, Payea MJ, Rossi M, Tsitsipatis D, Martindale JL, Piao Y, Mazan-Mamczarz K, Fan J, Cui CY, De S, Abdelmohsen K, de Cabo R, Gorospe M. A BDNF-TrkB autocrine loop enhances senescent cell viability. Nat Commun. 2022 Oct 20;13(1):6228. doi: 10.1038/s41467-022-33709-8. Erratum in: Nat Commun. 2022 Dec 7;13(1):7540. PMID: 36266274; PMCID: PMC9585019.

12. Wu GWY, Wolkowitz OM, Reus VI, Kang JI, Elnar M, Sarwal R, Flory JD, Abu-Amara D, Hammamieh R, Gautam A, Doyle FJ 3rd, Yehuda R, Marmar CR, Jett M, Mellon SH; SBPBC. Serum brain-derived neurotrophic factor remains elevated after long long-term follow-up of combat veterans with chronic post-traumatic stress disorder. Psychoneuroendocrinology. 2021 Jul 22;134:105360. doi:

10.1016/j.psyneuen.2021.105360. Epub ahead of print. PMID: 34757255.

13. Farkas CB, Dudás G, Babinszky GC, Földi L. Analysis of the Virus SARS-CoV-2 as a Potential Bioweapon in Light of International Literature. Mil Med. 2023 Mar 20;188(3-4):531-540. doi: 10.1093/milmed/usac123. PMID: 35569934; PMCID: PMC9384074

14. Molloy SS, Bresnahan PA, Leppla SH, Klimpel KR, Thomas G. Human furin is a calcium-dependent serine endoprotease that recognizes the sequence Arg-X-X-Arg and efficiently cleaves anthrax toxin protective antigen. J Biol Chem. 1992 Aug 15;267(23):16396-402. PMID: 1644824.

15. d'Adda di Fagagna, F. Living on a break: cellular senescence as a DNA-damage response. Nat Rev Cancer 8, 512–522 (2008). https://doi.org/10.1038/nrc2440

16. Xin M, Jin X, Cui X, Jin C, Piao L, Wan Y, Xu S, Zhang S, Yue X, Wang H, Nan Y, Cheng X. Dipeptidyl peptidase-4 inhibition prevents vascular aging in mice under chronic stress: Modulation of oxidative stress and inflammation. Chem Biol Interact. 2019 Dec 1;314:108842. doi: 10.1016/j.cbi.2019.108842.

17. Yao BC, Meng LB, Hao ML, Zhang YM, Gong T, Guo ZG. Chronic stress: a critical risk factor for atherosclerosis. J Int Med Res. 2019 Apr;47(4):1429-1440. doi: 10.1177/0300060519826820.

18. Mojtabavi H, Saghazadeh A, van den Heuvel L, Bucker J, Rezaei N. Peripheral blood levels of brain-derived neurotrophic factor in patients with post-traumatic stress disorder (PTSD): A systematic review and meta-analysis. PLoS One. 2020 Nov 5;15(11):e0241928. doi: 10.1371/journal.pone.0241928. PMID: 33152026; PMCID: PMC7644072.

19. Su S, Xiao Z, Lin Z, Qiu Y, Jin Y, Wang Z. Plasma brain-derived neurotrophic factor levels in patients who have post-traumatic stress disorder. Psychiatry Res. 2015 Sep 30;229(1-2):365-9. doi: 10.1016/j.psychres.2015.06.038.

20. Angelucci F, Veverova K, Katonová A, Vyhnalek M, Hort J. Plasminogen activator inhibitor-1 serum levels in frontotemporal lobar degeneration. J Cell Mol Med. 2024 Feb 22;28(5):e18013. doi: 10.1111/jcmm.18013.

21. Meselson M, Guillemin J, Hugh-Jones M, Langmuir A, Popova I, Shelokov A, Yampolskaya O. The Sverdlovsk anthrax outbreak of 1979. Science. 1994; 266:1202–1208.

22. Fromer M, Roussos P, Sieberts SK, Johnson JS, Kavanagh DH, Perumal TM, et al. Gene expression elucidates functional impact of polygenic risk for schizophrenia. Nat Neurosci. 2016;19(11):1442–1453. doi: 10.1038/nn.4399

23. Yang Y, He M, Tian X, Guo Y, Liu F, Li Y, et al. Transgenic overexpression of furin increases epileptic susceptibility. Cell Death Dis. 2018;9(11):1058. doi: 10.1038/s41419-018-1076-x.

24. Lin L, Zhou XF, Bobrovskaya L. Blockage of p75NTR ameliorates depressive-like behaviours of mice under chronic unpredictable mild stress. Behav Brain Res. 2021 Jan 1;396:112905. doi: 10.1016/j.bbr.2020.112905. Epub 2020 Sep 11. PMID: 32926907.

25. Moskaliuk VS, Kozhemyakina RV, Khomenko TM, Volcho KP, Salakhutdinov NF, Kulikov AV, Naumenko VS, Kulikova EA. On Associations between Fear-Induced Aggression, Bdnf Transcripts, and Serotonin Receptors in the Brains of Norway Rats: An Influence of Antiaggressive Drug TC-2153. Int J Mol Sci. 2023 Jan 4;24(2):983. doi: 10.3390/ijms24020983.

26. Malekan M, Nezamabadi SS, Samami E, Mohebalizadeh M, Saghazadeh A, Rezaei N. BDNF and its signaling in cancer. J Cancer Res Clin Oncol. 2023 Jun;149(6):2621-2636. doi: 10.1007/s00432-022-04365-8.

27. Cefis, M., Chaney, R., Quirié, A. et al. Endothelial cells are an important source of BDNF in rat skeletal muscle. Sci Rep 12, 311 (2022). https://doi.org/10.1038/s41598-021-03740-8.

28. Hofhansel, L., Weidler, C., Votinov, M. et al. Morphology of the criminal brain: gray matter reductions are linked to antisocial behavior in offenders. Brain Struct Funct 225, 2017–2028 (2020). https://doi.org/10.1007/s00429-020-02106-6

29. Chester DS, Lynam DR, Milich R, DeWall CN. Physical aggressiveness and gray matter deficits in ventromedial prefrontal cortex. Cortex. 2017 Dec;97:17-22. doi: 10.1016/j.cortex.2017.09.024. Epub 2017 Oct 7. PMID: 29073459; PMCID: PMC5716918.

30. Bernot D, Stalin J, Stocker P, Bonardo B, Scroyen I, Alessi MC, Peiretti F. Plasminogen activator inhibitor 1 is an intracellular inhibitor of furin proprotein convertase. J Cell Sci. 2011 Apr 15;124(Pt 8):1224-30. doi: 10.1242/jcs.079889.

31. Bouarab, C., Roullot-Lacarrière, V., Vallée, M. et al. PAI-1 protein is a key molecular effector in the transition from normal to PTSD-like fear memory. Mol Psychiatry 26, 4968–4981 (2021). https://doi.org/10.1038/s41380-021-01024-1

32. Elmi S, Sahu G, Malavade K, Jacob T. Role of tissue plasminogen activator and plasminogen activator inhibitor as potential biomarkers in psychosis. Asian J Psychiatr. 2019 Jun;43:105-110. doi: 10.1016/j.ajp.2019.05.021.

33. Green MJ, Matheson SL, Shepherd A, Weickert CS, Carr VJ. Brain-derived neurotrophic factor levels in schizophrenia: a systematic review with meta-analysis. Mol Psychiatry. 2011 Sep;16(9):960-72. doi: 10.1038/mp.2010.88. Epub 2010 Aug 24. PMID: 20733577.

34. Lin, C.-H., Chen, C.-C., Chou, C.-M., Wang, C.-Y., Hung, C.-C., Chen, J.Y., Chang, H.-W., Chen, Y.-C., Yeh, G.C. and Lee, Y.-H. (2009), Knockdown of the aryl hydrocarbon receptor attenuates excitotoxicity and enhances NMDA-induced BDNF expression in cortical neurons. Journal of Neurochemistry, 111: 777-789. https://doi.org/10.1111/j.1471-4159.2009.06364.x

35. Zmijewski JW, Jope RS. Nuclear accumulation of glycogen synthase kinase-3 during replicative senescence of human fibroblasts. Aging Cell. 2004 Oct;3(5):309-17. doi: 10.1111/j.1474-9728.2004.00117.x. PMID: 15379854; PMCID: PMC1931580.

36. Stankovic I, Notaras M, Wolujewicz P, Lu T, Lis R, Ross ME, Colak D. Schizophrenia endothelial cells exhibit higher permeability and altered angiogenesis patterns in patient-derived organoids. Transl Psychiatry. 2024 Jan 23;14(1):53. doi: 10.1038/s41398-024-02740-2. PMID: 38263175; PMCID: PMC10806043.

37. Cheemala A, Kimble AL, Tyburski JD, Leclair NK, Zuberi AR, Murphy M, Jellison ER, Reese B, Hu X, Lutz CM, Yan R, Murphy PA. Loss of Endothelial TDP-43 Leads to Blood Brain Barrier Defects in Mouse Models of Amyotrophic Lateral Sclerosis and Frontotemporal Dementia. bioRxiv [Preprint]. 2023 Dec 14:2023.12.13.571184. doi: 10.1101/2023.12.13.571184.

38. Moreira CG, Russell R, Mishra AA, Narayanan S, Ritchie JM, Waldor MK, Curtis MM, Winter SE, Weinshenker D, Sperandio V. Bacterial Adrenergic Sensors Regulate Virulence of Enteric Pathogens in the Gut. mBio. 2016 Jun 7;7(3):e00826-16. doi: 10.1128/mBio.00826-16.

39. Herda LR, Felix SB, Boege F. Drug-like actions of autoantibodies against receptors of the autonomous nervous system and their impact on human heart function. Br J Pharmacol. 2012 Jun;166(3):847-57. doi: 10.1111/j.1476-5381.2012.01828.x.

40. Morozova A, Zorkina Y, Pavlov K, Pavlova O, Abramova O, Ushakova V, Mudrak AV, Zozulya S, Otman I, Sarmanova Z, Klyushnik T, Reznik A, Kostyuk G, Chekhonin V. Associations of Genetic Polymorphisms and Neuroimmune Markers With Some Parameters of Frontal Lobe Dysfunction in Schizophrenia. Front Psychiatry. 2021 May 7;12:655178. doi: 10.3389/fpsyt.2021.655178.

41. Jiang, H., Li, X., Chen, S. et al. Plasminogen Activator Inhibitor-1 in depression: Results from Animal and Clinical Studies. Sci Rep 6, 30464 (2016). https://doi.org/10.1038/srep30464

42. Bouarab, C., Roullot-Lacarrière, V., Vallée, M. et al. PAI-1 protein is a key molecular effector in the transition from normal to PTSD-like fear memory. Mol Psychiatry 26, 4968–4981 (2021). https://doi.org/10.1038/s41380-021-01024-1

43. Elmi S, Sahu G, Malavade K, Jacob T. Role of tissue plasminogen activator and plasminogen activator inhibitor as potential biomarkers in psychosis. Asian J Psychiatr. 2019 Jun;43:105-110. doi: 10.1016/j.ajp.2019.05.021.

44. Party H, Dujarrier C, Hébert M, Lenoir S, Martinez de Lizarrondo S, Delépée R, Fauchon C, Bouton MC, Obiang P, Godefroy O, Save E, Lecardeur L, Chabry J, Vivien D, Agin V. Plasminogen Activator Inhibitor-1 (PAI-1) deficiency predisposes to depression and resistance to treatments. Acta Neuropathol Commun. 2019 Oct 14;7(1):153. doi: 10.1186/s40478-019-0807-2.

45. Yenilmez C, Ozdemir Koroglu Z, Kurt H, Yanas M, Colak E, Degirmenci I, Gunes HV. A study of the possible association of

plasminogen activator inhibitor type 1 4G/5G insertion/deletion polymorphism with susceptibility to schizophrenia and in its subtypes. J Clin Pharm Ther. 2017 Feb;42(1):103-107. doi: 10.1111/jcpt.12470.

46. Craddock TJ, Tuszynski JA, Hameroff S. Cytoskeletal signaling: is memory encoded in microtubule lattices by CaMKII phosphorylation? PLoS Comput Biol. 2012;8(3):e1002421. doi: 10.1371/journal.pcbi.1002421. Epub 2012 Mar 8. PMID: 22412364; PMCID: PMC3297561.

47. Le TH, Oh JM, Rami FZ, Li L, Chun SK, Chung YC. Effects of Social Defeat Stress on Microtubule Regulating Proteins and Tubulin Polymerization. Clin Psychopharmacol Neurosci. 2024 Feb 29;22(1):129-138. doi: 10.9758/cpn.23.1077. Epub 2023 Aug 10. PMID: 38247419; PMCID: PMC10811395.

48. Al Abed AS, Ducourneau EG, Bouarab C, Sellami A, Marighetto A, Desmedt A. Preventing and treating PTSD-like memory by trauma contextualization. Nat Commun. 2020 Aug 24;11(1):4220. doi: 10.1038/s41467-020-18002-w. PMID: 32839437; PMCID: PMC7445258.

49. Liester MB. Personality changes following heart transplantation: The role of cellular memory. Med Hypotheses. 2020 Feb;135:109468. doi: 10.1016/j.mehy.2019.109468. Epub 2019 Oct 31. PMID: 31739081.

50. Carter, B.; Khoshnaw, L.; Simmons, M.; Hines, L.; Wolfe, B.; Liester, M. Personality Changes Associated with Organ Transplants. Transplantology 2024, 5, 12-26. https://doi.org/10.3390/transplantology5010002

51. Bunzel B, Schmidl-Mohl B, Grundböck A, Wollenek G. Does changing the heart mean changing personality? A retrospective

inquiry on 47 heart transplant patients. Qual Life Res. 1992 Aug;1(4):251-6. doi: 10.1007/BF00435634. PMID: 1299456.

52. Al-Juhani A, Imran M, Aljaili ZK, Alzhrani MM, Alsalman RA, Ahmed M, Ali DK, Fallatah MI, Yousuf HM, Dajani LM. Beyond the Pump: A Narrative Study Exploring Heart Memory. Cureus. 2024 Apr 30;16(4):e59385. doi: 10.7759/cureus.59385. PMID: 38694651; PMCID: PMC11061817.

53. Al-Juhani A, Imran M, Aljaili ZK, Alzhrani MM, Alsalman RA, Ahmed M, Ali DK, Fallatah MI, Yousuf HM, Dajani LM. Beyond the Pump: A Narrative Study Exploring Heart Memory. Cureus. 2024 Apr 30;16(4):e59385. doi: 10.7759/cureus.59385. PMID: 38694651; PMCID: PMC11061817.

54. Guadagna S, Esiri MM, Williams RJ, Francis PT. Tau phosphorylation in human brain: relationship to behavioral disturbance in dementia. Neurobiol Aging. 2012 Dec;33(12):2798-806. doi: 10.1016/j.neurobiolaging.2012.01.015.

55. Grube M. Violent behavior in cancer patients--a rarely addressed phenomenon in oncological treatment. J Interpers Violence. 2012 Jul;27(11):2163-82. doi: 10.1177/0886260511431434. PMID: 22767207.

56. Niu R, Xue X, Zhao Y, Sun Z, Yan X, Li X, Feng C, Wang J. Effects of fluoride on microtubule ultrastructure and expression of Tubα1a and Tubβ2a in mouse hippocampus. Chemosphere. 2015 Nov;139:422-7. doi: 10.1016/j.chemosphere.2015.07.011. Epub 2015 Jul 30. PMID: 26232646.

57. Baharikhoob P, Kolla NJ. Microglial Dysregulation and Suicidality: A Stress-Diathesis Perspective. Front Psychiatry. 2020 Aug 11;11:781. doi: 10.3389/fpsyt.2020.00781.

58. Rodrigues FR, Papanikolaou A, Holeniewska J, Phillips KG, Saleem AB, Solomon SG. Altered low-frequency brain rhythms precede changes in gamma power during tauopathy. iScience. 2022 Sep 28;25(10):105232. doi: 10.1016/j.isci.2022.105232.

59. Sfera A, Osorio C, Rahman L, Zapata-Martín Del Campo CM, Maldonado JC, Jafri N, Cummings MA, Maurer S, Kozlakidis Z. PTSD as an Endothelial Disease: Insights From COVID-19. Front Cell Neurosci. 2021 Oct 29;15:770387. doi: 10.3389/fncel.2021.770387. PMID: 34776871; PMCID: PMC8586713.

60. Sfera, A.; Anton, J.J.; Imran, H.; Kozlakidis, Z.; Klein, C.; Osorio, C. Of Soldiers and Their Ghosts: Are We Ready for a Review of PTSD Evidence? BioMed 2023, 3, 484-506. https://doi.org/10.3390/biomed3040039

61. Yoon, J.H.; Seo, Y.; Jo, Y.S.; Lee, S.; Cho, E.; Cazenave-Gassiot, A.; Shin, Y.S.; Moon, M.H.; An, H.J.; Wenk, M.R.; et al. Brainlipidomics: From functional landscape to clinical significance. Sci. Adv. 2022, 8, eadc9317. [CrossRef]

62. Nicolson, G.L.; Ash, M.E. Lipid Replacement Therapy: A natural medicine approach to replacing damaged lipids in cellularmembranes and organelles and restoring function. Biochim. Biophys. Acta 2014, 1838, 1657–1679. [CrossRef] [PubMed]170.

63. Horn, A.; Jaiswal, J.K. Structural and signaling role of lipids in plasma membrane repair. Curr. Top. Membr. 2019, 84, 67–98.172.

64. Hamsanathan, S.; Gurkar, A.U. Lipids as Regulators of Cellular Senescence. Front. Physiol. 2022, 13, 796850.

65. An S, Cho SY, Kang J, Lee S, Kim HS, Min DJ, Son E, Cho KH. Inhibition of 3-phosphoinositide-dependent protein kinase 1 (PDK1) can revert cellular senescence in human dermal fibroblasts. Proc Natl

Acad Sci U S A. 2020 Dec 8;117(49):31535-31546. doi: 10.1073/pnas.1920338117. Epub 2020 Nov 23. PMID: 33229519; PMCID: PMC7733858.

66. Emamian ES. AKT/GSK3 signaling pathway and schizophrenia. Front Mol Neurosci. 2012 Mar 15;5:33. doi: 10.3389/fnmol.2012.00033.

67. Bellavite P, Fazio S, Affuso F. A Descriptive Review of the Action Mechanisms of Berberine, Quercetin and Silymarin on Insulin Resistance/Hyperinsulinemia and Cardiovascular Prevention. Molecules. 2023 Jun 1;28(11):4491. doi: 10.3390/molecules28114491. PMID: 37298967; PMCID: PMC10254920.

68. Xia QS, Wu F, Wu WB, Dong H, Huang ZY, Xu L, Lu FE, Gong J. Berberine reduces hepatic ceramide levels to improve insulin resistance in HFD-fed mice by inhibiting HIF-2α. Biomed Pharmacother. 2022 Jun;150:112955. doi: 10.1016/j.biopha.2022.112955.

69. Agnarelli, A., Natali, M., Garcia-Gil, M. et al. Cell-specific pattern of berberine pleiotropic effects on different human cell lines. Sci Rep 8, 10599 (2018). https://doi.org/10.1038/s41598-018-28952-3

70. Dang Y, An Y, He J, Huang B, Zhu J, Gao M, Zhang S, Wang X, Yang B, Xie Z. Berberine ameliorates cellular senescence and extends the lifespan of mice via regulating p16 and cyclin protein expression. Aging Cell. 2020 Jan;19(1):e13060. doi: 10.1111/acel.13060.

71. Lee B, Shim I, Lee H, Hahm DH. Berberine alleviates symptoms of anxiety by enhancing dopamine expression in rats with post-traumatic stress disorder. Korean J Physiol Pharmacol. 2018 Mar;22(2):183-192. doi: 10.4196/kjpp.2018.22.2.183.

72. Wen X, Zhou X, Guo L. Berberine Inhibits Endothelial Cell Proliferation via Repressing ERK1/2 Pathway. Natural Product Communications. 2023;18(3). doi:10.1177/1934578X231152690

73. Qattan M.Y., Khan M.I., Alharbi S.H., Verma A.K., Al-Saeed F.A., Abduallah A.M., Al Areefy A.A. Therapeutic Importance of Kaempferol in the Treatment of Cancer through the Modulation of Cell Signalling Pathways. Molecules. 2022;27:8864. doi: 10.3390/molecules27248864. [PMC free article] [PubMed] [CrossRef] [Google Scholar]

74. Maurya A.K., Vinayak M. PI-103 and Quercetin Attenuate PI3K-AKT Signaling Pathway in T-Cell Lymphoma Exposed to Hydrogen Peroxide. PLoS ONE. 2016;11:e0160686. doi: 10.1371/journal.pone.0160686. [PMC free article] [PubMed] [CrossRef] [Google Scholar]

75. Singh S., Srivastava P. Molecular Docking Studies of Myricetin and Its Analogues against Human PDK-1 Kinase as Candidate Drugs for Cancer. Comput. Mol. Biosci. 2015;5:20. doi: 10.4236/cmb.2015.52004. [CrossRef] [Google Scholar]

76. Qin J., Fu M., Wang J., Huang F., Liu H., Huangfu M., Yu D., Liu H., Li X., Guan X., et al. PTEN/AKT/mTOR signaling med ates anticancer effects of epigallocatechin-3-gallate in ovarian cancer. Oncol. Rep. 2020;43:1885–1896. doi: 10.3892/or.2020.7571. [PMC free article] [PubMed] [CrossRef] [Google Scholar]

77. Zughaibi T.A., Suhail M., Tarique M., Tabrez S. Targeting PI3K/Akt/mTOR Pathway by Different Flavonoids: A Cancer Chemopreventive Approach. Int. J. Mol. Sci. 2021;22:12455. doi: 10.3390/ijms222212455. [PMC free article] [PubMed] [CrossRef] [Google Scholar]

78. Liu X., Yao Z. Chronic over-nutrition and dysregulation of GSK3 in diseases. Nutr. Metab. 2016;13:49. doi: 10.1186/s12986-016-0108-8. [PMC free article] [PubMed] [CrossRef] [Google Scholar]

79. Issinger O.G., Guerra B. Phytochemicals in cancer and their effect on the PI3K/AKT-mediated cellular signalling. Biomed. Pharmacother. 2021;139:111650. doi: 10.1016/j.biopha.2021.111650. [PubMed] [CrossRef] [Google Scholar]

80. Guerra B., Issinger O.G. Natural Compounds and Derivatives as Ser/Thr Protein Kinase Modulators and Inhibitors. Pharmaceuticals. 2019;12:4. doi: 10.3390/ph12010004. [PMC free article] [PubMed] [CrossRef] [Google Scholar]i

Chapter 17
The Curse of Geography

The prevalence of suicide attempts and completed suicide rates in people with depression and schizophrenia are higher in North America and Northern Europe compared to the equatorial regions of the world. This is likely due to:

1. Fewer hours of sunshine with lower levels of vitamin D at higher latitude.

2. Higher incidence of viral infections (ex., Maternal influenza during pregnancy has been associated with an increased risk of schizophrenia in offspring).

3. Microbiome differences.

4. Supplementation with vitamin D3 and treatment with natural aryl hydrocarbon receptor (AhR) antagonists could avert not only neuropsychiatric disorders but also cancer.

A recent study has examined research data from 1982 to 2020, showing that the worldwide prevalence of suicide increases with the distance from the equator. The authors concluded that low vitamin D levels caused by insufficient sunlight exposure likely affect the CNS myelin repair, contributing to higher suicide rates.

Previous studies have highlighted the relationship between climatological factors and suicide. However, the arrival of COVID-19 has put this correlation in proper perspective (1) (2) (3) (4). For example, COVID-19 mortality rates are lower south of 35 degrees North.

AhR is activated by ligands, including tryptophan photooxidation products and vitamin D3, the active form of vitamin D (5) (6) (7) (8). Many viruses, such as SARS-CoV-2, also activate AhR (9) (10) (11). Moreover, the anti-suicidal properties of the antipsychotic clozapine, an AhR ligand, are well-established (12).

The gut microbes metabolize tryptophan and bind AhR along with serotonin and melatonin, linking this receptor to neuropsychiatric disorders (13). Furthermore, AhR is an integral part of the circadian clock, the molecular machinery of the sleep-wake cycle, which, under pathological circumstances, can lead to many illnesses, including cancer, MDD, multiple sclerosis (MS), and SCZ (14) (15) (16) (17).

In the following sections of this chapter, I will take a closer look at the role of climatological factors in neuropathology, including suicide. Moreover, it will also highlight the role of AhR as a receptor for solar electromagnetic radiation, as well as a potential target for MDD, suicidal behavior, and SCZ.

Suicide and AhR

Suicide is the second leading cause of mortality in adults, contributing worldwide to more than 800,000 deaths per year (18). Despite improved MDD treatments over the past decade, the incidence of suicidal behavior has remained largely unaffected. It has increased in adolescents and is currently the third leading cause of death in that group (19) (20).

In the gut, tryptophan is absorbed via broad neutral amino acid transporter 1 (B0AT1), a protein that partners with angiotensin-converting enzyme 2 (ACE-2), the entry portal of the SARS-CoV-2 virus. This pathogen disrupts the intestinal barrier by inducing cellular senescence in IECs and endothelial cells (ECs). At the same time, SARS-CoV-2 impairs tryptophan absorption by occupying ACE-2 (21) (Fig. 1). This facilitates microbial translocation into the host systemic circulation and, from there, into the brain (Fig.1).

Several studies have documented the existence of a brain microbiome and virome (viral microbiome), microorganisms that do not actively replicate in the CNS but thrive in a dormant state until the conditions for replication become favorable (21-22).

Microbial DNA and lipopolysaccharide (LPS), a component of Gram-negative bacteria, were detected in the brains of patients with AD, constituting proof of the concept of microbial translocation (23) (24) (25) (26) (27).

The distance from the equator and low temperatures have been associated with gut barrier disruption and increased microbial translocation into host tissues (28). Certain microbial species, previously associated with suicide, were found to exhibit latitudinal variation, likely accounting for the increase of this pathology in Northern countries (29) (30). For example, *Acinetobacter*, a microbe thriving at higher latitudes, expresses myelin-mimicking proteins, likely explaining the increased prevalence of both multiple sclerosis (MS) and suicide in Northern countries (31) (32) (33). Furthermore, tryptophan depletion activates the proinflammatory kynurenine pathway associated with increased suicide rates (34) (35). Aberrant activation of the proinflammatory kynurenine pathway was demonstrated in MDD and suicidal behavior, linking these pathologies to impaired tryptophan metabolism (34) (36).

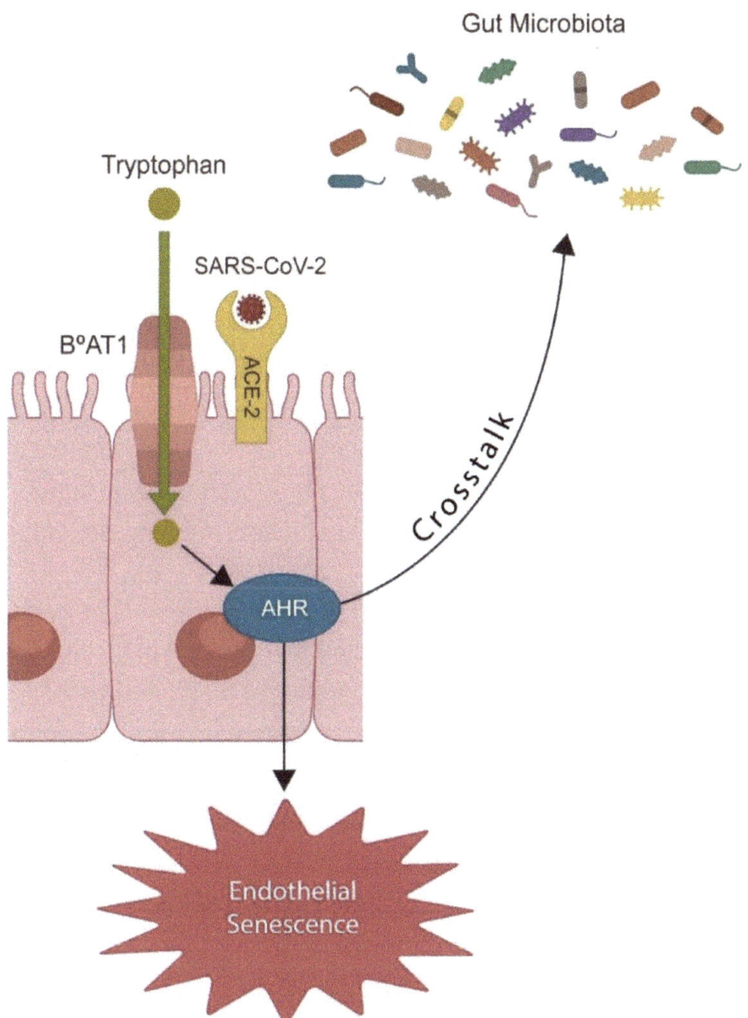

Fig. 17.1 shows how ACE-2 works with the tryptophan transporter B0AT1. When the SARS-CoV-2 virus attaches to ACE-2, it induces cellular senescence in IECs and ECs, increasing the barrier permeability. This also disrupts tryptophan absorption and activates AhR. Under normal circumstances, tryptophan metabolites generated by microbiota alter AhR. These pathologies enable microbial migration from the gut into the systemic circulation.

Other latitude-dependent disorders

Aside from neuropsychiatric disorders, the curse of geography also extends to several cancers, connecting excessive AhR activation with tumorigenesis. The inactivated AhR resides in the cytosol; however, when activated, it enters the nucleus, acting as a transcription factor, altering the expression of many genes, including those in charge of the cell cycle, and promoting malignant transformation. For this reason, inhibitory AhR ligands, including microbial metabolites, vitamin D3, and tryptophan photoproducts, are currently being evaluated as chemotherapy (37). In favor of this paradigm is the fact that breast cancer and colorectal carcinoma are more prevalent in Northern countries. On the other hand, AhR inhibitors, such as BAY 2416964, are currently being developed as anticancer drugs (38) (39) (40) (41) (42) (43).

Aside from affective disorders and suicide, the prevalence of several other neuropsychiatric conditions, including SCZ, ASD, and MS, is lower near the equator and increases with higher latitudes, implicating AhR activation in these pathologies (44) (45) (46). Pyridopyrimidinone is a patented AhR antagonist with a favorable profile for neuropsychiatry and may become the first AhR inhibitor to be used in neuropsychiatry (WO-2021102288-A1) (47).

Microbial migration outside the GI tract

In our previous work on microbial translocation disorders, we discussed antibodies against gut microbes and their components that are often misconstrued as autoantibodies (48) (49). However, restoration of gut barrier function may be beneficial for autoimmune disorders. For example, Baicalein, a protector of gut barrier function, has been patented for autoimmune disorders, linking this pathology to microbial translocation (CN101491533B) (50) (51).

Other latitude-related autoimmune disorders, such as IBDs, were associated with increased rates of suicide, linking this pathology to a dysfunctional gut barrier (52) (53) (54). In addition, bacterial translocation markers, including circulatory LBP, sCD14, and intestinal fatty-acid binding protein (I-FABP), were found elevated in suicide attempters, connecting once again neuropathology to gut barrier disruption (55).

As commensal microbiota express proteins identical to those of the human host, their translocation can activate the immune system, triggering pathology (56) (57) (58) (59). For example, *Escherichia coli (E. coli)* expresses glutamate receptors B and D (GluR-B and GluR-D), which, upon translocation, could elicit anti-N-methyl-d-aspartate-receptor (NMDAR) antibodies, immunoglobulins previously associated with suicidal behavior and SCZ (56) (60). Moreover, *Bacteroides species and Pseudomonas fluorescens* produce γ-aminobutyric acid (GABA) and GABA-binding proteins, which could elicit anti-GABA antibodies, molecules also connected to suicidal behavior (61-62).

Allergic disorders and suicide

A 2008 study by Postolache TT et al. found that several allergic conditions increase the suicide risk, linking this pathology to type II hypersensitivity (63) (64) (65). In addition, as hypersensitivity reactions are more common at higher latitudes, suicidal behavior in those areas may be due to a combination of factors, including atopic phenotypes (66) (67).

In 2010, mucosa-anchored group 2 innate lymphoid cells (ILC2s) were discovered and were found to be implicated in anthelminthic immunity and asthma (68). As ILC2 regulates oligodendrocytes and myelin generation, they were involved in neuropathology, including

MDD and suicide (69) (70) (71). Demyelinating disorders, such as MS or the related condition neuromyelitis optica, have been associated with increased suicidal behavior, connecting type II hypersensitivity to these pathologies (72) (73) (74) (75). For example, upregulation of ILC2-associated interleukin-4 (IL-4) and IL-13 was implicated in suicide by earlier studies, further connecting this condition to dysfunctional myelin (76).

Mast cells (MCs), known for allergy-mediated histamine release in type I hypersensitivity, also affect emotional regulation and cognition, linking allergic reactions to neuropathology (77). These cells have been known for forming extracellular traps (ET), also known as ETosis, a phenomenon involving externalization of antimicrobial peptides (AMPs), histone proteins, and DNA, upregulating the extracellular cell-free DNA (cfDNA), a marker of neuropathology, including suicide (78) (79). Interestingly, vitamin D inhibits NETosis, lowering cfDNA and revealing the antiallergic properties of this molecule (80) (81).

Conclusions

Many human diseases have been associated with colder climates and higher latitudes, indicating that insufficient sunlight, hypovitaminosis D, and low tryptophan photoproducts likely contribute to these pathologies.

Tryptophan photooxidation and conversion of pre-vitamin D3 via UV radiation into the active vitamin D3 indicate that despite the separation of modern societies from nature, humans continue to depend on the environment for survival.

Suicide, conceptualized as a pathology of insufficient sunlight exposure, is further proof that human biology is highly intertwined with the surrounding world and the universe. AhR, like chlorophyll in plants, functions as a liaison with the outer world, maintaining the photo-homeostasis of circadian, seasonal, and geographic changes. Therefore, a better understanding of AhR, the master regulator of geo-adaptation, will help design better treatments for mental illness, cancer, and other poorly understood disorders.

Chapter 17 References:

1. Björkstén, K.S., Kripke, D.F. & Bjerregaard, P. Accentuation of suicides but not homicides with rising latitudes of Greenland in the sunny months. BMC Psychiatry 9, 20 (2009). https://doi.org/10.1186/1471-244X-9-20

2. Davis GE, Lowell WE. Evidence that latitude is directly related to variation in suicide rates. Can J Psychiatry. 2002 Aug;47(6):572-4. doi: 10.1177/070674370204700611.

3. Gombash SE, Lee PW, Sawdai E, Lovett-Racke AE. Vitamin D as a Risk Factor for Multiple Sclerosis: Immunoregulatory or Neuroprotective? Front Neurol. 2022 May 16;13:796933. doi: 10.3389/fneur.2022.796933.

4. Gomez-Pinedo U, Cuevas JA, Benito-Martín MS, Moreno-Jiménez L, Esteban-Garcia N, Torre-Fuentes L, Matías-Guiu JA, Pytel V, Montero P, Matías-Guiu J. Vitamin D increases remyelination by promoting oligodendrocyte lineage differentiation. Brain Behav. 2020 Jan;10(1):e01498. doi: 10.1002/brb3.1498

5. Rhodes JM, Subramanian S, Laird E, Kenny RA. Editorial: low population mortality from COVID-19 in countries south of latitude 35 degrees North supports vitamin D as a factor determining severity. Aliment Pharmacol Ther. 2020 Jun;51(12):1434-1437. doi: 10.1111/apt.15777.

6. Oberg M, Bergander L, Håkansson H, Rannug U, Rannug A. Identification of the tryptophan photoproduct 6-formylindolo[3,2-b]carbazole, in cell culture medium, as a factor that controls the background aryl hydrocarbon receptor activity. Toxicol Sci. 2005 Jun;85(2):935-43. doi: 10.1093/toxsci/kfi154.

7. Rannug A, Rannug U, Rosenkranz HS, Winqvist L, Westerholm R, Agurell E, Grafström AK. Certain photooxidized derivatives of

tryptophan bind with very high affinity to the Ah receptor and are likely to be endogenous signal substances. J Biol Chem. 1987 Nov 15;262(32):15422-7.

8. Diani-Moore S, Labitzke E, Brown R, Garvin A, Wong L, Rifkind AB. Sunlight generates multiple tryptophan photoproducts eliciting high efficacy CYP1A induction in chick hepatocytes and in vivo. Toxicol Sci. 2006 Mar;90(1):96-110. doi: 10.1093/toxsci/kfj065.

9. Giovannoni, F., Li, Z., Remes-Lenicov, F. et al. AHR signaling is induced by infection with coronaviruses. Nat Commun 12, 5148 (2021). https://doi.org/10.1038/s41467-021-25412-x

10. Hu, J., Ding, Y., Liu, W. et al. When AHR signaling pathways meet viral infections. Cell Commun Signal 21, 42 (2023). https://doi.org/10.1186/s12964-023-01058-8

11. Takami M, Fujimaki K, Nishimura MI, Iwashima M. Cutting Edge: AhR Is a Molecular Target of Calcitriol in Human T Cells. J Immunol. 2015 Sep 15;195(6):2520-3. doi: 10.4049/jimmunol.1500344. Epub 2015 Aug 14. PMID: 26276877; PMCID: PMC4561210.

12. Fehsel K, Schwanke K, Kappel BA, Fahimi E, Meisenzahl-Lechner E, Esser C, Hemmrich K, Haarmann-Stemmann T, Kojda G, Lange-Asschenfeldt C. Activation of the aryl hydrocarbon receptor by clozapine induces preadipocyte differentiation and contributes to endothelial dysfunction. J Psychopharmacol. 2022 Feb;36(2):191-201. doi: 10.1177/02698811211055811.

13. Song Y, Slominski RM, Qayyum S, Kim TK, Janjetovic Z, Raman C, Tuckey RC, Song Y, Slominski AT. Molecular and structural basis of interactions of vitamin D3 hydroxyderivatives with aryl hydrocarbon receptor (AhR): An integrated experimental and

computational study. Int J Biol Macromol. 2022 Jun 1;209(Pt A):1111-1123. doi: 10.1016/j.ijbiomac.2022.04.048.

14. Manzella CR, Ackerman M, Singhal M, Ticho AL, Ceh J, Alrefai WA, Saksena S, Dudeja PK, Gill RK. Serotonin Modulates AhR Activation by Interfering with CYP1A1-Mediated Clearance of AhR Ligands. Cell Physiol Biochem. 2020 Feb 5;54(1):126-141. doi: 10.33594/000000209.

15. Tischkau SA. Mechanisms of circadian clock interactions with aryl hydrocarbon receptor signalling. Eur J Neurosci. 2020 Jan;51(1):379-395. doi: 10.1111/ejn.14361.

16. Benedetti F, Riccaboni R, Dallaspezia S, Locatelli C, Smeraldi E, Colombo C. Effects of CLOCK gene variants and early stress on hopelessness and suicide in bipolar depression. Chronobiol Int. 2015;32(8):1156-61. doi: 10.3109/07420528.2015.1060603.

17. Schubert KO, Föcking M, Cotter DR. Proteomic pathway analysis of the hippocampus in schizophrenia and bipolar affective disorder implicates 14-3-3 signaling, aryl hydrocarbon receptor signaling, and glucose metabolism: potential roles in GABAergic interneuron pathology. Schizophr Res. 2015 Sep;167(1-3):64-72. doi: 10.1016/j.schres.2015.02.002

18. Brundin, L., Bryleva, E. & Thirtamara Rajamani, K. Role of Inflammation in Suicide: From Mechanisms to Treatment. Neuropsychopharmacol 42, 271–283 (2017). https://doi.org/10.1038/npp.2016.116

19. Zalsman G. Genetics of Suicidal Behavior in Children and Adolescents. In: Dwivedi Y, editor. The Neurobiological Basis of Suicide. Boca Raton (FL): CRC Press/Taylor & Francis; 2012.

20. Dong F, Perdew GH. The aryl hydrocarbon receptor as a mediator of host-microbiota interplay. Gut Microbes. 2020 Nov 9;12(1):1859812. doi: 10.1080/19490976.2020.1859812.

21. Zhang Y, Yan R, Zhou Q. ACE2, B0AT1, and SARS-CoV-2 spike protein: Structural and functional implications. Curr Opin Struct Biol. 2022 Jun;74:102388. doi: 10.1016/j.sbi.2022.102388.

22. Link CD. Is There a Brain Microbiome? Neurosci Insights. 2021 May 27;16:26331055211018709. doi: 10.1177/26331055211018709.

23. Pretorius L, Kell DB, Pretorius E. Iron Dysregulation and Dormant Microbes as Causative Agents for Impaired Blood Rheology and Pathological Clotting in Alzheimer's Type Dementia. Front Neurosci. 2018 Nov 16;12:851. doi: 10.3389/fnins.2018.00851.

24. Westfall S, Dinh DM, Pasinetti GM. Investigation of Potential Brain Microbiome in Alzheimer's Disease: Implications of Study Bias. J Alzheimers Dis. 2020;75(2):559-570. doi: 10.3233/JAD-191328. PMID: 32310171.

25. Zhao Y, Cong L, Lukiw WJ. Lipopolysaccharide (LPS) Accumulates in Neocortical Neurons of Alzheimer's Disease (AD) Brain and Impairs Transcription in Human Neuronal-Glial Primary Co-cultures. Front Aging Neurosci. 2017 Dec 12;9:407. doi: 10.3389/fnagi.2017.00407.

26. Russ TC, Murianni L, Icaza G, Slachevsky A, Starr JM. Geographical Variation in Dementia Mortality in Italy, New Zealand, and Chile: The Impact of Latitude, Vitamin D, and Air Pollution. Dement Geriatr Cogn Disord. 2016;42(1-2):31-41. doi: 10.1159/000447449.

27. Evatt ML, Delong MR, Khazai N, Rosen A, Triche S, Tangpricha V. Prevalence of vitamin d insufficiency in patients with Parkinson

disease and Alzheimer disease. Arch Neurol. 2008 Oct;65(10):1348-52. doi: 10.1001/archneur.65.10.1348.

28. Guo J, Hu H, Chen Z, Xu J, Nie J, Lu J, Ma L, Ji H, Yuan J, Xu B. Cold Exposure Induces Intestinal Barrier Damage and Endoplasmic Reticulum Stress in the Colon via the SIRT1/Nrf2 Signaling Pathway. Front Physiol. 2022 Apr 20;13:822348. doi: 10.3389/fphys.2022.822348.

29. Taylor BV, Lucas RM, Dear K, Kilpatrick TJ, Pender MP, van der Mei IA, Chapman C, Coulthard A, Dwyer T, McMichael AJ, Valery PC, Williams D, Ponsonby AL. Latitudinal variation in incidence and type of first central nervous system demyelinating events. Mult Scler. 2010 Apr;16(4):398-405. doi: 10.1177/1352458509359724.

30. Dikongué E, Ségurel L. Latitude as a co-driver of human gut microbial diversity? Bioessays. 2017 Mar;39(3). doi: 10.1002/bies.201600145. Epub 2017 Jan 13. PMID: 28083908.

31. Ebringer A, Rashid T, Wilson C. The role of Acinetobacter in the pathogenesis of multiple sclerosis examined by using Popper sequences. Med Hypotheses. 2012 Jun;78(6):763-9. doi: 10.1016/j.mehy.2012.02.026

32. Hughes LE, Smith PA, Bonell S, Natt RS, Wilson C, Rashid T, Amor S, Thompson EJ, Croker J, Ebringer A. Cross-reactivity between related sequences found in Acinetobacter sp., Pseudomonas aeruginosa, myelin basic protein and myelin oligodendrocyte glycoprotein in multiple sclerosis. J Neuroimmunol. 2003 Nov;144(1-2):105-15. doi: 10.1016/s0165-5728(03)00274-1.

33. Ali P, Chen F, Hassan F, Sosa A, Khan S, Badshah M, Shah AA. Bacterial community characterization of Batura Glacier in the Karakoram Range of Pakistan. Int Microbiol. 2021 May;24(2):183-196. doi: 10.1007/s10123-020-00153-x.

34. Messaoud A, Mensi R, Douki W, Neffati F, Najjar MF, Gobbi G, Valtorta F, Gaha L, Comai S. Reduced peripheral availability of tryptophan and increased activation of the kynurenine pathway and cortisol correlate with major depression and suicide. World J Biol Psychiatry. 2019 Nov;20(9):703-711. doi: 10.1080/15622975.2018.1468031.

35. Dehhaghi M, Kazemi Shariat Panahi H, Guillemin GJ. Microorganisms, Tryptophan Metabolism, and Kynurenine Pathway: A Complex Interconnected Loop Influencing Human Health Status. Int J Tryptophan Res. 2019 Jun 19;12:1178646919852996. doi: 10.1177/1178646919852996.

36. Almulla, A.F.; Thipakorn, Y.; Vasupanrajit, A.; Tunvirachaisakul, C.; Oxenkrug, G.; Al-Hakeim, H.K.; Maes, M. The Tryptophan Catabolite or Kynurenine Pathway in a Major Depressive Episode with Melancholia, Psychotic Features and Suicidal Behaviors: A Systematic Review and Meta-Analysis. Cells 2022, 11, 3112. https://doi.org/10.3390/cells11193112

37. Dietrich C, Kaina B. The aryl hydrocarbon receptor (AhR) is used to regulate cell-cell contact and tumor growth. Carcinogenesis. 2010 Aug;31(8):1319-28. doi: 10.1093/carcin/bgq028. Epub 2010 Jan 27. PMID: 20106901; PMCID: PMC6276890.

38. Sun L. Recent advances in the development of AHR antagonists in immuno-oncology. RSC Med Chem. 2021 Apr 6;12(6):902-914. doi: 10.1039/d1md00015b. PMID: 34223158; PMCID: PMC8221258.

39. Bilinski K, Byth K, Boyages J.Association between Latitude and Breast Cancer Incidence in Mainland Australian Women. Journal of Cancer Research (2014) Volume 2014 | Article ID 149865 | https://doi.org/10.1155/2014/149865

40. Moan J, Porojnicu A, Lagunova Z, Berg JP, Dahlback A. Colon cancer: prognosis for different latitudes, age groups and seasons in Norway. J Photochem Photobiol B. 2007 Dec 14;89(2-3):148-55. doi: 10.1016/j.jphotobiol.2007.09.003.

41. Carlberg C, Velleuer E. Vitamin D and the risk for cancer: A molecular analysis. Biochem Pharmacol. 2022 Feb;196:114735. doi: 10.1016/j.bcp.2021.114735.

42. Powell JB, Goode GD, Eltom SE. The Aryl Hydrocarbon Receptor: A Target for Breast Cancer Therapy. J Cancer Ther. 2013 Sep;4(7):1177-1186. doi: 10.4236/jct.2013.47137.

43. Xie G, Raufman JP. Role of the Aryl Hydrocarbon Receptor in Colon Neoplasia. Cancers (Basel). 2015 Jul 31;7(3):1436-46. doi: 10.3390/cancers7030847. PMID: 26264025; PMCID: PMC4586780.

44. Kinney DK, Teixeira P, Hsu D, Napoleon SC, Crowley DJ, Miller A, Hyman W, Huang E. Relation of schizophrenia prevalence to latitude, climate, fish consumption, infant mortality, and skin color: a role for prenatal vitamin d deficiency and infections? Schizophr Bull. 2009 May;35(3):582-95. doi: 10.1093/schbul/sbp023.

45. Syed S, Moore KA, March E. A review of prevalence studies of Autism Spectrum Disorder by latitude and solar irradiance impact. Med Hypotheses. 2017 Nov;109:19-24. doi: 10.1016/j.mehy.2017.09.012.

46. Boccuto L, Chen CF, Pittman AR, Skinner CD, McCartney HJ, Jones K, Bochner BR, Stevenson RE, Schwartz CE. Decreased tryptophan metabolism in patients with autism spectrum disorders. Mol Autism. 2013 Jun 3;4(1):16. doi: 10.1186/2040-2392-4-16.

47. Villemure E, Volgraf M, Jiang Y, Wu G, Ly CQ, Yuen PW, Lu A, Luo X, Liu M, Zhang S, Lupardus PJ, Wallweber HJ, Liederer BM, Deshmukh G, Plise E, Tay S, Wang TM, Hanson JE, Hackos DH,

Scearce-Levie K, Schwarz JB, Sellers BD. GluN2A-Selective Pyridopyrimidinone Series of NMDAR Positive Allosteric Modulators with an Improved in Vivo Profile. ACS Med Chem Lett. 2016 Oct 31;8(1):84-89. doi: 10.1021/acsmedchemlett.6b00388.

48. Sfera, A.; Hazan, S.; Klein, C.; del Campo, C.M.Z.-M.; Sasannia, S.; Anton, J.J.; Rahman, L.; Andronescu, C.V.; Sfera, D.O.; Kozlakidis, Z.; Nicolson, G.L. Microbial Translocation Disorders: Assigning an Etiology to Idiopathic Illnesses. Appl. Microbiol. 2023, 3, 212-240. https://doi.org/10.3390/applmicrobiol3010015

49. Carneiro-Filho BA, Lima IP, Araujo DH, Cavalcante MC, Carvalho GH, Brito GA, Lima V, Monteiro SM, Santos FN, Ribeiro RA, Lima AA. Intestinal barrier function and secretion in methotrexate-induced rat intestinal mucositis. Dig Dis Sci. 2004 Jan;49(1):65-72. doi: 10.1023/b:ddas.0000011604.45531.2c. PMID: 14992437.

50. Bae, M. - J., Shin, H. S., See, H. - J., Jung, S. Y., Kwon, D. - A., & Shon, D. - H. (2016). Baicalein induces CD4+Foxp3+ T cells and enhances intestinal barrier function in a mouse model of food allergy. Scientific Reports, 6(1), 32225. https://doi.org/10.1038/srep32225

51. Dehhaghi M, Kazemi Shariat Panahi H, Heng B, Guillemin GJ. The Gut Microbiota, Kynurenine Pathway, and Immune System Interaction in the Development of Brain Cancer. Front Cell Dev Biol. 2020 Nov 19;8:562812. doi: 10.3389/fcell.2020.562812.

52. Stein AC, Gaetano JN, Jacobs J, Kunnavakkam R, Bissonnette M, Pekow J. Northern Latitude but Not Season Is Associated with Increased Rates of Hospitalizations Related to Inflammatory Bowel Disease: Results of a Multi-Year Analysis of a National Cohort. PLoS One. 2016 Aug 31;11(8):e0161523. doi: 10.1371/journal.pone.0161523

53. Ludvigsson JF, Olén O, Larsson H, Halfvarson J, Almqvist C, Lichtenstein P, Butwicka A. Association Between Inflammatory Bowel Disease and Psychiatric Morbidity and Suicide: A Swedish Nationwide Population-Based Cohort Study With Sibling Comparisons. J Crohns Colitis. 2021 Nov 8;15(11):1824-1836. doi: 10.1093/ecco-jcc/jjab039.

54. Xiong Q, Tang F, Li Y, Xie F, Yuan L, Yao C, et al. Association of inflammatory bowel disease with suicidal ideation, suicide attempts, and suicide: A systematic review and meta-analysis. J Psychosom Res. 2022 Sep;160:110983. doi: 10.1016/j.jpsychores.2022.110983.

55. Ohlsson L, Gustafsson A, Lavant E, Suneson K, Brundin L, Westrin Å, Ljunggren L, Lindqvist D. Leaky gut biomarkers in depression and suicidal behavior. Acta Psychiatr Scand. 2019 Feb;139(2):185-193. doi: 10.1111/acps.12978. Epub 2018 Nov 1. Erratum in: Acta Psychiatr Scand. 2020 Nov;142(5):423. PMID: 30347427; PMCID: PMC6587489.

56. Proal AD, Albert PJ, Marshall TG. The human microbiome and autoimmunity. Curr Opin Rheumatol. 2013 Mar;25(2):234-40. doi: 10.1097/BOR.0b013e32835cedbf. PMID: 23370376.

57. Zhang, X., Lang, Y., Sun, L. et al. Clinical characteristics and prognostic analysis of anti-gamma-aminobutyric acid-B (GABA-B) receptor encephalitis in Northeast China. BMC Neurol 20, 1 (2020). https://doi.org/10.1186/s12883-019-1585-y

58. Arvola M, Keinänen K. Characterization of the ligand-binding domains of glutamate receptor (GluR)-B and GluR-D subunits expressed in Escherichia coli as periplasmic proteins. J Biol Chem. 1996 Jun 28;271(26):15527-32. doi: 10.1074/jbc.271.26.15527.

59. Zhang L, Sander JW, Zhang L, Jiang XY, Wang W, Shuang K, et all. Suicidality is a common and serious feature of anti-N-methyl-D-

aspartate receptor encephalitis. J Neurol. 2017Dec;264(12):2378-2386. doi: 10.1007/s00415-017-8626-5.

60. Neugebauer R, Betz H, Kuhse J. Expression of a soluble glycine binding domain of the NMDA receptor in Escherichia coli. Biochem Biophys Res Commun. 2003 Jun 6;305(3):476-83. doi: 10.1016/s0006-291x(03)00768-x. PMID: 12763017.

61. Dagorn A, Chapalain A, Mijouin L, Hillion M, Duclairoir-Poc C, Chevalier S, Taupin L, Orange N, Feuilloley MG. Effect of GABA, a bacterial metabolite, on Pseudomonas fluorescens surface properties and cytotoxicity. Int J Mol Sci. 2013 Jun 6;14(6):12186-204. doi: 10.3390/ijms140612186.

62. Yin H, Pantazatos SP, Galfalvy H, Huang YY, Rosoklija GB, Dwork AJ, Burke A, Arango V, Oquendo MA, Mann JJ. A pilot integrative genomics study of GABA and glutamate neurotransmitter systems in suicide, suicidal behavior, and major depressive disorder. Am J Med Genet B Neuropsychiatr Genet. 2016 Apr;171B(3):414-426. doi: 10.1002/ajmg.b.32423.63.

63. Postolache, T.T., Komarow, H. & Tonelli, L.H. Allergy: A risk factor for suicide?. Curr Treat Options Neurol 10, 363–376 (2008). https://doi.org/10.1007/s11940-008-0039-4

64. Han CH, Chung JH. Asthma and other allergic diseases in relation to suicidal behavior among South Korean adolescents. J Psychosom Res. 2018 Dec;115.94-100. doi: 10.1016/j.jpsychores.2018.10.015.

65. Amritwar AU, Lowry CA, Brenner LA, Hoisington AJ, Hamilton R, Stiller JW, Postolache TT. Mental Health in Allergic Rhinitis: Depression and Suicidal Behavior. Curr Treat Options Allergy. 2017 Mar;4(1):71-97. doi: 10.1007/s40521-017-0110-z

66. Krstić G. Asthma prevalence associated with geographical latitude and regional insolation in the United States of America and

Australia. PLoS One. 2011 Apr 8;6(4):e18492. doi: 10.1371/journal.pone.0018492. PMID: 21494627; PMCID: PMC3072993.

67. Osborne NJ, Ukoumunne OC, Wake M, Allen KJ. Prevalence of eczema and food allergy is associated with latitude in Australia. J Allergy Clin Immunol. 2012 Mar;129(3):865-7. doi: 10.1016/j.jaci.2012.01.037..

68. Maazi H, Akbari O. Type two innate lymphoid cells: the Janus cells in health and disease. Immunol Rev. 2017 Jul;278(1):192-206. doi: 10.1111/imr.12554. PMID: 28658553; PMCID: PMC5492968.

69. Kobayashi T, Motomura Y, Moro K. The discovery of group 2 innate lymphoid cells has changed the concept of type 2 immune diseases. Int Immunol. 2021 Nov 25;33(12):705-709. doi: 10.1093/intimm/dxab063

70. Barichello T. The role of innate lymphoid cells (ILCs) in mental health. Discov Ment Health. 2022;2(1):2. doi: 10.1007/s44192-022-00006-1.

71. Sadeghi Hassanabadi N, Broux B, Marinović S, Gotthardt D. Innate Lymphoid Cells - Neglected Players in Multiple Sclerosis. Front Immunol. 2022 Jun 17;13:909275. doi: 10.3389/fimmu.2022.909275.

72. Pompili M, Forte A, Palermo M, Stefani H, Lamis DA, Serafini G, Amore M, Girardi P. Suicide risk in multiple sclerosis: a systematic review of current literature. J Psychosom Res. 2012 Dec;73(6):411-7. doi: 10.1016/j.jpsychores.2012.09.011.

73. Fredrikson S, Cheng Q, Jiang GX, Wasserman D. Elevated suicide risk among patients with multiple sclerosis in Sweden. Neuroepidemiology. 2003 Mar-Apr;22(2):146-52. doi: 10.1159/000068746. PMID: 12629281.

74. Rolf L, Sikkema T, Krudde J, van Harten B. Wittestofafwijkingen na
een zelfmoordpoging [White matter abnormalities following
attempted suicide]. Ned Tijdschr Geneeskd. 2013;157(41):A6526.
Dutch. PMID: 24103138.

75. Fernández VC, Alonso N, Melamud L, Villa AM. Psychiatric
comorbidities and suicidality among patients with neuromyelitis
optica spectrum disorders in Argentina. Mult Scler Relat Disord.
2018 Jan;19:40-43. doi: 10.1016/j.msard.2017.11.002.

76. Tonelli LH, Stiller J, Rujescu D, Giegling I, Schneider B, Maurer K,
Schnabel A, Möller HJ, Chen HH, Postolache TT. Elevated cytokine
expression in the orbitofrontal cortex of victims of suicide. Acta
Psychiatr Scand. 2008 Mar;117(3):198-206. doi: 10.1111/j.1600-
0447.2007.01128.x.

77. Traina G. Mast Cells in Gut and Brain and Their Potential Role as an
Emerging Therapeutic Target for Neural Diseases. Front Cell
Neurosci. 2019 Jul 30;13:345. doi: 10.3389/fncel.2019.00345.

78. Chen LY, Qi J, Xu HL, Lin XY, Sun YJ, Ju SQ. The Value of Serum
Cell-Free DNA Levels in Patients With Schizophrenia. Front
Psychiatry. 2021 Mar 30;12:637789. doi:
10.3389/fpsyt.2021.637789.

79. Lindqvist D, Fernström J, Grudet C, Ljunggren L, Träskman-Bendz
L, Ohlsson L, Westrin Å. Increased plasma levels of circulating cell-
free mitochondrial DNA in suicide attempters: associations with
HPA-axis hyperactivity. Transl Psychiatry. 2016 Dec 6;6(12):e971.
doi: 10.1038/tp.2016.236.

80. Mirzakhani H, Al-Garawi A, Weiss ST, Litonjua AA. Vitamin D and
the development of allergic disease: how important is it? Clin Exp
Allergy. 2015 Jan;45(1):114-25. doi: 10.1111/cea.12430.

81. Handono K, Sidarta YO, Pradana BA, Nugroho RA, Hartono IA, Kalim H, Endharti AT. Vitamin D prevents endothelial damage induced by increased neutrophil extracellular traps formation in patients with systemic lupus erythematosus. Acta Med Indones. 2014 Jul;46(3):189

Chapter 18
Treatment Strategies for Pathological Cell-Cell Fusion

> Cell-cell fusion or syncytia formation can happen spontaneously in normal aging or pathologically in viral infections, human endogenous retroviruses (HERVs) activation, or in neurodegenerative/neuropsychiatric disorders.
>
> Neurons can fuse with each other or with glial cells, triggering senescence that eventually leads to neurocognitive disorders or negative symptoms of schizophrenia.
>
> There are numerous natural and synthetic compounds for the treatment of cell-cell fusion discussed in this chapter.

A growing body of epidemiological and research data has associated neurotropic viruses with accelerated brain aging and increased risk of neuropsychiatric pathology.

Many viruses replicate optimally in senescent cells, as they offer a hospitable microenvironment with persistently elevated cytosolic calcium, abundant intracellular iron, and low interferon type I. As cell-cell fusion is a major driver of cellular senescence, many viruses have developed the ability to induce this phenotype by forming syncytia. Cell-cell fusion is associated with both premature cellular senescence and immunosuppression, enabling viruses to evade host defenses.

The COVID-19 pandemic has emphasized the connection between pathogens, cancer, and neuropsychiatric disorders, suggesting the possibility of common treatments. For example, the anticancer effects of Ivermectin and other antiparasitic drugs has been discovered when studying the ingress of SARS-CoV-2 virus into host cells.

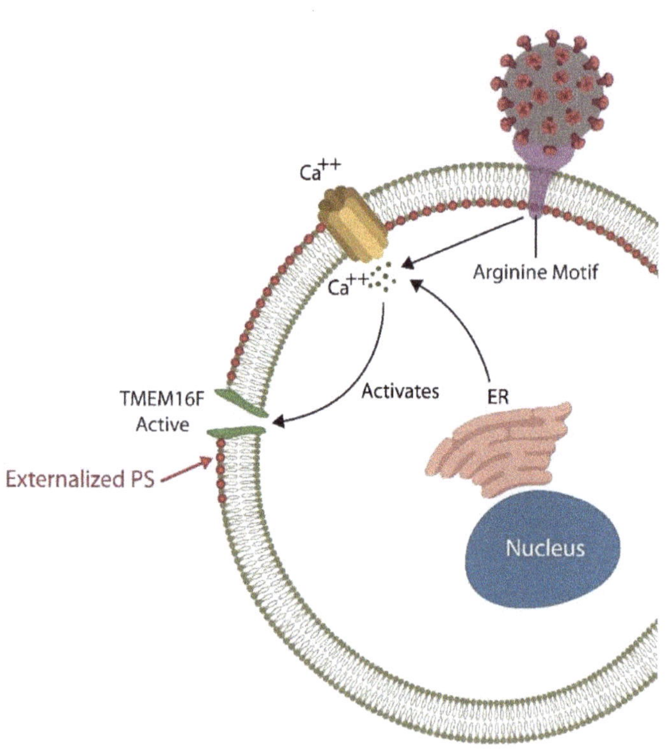

Fig. 18.1 Exogenous viruses, including SARS-CoV-2, enter host cells by attaching to the plasma membrane via arginine motif, Proline-Arginine-Arginine-Alanine-Arginine (PRRAR), beginning the 3 steps fusion process: (1) cytosolic Ca2+ upregulation (via extracellular import from the extracellular compartment or endoplasmic reticulum release) (2) TMEM16F activation and (3) phosphatidylserine (PS) externalization (ePS). Cells undergo fusion or cell death, depending on extracellular pH.

Arginase inhibitors

Arginine is both beneficial and detrimental to COVID-19. Useful because it generates neuroprotective nitric oxide (NO), and harmful because it also makes toxic peroxynitrite (ONOO−) (1) (2).

Novel SARS-CoV-2 studies have revealed a paradox: arginine supplementation and depletion have benefitted some COVID-19 patients, opening a debate on the best treatment strategy (3) (4). These contradictory findings can be reconciled to some extent, as arginine may be helpful and detrimental depending on the amount of arginase. Increased arginase depletes both arginine and NO, predisposing to COVID-19 critical illness and neurodegeneration (5) (6). Therefore, patients with elevated arginase levels would likely benefit from NO supplementation (but not arginine, as this may upregulate the ornithine/urea pathway) (7) (8). On the other hand, NO and arginine supplementation may be detrimental to patients with excessive peroxynitrite as it may upregulate oxidative stress (9). For this reason, arginase inhibitors (augment NO and lower peroxynitrite) may be a better therapeutic strategy than arginine depletion or supplementation (10).

Natural arginase inhibitors, diamino and α-amino acids, and flavonoid compounds, such as the plant extract (2S)-5,2′5′-trihydroxy-7,8-dimethoxy flavanone, may be beneficial for patients with COVID-19 and neurodegenerative disorders (11) (12) (13) (14).

Synthetic arginase inhibitors are broad-spectrum anthelmintics, including imidazothiazoles and their derivatives levamisole, oxazolopyridine, and aza benzimidazole, which have been found to possess antiviral, anticancer, and anti-neurodegenerative properties (15) (16). Imidazothiazoles have not been adequately studied but are promising as blockers of almost all viruses and for being neuroprotective.

Calcium channel blockers (CCBs)

Recent studies have reported that calcium channel blockers (CCBs) can ameliorate COVID-19 pathology, decreasing morbidity and mortality (17). Drugs, including amlodipine, nifedipine, nimodipine, and memantine, were demonstrated to be efficacious against SARS-CoV-2 virus and AD, revealing a related pathogenesis (18) (19)

Natural CCB compounds, bisbenzylisoquinoline alkaloid, neferine, and its analogs liensinine and isoliensinine, inhibit Ca^{2+} mediated cell-cell fusion, suggesting restoration of host antiviral immunity (20). Artemisia annua extract, artemisinin, blocks several voltage-gated ion channels, including NMDA, indicating potential antiviral and anti-neurodegenerative properties (21). Indeed, studies in rodents and cultured human neurons have shown that artemisinin ameliorates neurodegenerative pathology, emphasizing the role of dysfunctional Ca^{2+} signaling in these conditions (22).

Muscarinic acetylcholine receptors (mAChR) antagonists lower cytosolic Ca^{2+}, averting trophic conversion into neurotoxic astrocytes, suggesting a role in neurodegenerative disorders and SCZ (23). Indeed, M1 and M3 muscarinic receptor antagonists were shown to reverse the cocaine-induced astrocytic neurotoxicity, emphasizing their neuroprotective effects (24) (25).

TMEM16F inhibitors

TMEM16F inhibitors, an essential class of cell-cell fusion blockers, include a variety of agents, ranging from anthelmintic drugs to psychotropics and anticancer compounds. Recent studies have suggested that viruses and malignancies invade human cells by identical pathways, emphasizing that antiviral and anticancer drugs are related. For example, Ivermectin, a macrolide anthelmintic with antiviral properties, is also an effective tumor suppressor, suggesting similar action mechanisms (26) (27). Another example, TMEM16F inhibitor niclosamide and its analogs nitazoxanide, hexachlorophene, and dichlorophen, present with intriguing anthelmintic, anticancer, and anti-amyotrophic lateral sclerosis (ALS) properties, indicating similar pathogenesis (28). Indeed, as these agents target S100A4, a protein involved in SCZ and inhibited by the phenothiazine class of antipsychotic drugs, a common pathogenetic mechanism is highlighted (29) (30), in addition, since S100A4 has also been implicated in tumorigenesis, it may be the common denominator between viral illness, cancer, and neuropsychiatric disorders (32) (33).

Recent in silico studies have shown that several psychotropic drugs, including trifluoperazine and SSRIs, block TMEM-16F, explaining their antiviral and anti-syncytial properties (33) (34).

<u>Natural TMEM16F inhibitors</u>, including the polyphenol Epigallocatechin gallate, have antiviral, anti-neurodegenerative, and anti-cancer properties, emphasizing once more a joint action mechanism (35) (37) (38). Another polyphenol, tannic acid, may or may not downregulate TMEM16F as two different studies found conflicting results, indicating that more research is needed in this area (39).

Senolytic drugs

Senolytic drugs enhance the elimination of senescent, infected, or cancer cells, preventing their accumulation.

Several senolytic drugs with established antiviral properties, including hydroxychloroquine and related agents, lower β-galactosidase, a well-known senescence marker, indicating efficacy against virus-induced senescence (40). Interestingly, extensive observational studies showed that hydroxychloroquine may ameliorate AD symptoms, suggesting that senescent cell clearance may be a helpful strategy against neurodegenerative disorders (41) (42). Other senolytic agents with antiviral properties, such as azithromycin, minocycline, and roxithromycin, were deemed beneficial to COVID-19 patients as they selectively eliminate senescent and virus-infected cells (43) (44) (45). Indeed, several senolytic antibiotics, including tetracyclines, have demonstrated anti-neurodegenerative properties in preclinical studies, emphasizing the link between viruses and neurodegeneration (46) (47).

The natural senolytic agent quercetin, an effective antiviral and anti-neurodegeneration compound, is currently in clinical trials for COVID-19 (48) (49) (NCT05037240). Quercetin was found to preempt the development of neuronal damage and possess anticancer and anti-inflammatory properties (50).

A novel senolytic vaccine, recently tested in progeroid mice, may usher in a new era in senolytic interventions as it opens the possibility of preventing the development of neurodegenerative disorders, viral infections, and possibly cancer (51) (52). Furthermore, an antibody-drug conjugate against a membrane senescence marker was demonstrated to clear senescent and virus-infected cells, emphasizing a new senolytic strategy (53).

Microtubule stabilizing agents (MSA)

MSAs are compounds that attach to the microtubules, preventing their disassembly. Most drugs targeting microtubules are anticancer agents that may also possess anti-neurodegenerative and antiviral effects (54) (55) (56) (57). Many of these drugs demonstrated beneficial effects in animal models. However, those tested in humans are few and include TPI-287 and NAP (Davunetide CP201), an intranasal neuropeptide (NAPVSIPQ) (NAP) (NCT01966666) (58). These MSAs have not reached the clinic. However, activity-dependent neuroprotective protein (ADNP), derived from NAP, remains a potential hope and is scheduled for future clinical trials (59) (60) (61). A recent addition to MSAs, sabizabulin, is currently in clinical trials as an antiviral drug, suggesting a possible benefit in tauopathies (NCT04388826) (63).

<u>Natural MSA compounds</u>, CNDR-51549 and CNDR51555 (US patent: US20170173016 A1) were found to cross the BBB, indicating potential benefit in tauopathies (64). Another compound, CNDR-51657, was demonstrated to downregulate the hyperphosphorylated tau, suggesting a preventive potential (65). Another natural MSA compound and Tacca extract, taccalonolides, may benefit AD patients by augmenting tubulin polymerization, reversing the effect of play (66) (67). Interestingly, studies from the 1970s observed that lithium was an MSA, raising exciting questions about its established antiviral and neuroprotective properties (68) (69) (70). Indeed, lithium reverses tau-induced astrocytic senescence and enhances T-cell function, suggesting it also possesses senolytic properties (71) (72). This is significant, as lithium can reverse the virus-induced damage of tubulin, a key molecule in T-cell activation (73).

MSAs, many of which are plant extracts, are exciting compounds that require further research as antiviral and neuroprotective agents.

COMPOUND	REFERENCES
Natural arginase inhibitors	
diamino acids	11
α-amino acids S Clemente G	11
2S)-5,2′5′-trihydroxy-7,8-dimethoxy flavanone	11
Synthetic arginase inhibitors	
Imidazothiazoles: levamisole, oxazolopyridine, azabenzimidazole	15/16
Calcium channel blockers	
amlodipine, nifedipine, nimodipine, memantine	17/18
bisbenzylisoquinoline alkaloid	19
neferine, liensinine, isoliensinine	19
artemisinin	20
TMEM16F inhibitors	
Ivermectin	26/27
Niclosamide, nitazoxanide, hexachlorophene, and dichlorophen	28
trifluoperazine	29
serotonin reuptake inhibitors (SSRIs)	33

epigallocatechin gallate	35
Senolytic drugs	
hydroxychloroquine	41
azithromycin, minocycline, and roxithromycin	297/298
quercetin	50
senolytic vaccine	51/52
antibody–drug conjugates	63
Microtubule stabilizing agents	
TPI-287 (discontinued)	58
Davunetide (discontinued)	58
CNDR-51549	59
CNDR-51555	60
CNDR-51657	61
Sabizabulin	63
Taccalonolides	66/67
Lithium	73

Table 18.3 Potential anti-fusion therapeutic agents

Conclusions

Viruses augment infectivity by fusing host cells into multinucleated hybrid entities that engender cellular senescence, immunosuppression, or immune exhaustion that may predispose to neurodegenerative disorders. The study of physiological and pathological syncytia has emphasized the role of arginine, calcium signaling, TMEM16F, and the cytoskeleton in synaptic plasticity, memory, and cognition. These novel findings are likely to contribute to the development of new therapeutic strategies not only for neuropsychiatric conditions but also for cancer and viral infections.

A better understanding of physiological fusogens and their properties and function will lead to more focused interventions against autoimmune and placental disorders. Adequate HERV inhibition will likely improve the outcome of antiviral and antitumor drugs, opening the possibility of neurodegenerative disorders prevention. This is illustrated by the novel recombinant anti-HERV-W ENV antibody (GNbAC1), currently in clinical trials for MS, and a promising antiviral agent (NCT01639300) (73) (74). The same may be true of arginase, MSA, and TMEM16F inhibitors, drugs with multiple therapeutic targets.

The study of cell-cell fusion is in its infancy; therefore, a better understanding of the molecular underpinnings of syncytia formation will shed light on the cellular uptake of pathogens and oncogenes, opening novel avenues for preventive care.

Chapter 18 References:

Zhou, C., Ramaswamy, S., Johnson, D. et al. Novel Roles for Peroxynitrite in Angiotensin II and CaMKII Signaling. Sci Rep 6, 23416 (2016). https://doi.org/10.1038/srep23416

Paris D, Parker TA, Town T, Suo Z, Fang C, Humphrey J, Crawford F, Mullan M. Role of peroxynitrite in the vasoactive and cytotoxic effects of Alzheimer's beta-amyloid1-40 peptide. Exp Neurol. 1998 Jul;152(1):116-22. doi: 10.1006/exnr.1998.6828. PMID: 9682018.

1. Dominic P, Ahmad J, Bhandari R, Pardue S, Solorzano J, Jaisingh K, et al. Decreased availability of nitric oxide and hydrogen sulfide is a hallmark of COVID-19. Redox Biol. 2021 Jul;43:101982. doi: 10.1016/j.redox.2021.101982. Epub 2021 May 8. PMID: 34020311; PMCID: PMC8106525.

2. Grimes JM, Khan S, Badeaux M, Rao RM, Rowlinson SW, Carvajal RD. Arginine depletion as a therapeutic approach for patients with COVID-19. Int J Infect Dis. 2021;102:566-570. doi:10.1016/j.ijid.2020.10.100

3. Derakhshani A, Hemmat N, Asadzadeh Z, Ghaseminia M, Shadbad MA, Jadideslam G, et al. Arginase 1 (Arg1) as an Up-Regulated Gene in COVID-19 Patients: A Promising Marker in COVID-19 Immunopathy. J Clin Med. 2021 Mar 4;10(5):1051. doi: 10.3390/jcm10051051. PMID: 33806290; PMCID: PMC7961773.

4. Dean MJ, Ochoa JB, Sanchez-Pino MD, Zabaleta J, Garai J, Del Valle L, et al. Severe COVID-19 Is Characterized by an Impaired Type I Interferon Response and Elevated Levels of Arginase Producing Granulocytic Myeloid Derived Suppressor Cells. Front Immunol. 2021 Jul 14;12:695972. doi: 10.3389/fimmu.2021.695972. PMID: 34341659; PMCID: PMC8324422.

5. Lotz C, Muellenbach RM, Meybohm P, Mutlak H, Lepper PM, Rolfes CB, et all. Effects of inhaled nitric oxide in COVID-19-induced ARDS - Is it worthwhile? Acta Anaesthesiol Scand. 2021 May;65(5):629-632. doi: 10.1111/aas.13757. Epub 2020 Dec 20. PMID: 33296498.

6. Fang W, Jiang J, Su L, et al. The role of NO in COVID-19 and potential therapeutic strategies. Free Radic Biol Med. 2021;163:153-162. doi:10.1016/j.freeradbiomed.2020.12.008

7. Nguyen MC, Park JT, Jeon YG, Jeon BH, Hoe KL, Kim YM, et al. Arginase Inhibition Restores Peroxynitrite-Induced Endothelial Dysfunction via L-arginine-dependent endothelial Nitric Oxide Synthase Phosphorylation. Yonsei Med J. 2016 Nov;57(6):1329-38. doi: 10.3349/ymj.2016.57.6.1329. PMID: 27593859; PMCID: PMC5011263.

8. Clemente GS, van Waarde A, F Antunes I, Dömling A, H Elsinga P. Arginase as a Potential Biomarker of Disease Progression: A Molecular Imaging Perspective. Int J Mol Sci. 2020 Jul 25;21(15):5291. doi: 10.3390/ijms21155291. PMID: 32722521; PMCID: PMC7432485.

9. Girard-Thernier C, Pham TN, Demougeot C. The Promise of Plant-Derived Substances as Inhibitors of Arginase. Mini Rev Med Chem. 2015;15(10):798-808. doi: 10.2174/1389557515666150511153852. PMID: 25963565.

10. Minozzo BR, Fernandes D, Beltrame FL. Phenolic Compounds as Arginase Inhibitors: New Insights Regarding Endothelial Dysfunction Treatment. Planta Med. 2018 Mar;84(5):277-295. doi: 10.1055/s-0044-100398. Epub 2018 Jan 17. PMID: 29342480.

11. Li D, Zhang H, Lyons TW, Lu M, Achab A, Pu Q, Childers M, et al. Comprehensive Strategies to Bicyclic Prolines: Applications in the

Synthesis of Potent Arginase Inhibitors. ACS Med Chem Lett. 2021 Oct 13;12(11):1678-1688. doi: 10.1021/acsmedchemlett.1c00258. PMID: 34795856; PMCID: PMC8591728.

12. Arraki K, Totoson P, Decendit A, et al. Mammalian Arginase Inhibitory Activity of Methanolic Extracts and Isolated Compounds from Cyperus Species. Molecules. 2021;26(6):1694. Published 2021 Mar 18. doi:10.3390/molecules26061694

13. Weiss A, Touret F, Baronti C, et al. Niclosamide shows strong antiviral activity in a human airway model of SARS-CoV-2 infection and a conserved potency against the Alpha (B.1.1.7), Beta (B.1.351) and Delta variant (B.1.617.2). PLoS One. 2021;16(12):e0260958. Published 2021 Dec 2. doi:10.1371/journal.pone.0260958

14. Al-Horani RA, Kar S. Potential Anti-SARS-CoV-2 Therapeutics That Target the Post-Entry Stages of the Viral Life Cycle: A Comprehensive Review. Viruses. 2020;12(10):1092. Published 2020 Sep 26. doi:10.3390/v12101092

15. Straus MR, Bidon MK, Tang T, Jaimes JA, Whittaker GR, Daniel S. Inhibitors of L-Type Calcium Channels Show Therapeutic Potential for Treating SARS-CoV-2 Infections by Preventing Virus Entry and Spread. ACS Infect Dis. 2021 Oct 8;7(10):2807-2815. doi: 10.1021/acsinfecdis.1c00023. Epub 2021 Sep 9. PMID: 34498840; PMCID: PMC8442615.

16. Nimmrich V, Eckert A. Calcium channel blockers and dementia. Br J Pharmacol. 2013;169(6):1203-1210. doi:10.1111/bph.12240

17. Solaimanzadeh I. Nifedipine and Amlodipine Are Associated With Improved Mortality and Decreased Risk for Intubation and Mechanical Ventilation in Elderly Patients Hospitalized for COVID-19. Cureus. 2020 May 12;12(5):e8069. doi: 10.7759/cureus.8069. PMID: 32411566; PMCID: PMC7219014.

18. Minozzo BR, Fernandes D, Beltrame FL. Phenolic Compounds as Arginase Inhibitors: New Insights Regarding Endothelial Dysfunction Treatment. Planta Med. 2018 Mar;84(5):277-295. doi: 10.1055/s-0044-100398. Epub 2018 Jan 17. PMID: 29342480.

19. Qiao G, Li S, Yang B, Li B. Inhibitory effects of artemisinin on voltage-gated ion channels in intact nodose ganglion neurons of adult rats. Basic Clin Pharmacol Toxicol. 2007 Apr;100(4):217-24. doi: 10.1111/j.1742-7843.2006.00009.x. PMID: 17371525.

20. Zhao X, Li S, Gaur U, Zheng W. Artemisinin Improved Neuronal Functions in Alzheimer's Disease Animal Model 3xtg Mice and Neuronal Cells via Stimulating the ERK/CREB Signaling Pathway. Aging Dis. 2020 Jul 23;11(4):801-819. doi: 10.14336/AD.2019.0813. PMID: 32765947; PMCID: PMC7390534.

21. Takata N, Mishima T, Hisatsune C, Nagai T, Ebisui E, Mikoshiba K, et al. Astrocyte calcium signaling transforms cholinergic modulation to cortical plasticity in vivo. J Neurosci. 2011 Dec 7;31(49):18155-65. doi: 10.1523/JNEUROSCI.5289-11.2011. Erratum in: J Neurosci. 2012 Aug 29;32(35):12303. PMID: 22159127; PMCID: PMC6634158.

22. Garcia, R., Dati, L., Torres, L. et al. M1 and M3 muscarinic receptors may play a role in the neurotoxicity of anhydroecgonine methyl ester, a cocaine pyrolysis product. Sci Rep 5, 17555 (2015). https://doi.org/10.1038/srep17555

23. Calcutt NA, Smith DR, Frizzi K, Sabbir MG, Chowdhury SK, Mixcoatl-Zecuatl T, et al. Selective antagonism of muscarinic receptors is neuroprotective in peripheral neuropathy. J Clin Invest. 2017 Feb 1;127(2):608-622. doi: 10.1172/JCI88321. Epub 2017 Jan 17. PMID: 28094765; PMCID: PMC5272197.

24. Formiga FR, Leblanc R, de Souza Rebouças J, Farias LP, de Oliveira RN, Pena L. Ivermectin: an award-winning drug with expected antiviral activity against COVID-19. J Control Release. 2021 Jan 10;329:758-761. doi: 10.1016/j.jconrel.2020.10.009

25. Tang M, Hu X, Wang Y, Yao X, Zhang W, Yu C, et al. Ivermectin is a potential anticancer drug derived from an antiparasitic medication. Pharmacol Res. 2021 Jan;163:105207. doi: 10.1016/j.phrs.2020.105207. Epub 2020 Sep 21. PMID: 32971268; PMCID: PMC7505114.

26. Xu J, Shi PY, Li H, Zhou J. Broad Spectrum Antiviral Agent Niclosamide and Its Therapeutic Potential. ACS Infect Dis. 2020 May 8;6(5):909-915. doi: 10.1021/acsinfecdis.0c00052. Epub 2020 Mar 10. PMID: 32125140; PMCID: PMC7098069.

27. Peng XC, Zhang M, Meng YY, Liang YF, Wang YY, Liu XQ, et al. Cell-cell fusion as an essential mechanism of tumor metastasis (Review). Oncol Rep. 2021 Jul;46(1):145. doi: 10.3892/or.2021.8096. Epub 2021 Jun 3. PMID: 34080662.

28. D'Ambrosi N, Milani M, Apolloni S. S100A4 in the Physiology and Pathology of the Central and Peripheral Nervous System. Cells. 2021;10(4):798. Published 2021 Apr 2. doi:10.3390/cells10040798

29. Malashkevich VN, Dulyaninova NG, Ramagopal UA, Liriano MA, Varney KM, Knight D, et al. Phenothiazines inhibit S100A4 function by inducing protein oligomerization. Proc Natl Acad Sci U S A. 2010 May 11;107(19):8605-10. doi: 10.1073/pnas.0913660107. Epub 2010 Apr 26. PMID: 20421509; PMCID: PMC2889333.

30. Fei F, Qu J, Zhang M, Li Y, Zhang S. S100A4 in cancer progression and metastasis: A systematic review. Oncotarget. 2017;8(42):73219-73239. Published 2017 May 19. doi:10.18632/oncotarget.18016

31. Cavaliere, F., Fornarelli, A., Bertan, F. et al. The tricyclic antidepressant clomipramine inhibits neuronal autophagic flux. Sci Rep 9, 4881 (2019). https://doi.org/10.1038/s41598-019-40887-x

32. Bartels C, Wagner M, Wolfsgruber S, Ehrenreich H, Schneider A; Alzheimer's Disease Neuroimaging Initiative. Impact of SSRI Therapy on Risk of Conversion From Mild Cognitive Impairment to Alzheimer's Dementia in Individuals With Previous Depression. Am J Psychiatry. 2018 Mar 1;175(3):232-241. doi: 10.1176/appi.ajp.2017.17040404. Epub 2017 Nov 28. PMID: 29179578.

33. Millington-Burgess, S.L., Harper, M.T. Epigallocatechin gallate inhibits the release of extracellular vesicles from platelets without inhibiting phosphatidylserine exposure. Sci Rep 11, 17678 (2021). https://doi.org/10.1038/s41598-021-97212-8

34. Li J, Song D, Wang S, Dai Y, Zhou J, Gu J. Antiviral Effect of Epigallocatechin Gallate via Impairing Porcine Circovirus Type 2 Attachment to Host Cell Receptor. Viruses. 2020;12(2):176. Published 2020 Feb 4. doi:10.3390/v12020176

35. Du GJ, Zhang Z, Wen XD, et al. Epigallocatechin Gallate (EGCG) is the most effective cancer chemopreventive polyphenol in green tea. Nutrients. 2012;4(11):1679-1691. Published 2012 Nov 8. doi:10.3390/nu4111679

36. Ousingsawat, J., Wanitchakool, P., Schreiber, R. et al. Contribution of TMEM16F to pyroptotic cell death. Cell Death Dis 9, 300 (2018). https://doi.org/10.1038/s41419-018-0373-8

37. Le T, Le SC, Zhang Y, Liang P, Yang H. Evidence that polyphenols do not inhibit the phospholipid scramblase TMEM16F. J Biol Chem. 2020 Aug 28;295(35):12537-12544. doi:

10.1074/jbc.AC120.014872. Epub 2020 Jul 24. PMID: 32709749; PMCID: PMC7458812.

38. Van Gool WA , Weinstein HC , Scheltens P , et al . Effect of hydroxychloroquine on the progression of dementia in early Alzheimer's disease: an 18-month randomised, double-blind, placebo-controlled study. Lancet 2001;358:455–60.doi:10.1016/S0140-6736(01)05623-9

39. Lai SW, Kuo YH, Liao KF. Chronic hydroxychloroquine exposure and the risk of Alzheimer's disease. Ann Rheum Dis. 2021 Jul;80(7):e105. doi: 10.1136/annrheumdis-2019-216173. Epub 2019 Aug 21. PMID: 31434638.

40. Sargiacomo C, Sotgia F, Lisanti MP. COVID-19 and chronological aging: senolytics and other anti-aging drugs for the treatment or prevention of corona virus infection? Aging (Albany NY). 2020 Mar 30;12(8):6511-6517. doi: 10.18632/aging.103001. Epub 2020 Mar 30. PMID: 32229706; PMCID: PMC7202514.

41. Ozsvari B, Nuttall JR, Sotgia F, Lisanti MP. Azithromycin and Roxithromycin define a new family of "senolytic" drugs that target senescent human fibroblasts. Aging (Albany, NY). 2018 Nov 14;10(11):3294-3307. doi: 10.18632/aging.101633. PMID: 30428454; PMCID: PMC6286845.

42. Osorio C, Kanukuntla T, Diaz E, Jafri N, Cummings M, Sfera A. The Post-amyloid Era in Alzheimer's Disease: Trust Your Gut Feeling. Front Aging Neurosci. 2019 Jun 26;11:143. doi: 10.3389/fnagi.2019.00143. PMID: 31297054; PMCID: PMC6608545.

43. Forloni G, Colombo L, Girola L, Tagliavini F, Salmona M. Anti-amyloidogenic activity of tetracyclines: studies in vitro. FEBS Lett.

2001 Jan 5;487(3):404-7. doi: 10.1016/s0014-5793(00)02380-2. PMID: 11163366.

44. Diomede L, Cassata G, Fiordaliso F, Salio M, Ami D, et al. (2010) Tetracycline and its analogueues protect Caenorhabditis elegans from βamyloid-induced toxicity by targeting oligomers. Neurobiol Dis 40: 424-431.

45. Di Pierro F, Iqtadar S, Khan A, et al. Potential Clinical Benefits of Quercetin in the Early Stage of COVID-19: Results of a Second, Pilot, Randomized, Controlled and Open-Label Clinical Trial. Int J Gen Med. 2021;14:2807-2816. Published 2021 Jun 24. doi:10.2147/IJGM.S318949

46. Khan H, Ullah H, Aschner M, Cheang WS, Akkol EK. Neuroprotective Effects of Quercetin in Alzheimer's Disease. Biomolecules. 2019;10(1):59. Published 2019 Dec 30. doi:10.3390/biom10010059

47. Islam MS, Quispe C, Hossain R, et al. Neuropharmacological Effects of Quercetin: A Literature-Based Review. Front Pharmacol. 2021;12:665031. Published 2021 Jun 17. doi:10.3389/fphar.2021.665031

48. Vafadar A, Shabaninejad Z, Movahedpour A, et al. Quercetin and cancer: new insights into its therapeutic effects on ovarian cancer cells. Cell Biosci. 2020;10:32. Published 2020 Mar 10. doi:10.1186/s13578-020-00397-0

49. Yoshida S, Nakagami H, Hayashi H, Ikeda Y, Sun J, Tenma A, et al. The CD153 vaccine is a senotherapeutic option for preventing the accumulation of senescent T cells in mice. Nat Commun. 2020 May 18;11(1):2482. doi: 10.1038/s41467-020-16347-w. PMID: 32424156; PMCID: PMC7235045.

50. Suda, M., Shimizu, I., Katsuumi, G. et al. Senolytic vaccination improves normal and pathological age-related phenotypes and increases lifespan in progeroid mice. Nat Aging (2021). https://doi.org/10.1038/s43587-021-00151-2

51. Poblocka, M., Bassey, A.L., Smith, V.M. et al. Targeted clearance of senescent cells using an antibody-drug conjugate against a specific membrane marker. Sci Rep 11, 20358 (2021). https://doi.org/10.1038/s41598-021-99852-2

52. Sirakanyan S, Arabyan E, Hakobyan A, Hakobyan T, Chilingaryan G, Sahakyan H, et al. A new microtubule-stabilizing agent shows potent antiviral effects against African swine fever virus with no cytotoxicity. Emerg Microbes Infect. 2021 Dec;10(1):783-796. doi: 10.1080/22221751.2021.1902751. PMID: 33706677; PMCID: PMC8079068.

53. Fernandez-Valenzuela JJ, Sanchez-Varo R, Muñoz-Castro C, De Castro V, Sanchez-Mejias E, Navarro V, et al. Enhancing microtubule stabilization rescues cognitive deficits and ameliorates pathological phenotype in an amyloidogenic Alzheimer's disease model. Sci Rep. 2020 Sep 8;10(1):14776. doi: 10.1038/s41598-020-71767-4. PMID: 32901091; PMCID: PMC7479116.

54. Tsai RM, Miller Z, Koestler M, Rojas JC, Ljubenkov PA, Rosen HJ, et al. Reactions to Multiple Ascending Doses of the Microtubule Stabilizer TPI-287 in Patients With Alzheimer Disease, Progressive Supranuclear Palsy, and Corticobasal Syndrome: A Randomized Clinical Trial. JAMA Neurol. 2020 Feb 1;77(2):215-224. doi: 10.1001/jamaneurol.2019.3812. PMID: 31710340; PMCID: PMC6865783.

55. Hung SY, Fu WM. Drug candidates in clinical trials for Alzheimer's disease. J Biomed Sci. 2017;24(1):47. Published 2017 Jul 19. doi:10.1186/s12929-017-0355-7

56. Gozes I. The ADNP Syndrome and CP201 (NAP) Potential and Hope. Front Neurol. 2020 Nov 24;11:608444. doi: 10.3389/fneur.2020.608444. PMID: 33329371; PMCID: PMC7732499.

57. Santiago-Mujika E, Luthi-Carter R, Giorgini F, Kalaria RN, Mukaetova-Ladinska EB. Tubulin and Tubulin Posttranslational Modifications in Alzheimer's Disease and Vascular Dementia. Front Aging Neurosci. 2021;13:730107. Published 2021 Oct 29. doi:10.3389/fnagi.2021.730107

58. Al-Horani RA, Kar S. Potential Anti-SARS-CoV-2 Therapeutics That Target the Post-Entry Stages of the Viral Life Cycle: A Comprehensive Review. Viruses. 2020;12(10):1092. Published 2020 Sep 26. doi:10.3390/v12101092

59. Varidaki A, Hong Y, Coffey ET. Repositioning Microtubule Stabilizing Drugs for Brain Disorders. Front Cell Neurosci. 2018 Aug 8;12:226. doi: 10.3389/fncel.2018.00226. PMID: 30135644; PMCID: PMC6092511.

60. Malebari AM, Wang S, Greene TF, O'Boyle NM, Fayne D, Khan MF. Synthesis and Antiproliferative Evaluation of 3-Chloroazetidin-2-ones with Antimitotic Activity: Heterocyclic Bridged Analogues of Combretastatin A-4. Pharmaceuticals (Basel). 2021 Oct 31;14(11):1119. doi: 10.3390/ph14111119. PMID: 34832901; PMCID: PMC8624998.

61. Kovalevich, J., Cornec, A. S., Yao, Y., James, M., Crowe, A., Lee, V. M., et al. (2016). Characterization of the brain–penetrant pyrimidine–containing molecules with differential microtubule–stabilizing activities developed as potential therapeutic agents for Alzheimer's disease and related tauopathies. J. Pharmacol. Exp. Ther. 357, 432–450. doi: 10.1124/jpet.115.231175

62. Zhang B, Yao Y, Cornec AS, Oukoloff K, James MJ, Koivula P, et al. A brain-penetrant triazolopyrimidine enhances microtubule-stability, reduces axonal dysfunction and decreases tau pathology in a mouse tauopathy model. Mol Neurodegener. 2018 Nov 7;13(1):59. doi: 10.1186/s13024-018-0291-3. PMID: 30404654; PMCID: PMC6223064.

63. Chen X, Winstead A, Yu H, Peng J. Taccalonolides: A Novel Class of Microtubule-Stabilizing Anticancer Agents. Cancers (Basel). 2021 Feb 22;13(4):920. doi: 10.3390/cancers13040920. PMID: 33671665; PMCID: PMC7926778.

64. Murru A, Manchia M, Hajek T, et al. Lithium's antiviral effects: a potential drug for CoViD-19 disease?. Int J Bipolar Disord. 2020;8(1):21. Published 2020 May 20. doi:10.1186/s40345-020-00191-4

65. Matsunaga S, Kishi T, Annas P, Basun H, Hampel H, Iwata N. Lithium as a Treatment for Alzheimer's Disease: A Systematic Review and Meta-Analysis. J Alzheimers Dis. 2015;48(2):403-10. doi: 10.3233/JAD-150437. PMID: 26402004.

66. Bhattacharyya B, Wolff J. Stabilization of microtubules by lithium lithium-ion. Biochem Biophys Res Commun. 1976 Nov 22;73(2):383-90. doi: 10.1016/0006-291x(76)90719-1. PMID: 826253.

67. Olson A, Hussong SA, Kayed R, Galvan V. TAU-INDUCED ASTROCYTE SENESCENCE: A NOVEL MECHANISM FOR NEURONAL DYSFUNCTION IN ALZHEIMER'S DISEASE. Innov Aging. 2019;3(Suppl 1):S91-S92. Published 2019 Nov 8. doi:10.1093/geronimo/igz038.348

68. Kucharz EJ, Sierakowski S, Staite ND, Goodwin JS. Mechanism of lithium-induced augmentation of T-cell proliferation. Int J

Immunopharmacol. 1988;10(3):253-9. doi: 10.1016/0192-0561(88)90056-2. PMID: 3263331.

69. Viel T, Chinta S, Rane A, Chamoli M, Buck H, Andersen J. Microdose lithium reduces cellular senescence in human astrocytes - a potential pharmacotherapy for COVID-19? Aging (Albany, NY). 2020 Jun 13;12(11):10035-10040. doi: 10.18632/aging.103449. Epub 2020 Jun 13. PMID: 32534451; PMCID: PMC7346079

70. Kopf A, Kiermaier E. Dynamic Microtubule Arrays in Leukocytes and Their Role in Cell Migration and Immune Synapse Formation. Front Cell Dev Biol. 2021 Feb 9;9:635511. doi: 10.3389/fcell.2021.635511. PMID: 33634136; PMCID: PMC7900162.

71. Garcia-Montojo M, Nath A. HERV-W envelope expression in blood leukocytes as a marker of disease severity of COVID-19. EBioMedicine. 2021 May;67:103363. doi: 10.1016/j.ebiom.2021.103363. Epub 2021 May 13. PMID: 33993053; PMCID: PMC8116818.

72. Diebold M, Derfuss T. The monoclonal antibody GNbAC1: targeting human endogenous retroviruses in multiple sclerosis. Ther Adv Neurol Disord. 2019;12:1756286419833574. Published 2019 Mar 7. doi:10.1177/1756286419833574

Chapter 19
It's Ceramide Not Cholesterol

Life depends on the integrity of biological barriers, membranes that separate the human body from the outside environment, and the body compartments from each other.

Mental illness is likely driven by impaired tight junctions (TJs) due to dysfunctional AhR, allowing gut microbes to migrate via paracellular space into the systemic circulation, eventually reaching the brain. The body's immune response to translocated bacteria or their proteins engender the clinical picture of neuropsychiatric syndromes. In addition, AhR induces cellular senescence in IECs, altering the TJs and promoting more translocation. Moreover, AhR may shift tryptophan catabolism toward the kynurenine pathway, upregulating quinolinic acid, a toxin associated with SCZ, ASD, MDD, PTSD, and suicide. Interestingly, psychological stress may produce the same effect by activating IDO.

Microbe-activated AhR induces premature cellular senescence, further disrupting biological barriers. Cellular senescence promotes lipid oxidation, plasmalogen depletion, and toxic ceramide formation, causing neuronal death.

MLR and plasmalogen replacement therapy (PRT) eliminate oxidized membrane lipids, restoring membrane integrity and physiological properties to avert neuropathology.

The cell membrane lipid bilayer is said to be "asymmetric," meaning that the outer and inner leaflets are comprised of different lipid species. The main plasma membrane lipid categories are phospholipids, glycolipids, and cholesterol.

In this chapter, I will examine two cell membrane lipid species that are altered in SMI: ceramide and plasmalogens. I will also discuss supplementation with natural, healthy lipids via replacement with plasmalogens and other natural lipids.

Ceramide, an endogenous toxin

Ceramides are cell membrane phospholipids composed of sphingosine. They play a key role in the cellular response to stressors and extracellular stimuli.

In SCZ, phosphatidylcholine (PC) levels are low, and there is a significant increase in white matter ceramide, regardless of the antipsychotic treatment (1). Ceramides are obtained from three sources: the diet, de novo synthesis in human tissues, and production by gut commensal flora, such as *Bacteroidetes*. Indeed, oral cavity *Bacteroidetes* are more abundant in patients with SCZ than in healthy controls, emphasizing the microbial source of excessive ceramide in this disorder (2). Moreover, several studies have shown that inflammation can convert ceramide into a toxic form, leading to neuropathology (3).

Novel preclinical studies have shown that gut microbes can metabolize dietary PC into a toxin, trimethylamine-N-oxide (TMAO), a biomolecule implicated in atherosclerosis and SCZ. This is important not only for explaining the lower levels of PC in SCZ but also for the high prevalence of coronary artery disease in patients with SMI (4). Indeed, proinflammatory cytokines and inflammation likely account for the presence of TMAO in SCZ (5). Cytokines were previously shown to facilitate the formation of toxic ceramide species that cross the BBB, causing CNS pathology, including insulin resistance and oxidative stress (6).

Plasmalogens, the endogenous statins

Plasmalogens are a class of cell membrane glycerophospholipids characterized by a vinyl-ether bond, which confers this lipid's potent antioxidant properties, including the ability to protect from peroxidation the other lipids in the membrane bilayer (7). Plasmalogens maintain the biophysical properties of cell membranes, including shape, fluidity, and thickness, which are necessary for aligning cell surface receptors and proper neurotransmission. Interestingly, antipsychotic drugs with antioxidant properties, such as phenothiazines, can enter the lipid bilayer of cellular and mitochondrial membranes, acting synergistically with plasmalogens (8) (9). For this reason, decreased plasmalogen levels in plasma and platelets of patients with SCZ and mood disorders are considered biomarkers of SMI (10) (11).

Phenazines are a class of natural phenothiazines produced by marine and terrestrial microorganisms and some gut microbes, likely engendering an inbuilt antipsychotic system resembling endogenous opioids. In addition, these agents also exert antimicrobial, antiparasitic, neuroprotective, anti-inflammatory, and anticancer activities and are currently in clinical trials for some of these pathologies. There are over 100 different natural phenazines and about 6000 synthetic derivatives with antioxidant properties that can enter the cell membranes, rescuing the bilayer lipids (12). Moreover, a new class of antioxidant phenothiazines, developed primarily for cancer, can be utilized in SMI along with PRT (13).

PRT, with its potential to restore the physiologic levels of plasmalogen in cell and mitochondrial membranes via a natural compound, offers a promising avenue for lipid metabolism research. Alternate plasmalogen levels in several conditions, including normal aging, SCZ, chronic inflammation, and neurodegenerative and metabolic disorders, underscore the significance of this potential. The ability of PRT to be utilized along with other lipids provided by MLR further enhances its potential.

Plasmalogens, functioning like endogenous statins, offer a safe and preferable alternative. Their ability to lower cholesterol synthesis suggests the existence of an equilibrium between the two lipid species. Since plasmalogens are natural products devoid of statin side effects, such as hepatotoxicity and diabetes mellitus, they are a reassuring choice, particularly in psychiatric patients in which statins can cause aggressive behavior.

A recent study determined the optimal oral dose of PRT, comprised of docosahexaenoic acid (DHA) with 1-O-alkyl-2-acylglycerol (AAG) plasmalogen, as 900 to 3,600 mg/day over four months. The authors noted improved cognition and mobility in patients with neurocognitive disorders (16).

MLR refers to the oral intake of natural membrane lipid supplements to replace oxidized lipids in the cell membrane bilayer with natural glycerophospholipids.

Membrane injury by oxidative stress is common in numerous disorders and normal aging. MLR, with its potential to restore the physiological function of plasma membranes throughout the body, including the gut barrier and BBB, offers a promising therapeutic intervention. By lowering the permeability of epithelial and endothelial barriers, MLR shows the potential to avert microbial migration.

Viruses, including SARS-CoV-2, damage the cell membranes as they enter the intracellular compartment to replicate. Damaged membranes externalize phosphatidylserine (PS), a universal signal for phagocyte fusion or elimination. SARS-CoV-2-induced cellular senescence upregulates cytosolic iron, predisposing to lipid peroxidation and ferroptosis.

Ferroptosis is an iron-induced form of programmed cell death caused by the accumulation in the absence of glutathione peroxidase 4 (GPX4) (17). Oxidized lipids act as foreign molecules and activate the host pattern recognition receptors (PRR), triggering chronic inflammation, neuropathic pain, depression, and neurodegeneration. Rescue from ferroptosis can be achieved by lowering intracellular iron, increasing GPX4, or replacing the oxidized lipids in cell membranes. Several studies have shown that the SARS-CoV-2 virus upregulates intracellular iron by hijacking the host lysosomes and disrupting ferritin autophagy in these organelles. The lysosomal function would need to be restored to restore iron homeostasis, which is difficult now. The lack of effective treatments for lysosomal disorders illustrates this.

Enhanced lipid peroxidation and ferroptosis have been associated with several conditions, including myalgic encephalomyelitis /chronic fatigue syndrome (ME/CFS), Gulf War Illness (GWI), chronic pain, and neuropsychiatric disorders. Ferroptosis-disintegrating cells release alarmins, such as the high mobility group box 1 (HMGB1), known for disrupting the intestinal barrier and BBB (18).

Natural membrane supplementation with glycerophospholipids was demonstrated to restore biological barriers' homeostasis and limit microbial translocation (19). MLR aims to substitute ferroptosis-driving oxidized lipids with healthy glycerophospholipids.

Oxidized cell membrane lipids activate AhR, inhibiting Akt, which disinhibits glycogen synthase kinase three beta (GSK3β). Aberrant activation of GSK3β has been documented in various neuropsychiatric conditions, especially SCZ and bipolar disorder, as well as aggressive behavior in the context of SMI. For example, lithium, several antipsychotic drugs, and the natural compounds berberine and kaempferol inhibit GSK3β, suggesting that these herbal medicines exert antipsychotic properties without the adverse effects of conventional psychotropic drugs.

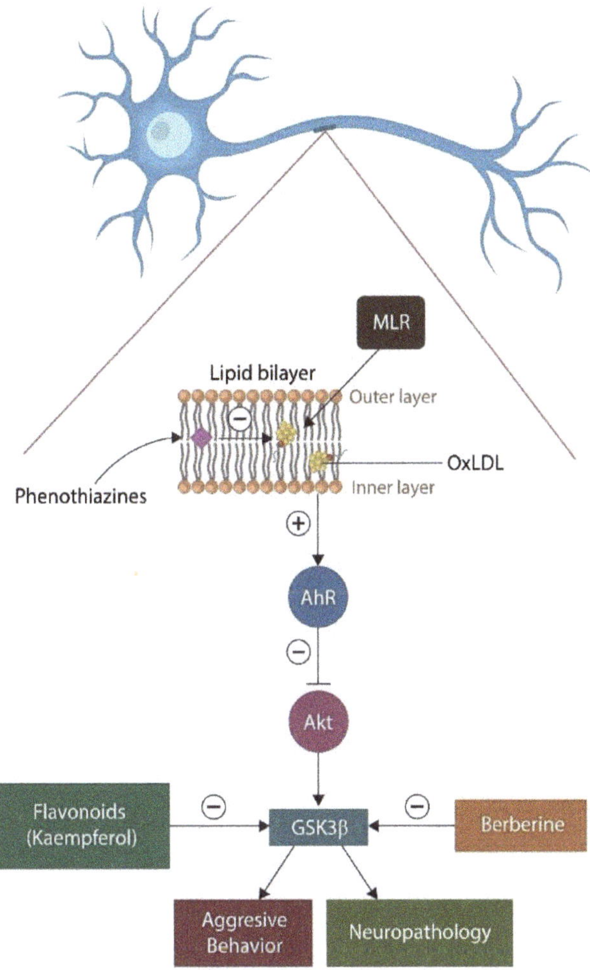

Fig. 19.1 The lipid bilayer of neuronal cells contains phospholipids, glycolipids, and cholesterol. Oxidized lipids disrupt the cell and mitochondrial membrane. Like MLR, phenothiazines exert antioxidant properties and enter the cell membranes, repairing the lipids. This averts AhR activation and GSK3β-mediated pathology. Kaempferol and Berberine inhibit GSK3β, acting in synergy with MLR and phenothiazines.

Mitochondrial membrane

Mitochondria have a unique microbe-like membrane on the organelle surface. This membrane, comprised of an inner and outer layer, has an intermembrane space containing mitochondrial matrix enzymes, mitochondrial ribosomes, tRNAs, mRNAs, and mitochondrial DNA (mtDNA). The inner membrane harbors the electron transport system and the oxidative phosphorylation (OXPHOS) machinery. The electron transport chain pumps protons into the intermembrane space, creating an electrochemical gradient that drives the OXPHOS and ATP synthesis.

Like the plasma membrane, the mitochondrial membrane contains an asymmetric lipid bilayer that contains phosphatidyl ethanolamine (PE), phosphatidylcholine (PC), and cardiolipin (CL). Cardiolipin (CL), a unique lipid found primarily in the mitochondrion, is crucial for maintaining the inner membrane fluidity and the transmembrane potential. In the CNS, cardiolipin is found in neurons and glial cells, where it maintains energy homeostasis and drives apoptosis when the cell is beyond repair. MLR restores optimal permeability of the gut barrier and BBB, averting microbial migration outside the GI tract and into the brain. Interestingly, anti-cardiolipin antibodies were documented in SCZ, while commensal flora, including *Muribaculum intestinal*, produces CL, suggesting that antibodies may be directed against the product of this microbe.

Mitochondria contain their mitochondrial AhR (mAhR), which is activated by the oxidized lipids, generating ROS that can lead to organelle demise.

Taken together, cellular and mitochondrial membranes contain an asymmetric lipid bilayer, increasing lipid peroxidation susceptibility in long-living, postmitotic cells, like neurons. Oxidized lipids activate AhR, ultimately disinhibiting GSK3β, leading to psychopathology and aggressive behaviors. Removal and replacing oxidized lipids with natural glycerophospholipids and plasmalogens prevents neuronal apoptosis and restores their function.

Chapter 19 References:

1. Schwarz E., Prabakaran S., Whitfield P., Major H., Leweke F. M., Keothe D., et al.. (2008). High throughput lipidomic profiling of schizophrenia and bipolar disorder brain tissue reveals alterations of free fatty acids, phosphatidylcholines, and ceramides. J. Proteome Res. 7, 4266–4277. 10.1021/pr800188y

2. Zhu, F., Ju, Y., Wang, W. et al. Metagenome-wide association of gut microbiome features for schizophrenia. Nat Commun 11, 1612 (2020). https://doi.org/10.1038/s41467-020-15457-9

3. Johnson, E.L., Heaver, S.L., Waters, J.L. et al. Sphingolipids produced by gut bacteria enter host metabolic pathways, impacting ceramide levels. Nat Commun 11, 2471 (2020). https://doi.org/10.1038/s41467-020-16274-w

4. Liu Y, Dai M. Trimethylamine N-Oxide Generated by the Gut Microbiota Is Associated with Vascular Inflammation: New Insights into Atherosclerosis. Mediators Inflamm. 2020 Feb 17;2020:4634172. doi: 10.1155/2020/4634172.

5. Nguyen TT, Kosciolek T, Daly RE, Vázquez-Baeza Y, Swafford A, Knight R, Jeste DV. Gut microbiome in Schizophrenia: Altered functional pathways related to immune modulation and atherosclerotic risk. Brain Behav Immun. 2021 Jan;91:245-256. doi: 10.1016/j.bbi.2020.10.003.

6. de la Monte SM. Triangulated mal-signaling in Alzheimer's disease: roles of neurotoxic ceramides, ER stress, and insulin resistance reviewed. J Alzheimers Dis. 2012;30 Suppl 2(0 2): S231-49. doi: 10.3233/JAD-2012-111727.

7. Almsherqi ZA. Potential Role of Plasmalogens in the Modulation of Biomembrane Morphology. Front Cell Dev Biol. 2021 Jul 21;9:673917. doi: 10.3389/fcell.2021.673917.

8. Bindoli A, Rigobello MP, Favel A, Galzigna L. Antioxidant action and photosensitizing effects of three different chlorpromazines. J Neurochem. 1988 Jan;50(1):138-41. doi: 10.1111/j.1471-4159.1988.tb13240.x. PMID: 3335839.

9. Egbujor MC, Tucci P, Buttari B, Nwobodo DC, Marini P, Saso L. Phenothiazines: Nrf2 activation and antioxidant effects. J Biochem Mol Toxicol. 2024 Mar;38(3):e23661.

10. Wood PL, Unfried G, Whitehead W, Phillipps A, Wood JA. Dysfunctional plasmalogen dynamics in the plasma and platelets of patients with schizophrenia. Schizophr Res. 2015 Feb;161(2-3):506-10. doi: 10.1016/j.schres.2014.11.032. Epub 2014 Dec 12. PMID: 25497441.

11. Fujino M, Fukuda J, Isogai H, Ogaki T, Mawatari S, Takaki A, Wakana C, Fujino T. Orally Administered Plasmalogens Alleviate Negative Mood States and Enhance Mental Concentration: A Randomized, Double-Blind, Placebo-Controlled Trial. Front Cell Dev Biol. 2022 Jun 2;10:894734. doi: 10.3389/fcell.2022.894734.

12. Yan J, Liu W, Cai J, Wang Y, Li D, Hua H, Cao H. Advances in Phenazines over the Past Decade: Review of Their Pharmacological Activities, Mechanisms of Action, Biosynthetic Pathways and Synthetic Strategies. Mar Drugs. 2021 Oct 27;19(11):610. doi: 10.3390/md19110610. PMID: 34822481; PMCID: PMC8620606.

13. Voronova O, Zhuravkov S, Korotkova E, Artamonov A, Plotnikov E. Antioxidant Properties of New Phenothiazine

Derivatives. Antioxidants (Basel). 2022 Jul 14;11(7):1371. doi: 10.3390/antiox11071371.

14. Mankidy R., Ahiahonu P. W., Ma H., Jayasinghe D., Ritchie S. A., Khan M. A., et al. (2010). Membrane Plasmalogen Composition and Cellular Cholesterol Regulation: A Structure Activity Study. Lipids Health Dis. 9 (1), 1–17. 10.1186/1476-511X-9-62

15. Sirtori CR. The pharmacology of statins. Pharmacol Res. 2014 Oct;88:3-11. doi: 10.1016/j.phrs.2014.03.002. Epub 2014 Mar 20. PMID: 24657242.

16. Goodenowe DB, Haroon J, Kling MA, Zielinski M, Mahdavi K, Habelhah B, Shtilkind L, Jordan S. Targeted Plasmalogen Supplementation: Effects on Blood Plasmalogens, Oxidative Stress Biomarkers, Cognition, and Mobility in Cognitively Impaired Persons. Front Cell Dev Biol. 2022 Jul 6;10:864842. doi: 10.3389/fcell.2022.864842.

17. Weiland A, Wang Y, Wu W, Lan X, Han X, Li Q, Wang J. Ferroptosis and Its Role in Diverse Brain Diseases. Mol Neurobiol. 2019 Jul;56(7):4880-4893. doi: 10.1007/s12035-018-1403-3.

18. Chen X, Zhao HX, Bai C, Zhou XY. Blockade of high-mobility group box 1 attenuates intestinal mucosal barrier dysfunction in experimental acute pancreatitis. Sci Rep. 2017 Jul 28;7(1):6799. doi: 10.1038/s41598-017-07094-y.

19. Nicolson GL, Ferreira de Mattos G, Ash M, Settineri R, Escribá PV. Fundamentals of Membrane Lipid Replacement: A Natural Medicine Approach to Repairing Cellular Membranes and Reducing Fatigue, Pain, and Other Symptoms While Restoring Function in Chronic Illnesses

and Aging. Membranes (Basel). 2021 Nov 29;11(12):944. Doi: 10.3390/membranes11120944.

Chapter 20
Lifestyle and Chronic Mental Illness

Can diet, exercise, and lifestyle coaching help patients with SCZ and MDD?

The short answer is yes, but it is challenging to implement these measures, especially in chronic patients with negative symptoms of SCZ. However, the main reason lifestyle medicine is underutilized in SMI is its acceptability by both patients and physicians as a treatment modality comparable to psychopharmacology or psychotherapy (1).

Numerous studies have documented that patients with SMI may be malnourished as they have poor dietary practices marked by increased intake of sodium, cholesterol, and higher saturated fats, as well as low fiber content (2). This is significant because typical Western adults consume 5–10 g of fiber daily instead of 35 or 50 g, which is considered optimal. Patients with SCZ consume an even lower amount of dietary fiber and are often deficient in SCFA (3). Fiber is an essential nutritional component because fermentation by specific gut microbes generates SCFA, such as acetate, propionate, or butyrate.

Butyrate is a new player in neuropsychiatry because of its ability to inhibit histone deacetylase (HDAC), an action identical to that of the mood stabilizer valproic acid used in the treatment of bipolar d/o and SCZ. Butyrate binds to several G protein-coupled receptors (GPCRs), including

GPR41, GPR43, and GPR109A. Moreover, butyrate is the primary energy source for IECs and averts microbial translocation by decreasing gut barrier permeability. Furthermore, SCFAs were shown to augment leptin production, a hormone decreased in neuropsychiatric conditions marked by impulsivity (4). Moreover, butyrate was found to protect against insulin resistance and inflammation, while propionate was demonstrated to lower cholesterol synthesis (5). GPR 43, the butyrate receptors, are expressed on adipocytes and associated with obesity. Moreover, GPR43 receptors regulate the function of innate lymphoid cells type 3 (ILC3), gut resident lymphocytes that produce IL-22, the "guardian" of the intestinal barrier (Fig. 20.1).

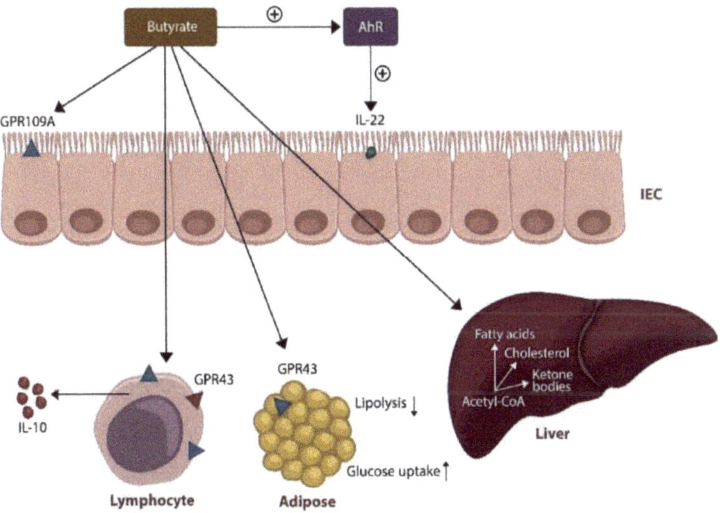

Fig. 20.1 Butyrate is synthesized and absorbed in the large intestine. Several receptors for butyrate have been identified, including GPR41, GPR43, and GPR109A. GPR43 is found in fatty tissues and immune cells. GPR109A is expressed in the colonic epithelium. A small portion of

butyrate is transported to the liver and metabolized into fatty acids, cholesterol, and ketone bodies. Butyrate activates AhR, a positive regulator of IL-22.

Novel studies have implicated butyrate in SCZ as butyrate-producing bacteria, such as *Butyricicoccus, Roseburia, and Faecalibacterium*, are less abundant in patients with this disorder. Others have suggested adding butyrate to the treatment regimen of SCZ patients (6). Butyrate is believed to exhibit antidepressant effects and may also improve sleep, learning, and cognition. Butyrate inhibited inflammatory microglia, decreasing neurotoxicity and the subsequent neuronal loss (7). As preclinical studies show, it also protects mitochondria and reduces lipid peroxidation and neuronal apoptosis via GPR41 (8).

GPR109A is the receptor for both niacin and butyrate, suggesting a molecular resemblance between the two ligands is implicated in SCZ (9). For example, in the 1950s, niacin was used to treat SCZ but fell from favor in the subsequent years. However, at least a subset of SCZ patients respond to niacin. Along this line, novel studies have linked niacin to mitochondrial rehabilitation and reactivation of OXPHOS.

It has been suggested that the obesity epidemic over the past decades may have been caused by excessive niacin consumption, resulting from the fortification (addition of niacin to food). This program started in the early 1940s. People should question niacin and all food "fortification "programs" implemented in the US and Western Europe throughout the 20th century. Consumer groups did not approve of most food fortifications like fluoride in drinking water. Currently, 94 countries have legislation to mandate niacin fortification of cereal grain. Global Alliance for Improved Nutrition (GAIN), established in Geneva in 2002, decides what "mandatory" nutrients are added to various food products worldwide.

Obesity is a form of paradoxical malnutrition, marked by decreased physical and mental performance, cognition, and emotion (10). It is believed that obesity is also connected to tryptophan metabolites and the AhR ligand kynurenine. Indeed, kynurenine and tryptophan concentrations were significantly higher in prediabetes and obesity, suggesting a marker value (11). Several studies have linked obesity to the aberrant AhR activation by tryptophan or its metabolites. It is well-established that AhR is abundantly expressed in biological barriers, including the gut barrier and BBB, and regulates xenobiotic metabolism, adaptive immunity, and the microbiome. In addition, neurotransmitters relevant for neuropsychiatry, including 5-HT, melatonin, and DA, are AhR ligands, making this receptor a key hub for nutritional psychiatry.

Malnutrition during pregnancy has been connected to SCZ in offspring, as seen during the Dutch hunger of 1944-1945. This tragic event has served as an unplanned experiment of perinatal causes of SCZ (12) (13). Other studies came from the 1950s during China's Great Leap Forward famine, often resulting in prepartum malnutrition and offspring with SCZ (14). These studies raise the question of how the fetus remembers the environment it was exposed to in the womb and develops SCZ decades later. These studies led to the development of epigenetics, the expression of genes in the absence of DNA changes. In other words, the environment controls which gene is expressed and which is silenced to adapt to specific situations. Along this line, some genes may only be active during development and permanently silenced afterward.

Aryl hydrocarbon receptor and nutritional psychiatry

Throughout human history, food has been a precious but cyclical commodity. The weather, crops, wars, and calamities generated famine cycles and plenty. Ensuring the constancy of feeding resources constituted a significant driver of brain development. It is, therefore, not surprising that nutrients influence behavior, a living remnant from the hunter-gatherer society. Even in less developed countries, the ancestral specter of famine remains alive and may contribute to overeating and weight gain. For example, obesity is most prevalent in countries with a per capita gross domestic product (GDP) of less than $5,000 (15).

Nutritional psychiatry is a novel and rapidly evolving field that studies dietary interventions, including nutritional supplementation as treatments for neuropsychiatric disorders. It has been established that the beneficial effects of dietary interventions and nutrients upregulate neurogenesis and lower oxidative stress, inflammation, and microbial translocation (16). Adult neurogenesis refers to the generation of new neurons from neural stem cells in the adult brain, a physiological process that takes place in the subgranular zone (SGZ) of the hippocampus and the subventricular zone (SVZ) of the lateral ventricles.

It is well known that obesity has reached epidemic proportions worldwide and that fiber intake in psychiatric patients is deficient compared to the recommended 35-50 grams a day. In contrast, the prevalence of obesity is four times higher than that of the general population (17). Nutritional psychiatry aims to lower SMI and correct malnutrition in these patients.

An equally important aim is lowering microbial translocation with foods that improve the function of TJs, as well as the molecular Velcro that keeps IECs together. These compounds include flavonoids, alkaloids, polyamines, probiotics, tannate, and non-flavonoid polyphenols (Table 20.1).

Category	Compound	References
Alkaloids	Berberine	18
Flavonoids	Kaempferol, Quercetin	19
Polyphenols (non-flavonoid)	Curcumin, Resveratrol	20
Amino Acid	Glutamine	21
Monounsaturated fatty acids,	Olive oil	22
Probiotics	Bifidobacteria and Lactobacillus	23
Tannate	Gelatine tannate	24
Polyamines	Putrescine, Spermidine	25

Table 20.1. Compounds that protect the gut barrier by upregulating tight junctions.

Taken together, patients with SMI have poor dietary practices and may be malnourished or obese (a form of malnutrition). Low-fiber diets result in low butyrate, which is antioxidant, anti-inflammatory, and a positive regulator of IL-22, the "guardian" of the gut barrier. Increased intestinal permeability and microbial translocation induce various pathologies, including SMI.

Nutritional approaches with specific compounds that rescue the gut barrier act as antipsychotic and antidepressant agents and should be utilized more often in psychiatric hospitals.

Chapter 20 References:

1. Richardson, K., Petukhova, R., Hughes, S. et al. The acceptability of lifestyle medicine for the treatment of mental illness: perspectives of people with and without lived experience of mental illness. BMC Public Health 24, 171 (2024). https://doi.org/10.1186/s12889-024-17683-y

2. Onaolapo OJ, Onaolapo AY. Nutrition, nutritional deficiencies, and schizophrenia: An association worthy of constant reassessment. World J Clin Cases. 2021 Oct 6;9(28):8295-8311. doi: 10.12998/wjcc.v9.i28.8295.

3. Slavin J. Fiber and prebiotics: mechanisms and health benefits. Nutrients (2013) 5(4):1417–35. 10.3390/nu5041417

4. Den Besten G, van Eunen K, Groen AK, Venema K, Reijngoud D-J, Bakker BM. The role of short-chain fatty acids in the interplay between diet, gut microbiota, and host energy metabolism. J Lipid Res (2013) 54(9):2325–40. 10.1194/jar.R036012

5. Simpson HL, Campbell BJ. Review article: dietary fibre-microbiota interactions. Aliment Pharmacol Ther (2015) 42(2):158–79. 10.1111/apt.13248

6. Kelly DL, Kane MA, Fraser CM, Sayer MA, Grant-Beurmann S, Liu T, Gold JM, Notarangelo FM, Vyas GR, Richardson CM, August SM, Kotnana B, Miller J, Liu F, Buchanan RW. Prebiotic Treatment Increases Serum Butyrate in People With Schizophrenia: Results of an Open-Label Inpatient Pilot Clinical Trial. J Clin Psychopharmacol. 2021 Mar-Apr 01;41(2):200-202. doi: 10.1097/JCP.0000000000001364.

7. Caetano-Silva, M.E., Rund, L., Hutchinson, N.T. et al. Inhibition of inflammatory microglia by dietary fiber and short-chain fatty acids. Sci Rep 13,

Conclusion

Although antidepressant drugs were available several decades, before the release of the first SSRI, Prozac, this particular drug marked a paradigm shift in regards to tolerability and efficacy.

In 1994, when "Prozac Nation" was published, Big Pharma was already marketing directly to the patient, trying to eliminate all obstacles on the road to the lifelong "serotonization" of the Nation. Indeed, not only did Big Pharma approach the patient directly (direct-to-consumer marketing), but they also normalized drug-taking behavior under the pretense of combating stigma. This was achieved by comparing SMI with hypertension or diabetes, conditions requiring life-long treatment that are stable for long intervals of time. While eliminating stigma may be helpful for the patients to realize that they are not facing these diseases alone, it also fills the coffers of Big Pharma.

Do SMI, such as SCZ and depression, need to be treated for life? The industry-sponsored studies say yes. Industry-subservient academia and the American Psychiatric Association cannot agree more.

The same is true of most psychotropic drugs. Chronic use of antipsychotic agents has been associated with mitochondrial loss and GMV reduction, but a conspiracy of silence has been at work when it comes to these issues. As academia has been silent, most practicing psychiatrists may not even be aware of the GMV loss documented by numerous neuroimaging studies over the past two decades.

Is it possible that antipsychotic maintenance therapy is the cause of brain parenchymal thinning? Since mitochondria and gray matter loss occur due to psychotic illness itself as well as because of treatment, maintenance therapy in SCZ may require non-DA blocking drugs or even dopamine replacement therapy.

Aside from its role in hedonic behavior, brain DA averts gray matter reduction. Thus, supplementation instead of blocking might attenuate the negative and cognitive symptoms of SCZ. Another option consists of muscarinic agonists (such as Emraclidine), devoid of gray matter adverse effects.

Decades of observation, research, innumerable treatment plans, and forensic Court hearings contributed to this book. All of these have convinced me that neurotransmitters working in the synaptic cleft do not comprise the primary etiopathogenesis of neuropsychiatric disorders. In addition, I have learned the following:

- Rather than only in neurons, memory is stored in the cellular cytoskeleton, especially the microtubules, in cells throughout the body.

- SCZ pathology starts with gray matter loss in the temporoparietal lobe and spreads in a prion-like manner through the entire brain, unaffected by the psychotropics.

- It is possible that viruses usurp the tau protein and use it to carry phosphorylated tau from cell to cell, spreading the infection, as documented in COVID-19.

- EP and premature brain aging are AhR-dependent defense mechanisms protecting against infection and cancer. Can cancer be cured by simply blocking the EP?

- Since psychosis and antipsychotics cause gray matter loss, maintenance therapy should not enhance this pathology by using dopamine-blocking agents as it is done presently.

- Statins should not be used in patients with SMI as they can trigger aggressive behavior. Plasmalogens, natural statins, should be prescribed instead.

- Fortification of grains with niacin has been the likely cause of obesity in the US and the world for the past several decades. The role of niacin in obesity should be studied more, and fortification should be discontinued.

- Water fluorination (started in the 1945) is the likely cause of the mental health crisis over the past 80 years. Fluoride alters phospholipid metabolism in cell/neuronal membranes, promoting behavioral and cognitive disturbances, including ASDs. There appears to be a synergism between serotonin and fluoride, as the latter augments the former.

- SSRIs work by trafficking mitochondria from astrocytes to neurons, increasing cellular energy. Increased synaptic serotonin is unlikely to affect MDD as it would downregulate the postsynaptic serotonergic receptors, attenuating the effect of this neurotransmitter.

- Loss of butyrate can cause depression and psychosis by facilitating microbial translocation. Supplementation with sodium butyrate can rehabilitate gut mucosa, preventing translocation.

- Antipsychotic drugs' mechanism of action is most likely biophysical and occurs at the level of plasma or mitochondrial membranes.

- Another potential antipsychotic mechanism may be the "killing" of translocated microbes via the antibiotic-like properties of these drugs.

- Many autoimmune disorders likely consist of immune responses to the proteins of translocated bacteria, totally changing the concept of autoimmunity.

The COVID-19 pandemic has clarified several unknowns in SMI, such as the importance of EP, iron, and ferroptosis; the role of polyamines, cell-cell fusion, cell membrane pathology, HERV activation, and cellular senescence was poorly defined before the pandemic. The virus spreading pathological tau protein from cell to cell in a prion-like manner is another intriguing discovery that links viruses to tauopathies. Tau is a stabilizer of tubulin in microtubules. Thus, phosphorylated tau detaches from the microtubules, causing the disintegration of these memory-storing structures.

Since these pathologies are involved in several neuropsychiatric conditions, significant advances in this field may occur abruptly across many diagnostic entities.

In this book, I discussed potential biophysical and biochemical treatment strategies utilizing natural and synthetic compounds and some forms of stimulation, including whole-body vibration and light entrainment, that could be of interest to both patients and clinicians.

Bibliography

A Colliva, S Vodret, W Bongiovanni, S Zacchigna, Cardiomyocyte fusion as a new mechanism contributing to pathological cardiac hypertrophy, Cardiovascular Research, Volume 118, Issue Supplement_1, June 2022, cvac066.092, https://doi.org/10.1093/cvr/cvac066.092

Massive A, Cavalli N, Mencarini L, Plach S, Sanders S. Early assessment of the relationship between the COVID-19 pandemic and births in high-income countries. Proc Natl Acad Sci USA. 2021 Sep 7;118(36):e2105709118. doi: 10.1073/pnas.2105709118.

AbdelMassih AF, Ye J, Kamel A, Mishriky F, Ismail HA, Ragab HA, El Qadi L, Malak L, Abdu M, El-Husseiny M, Ashraf M, Hafez N, AlShehry N, El-Husseiny N, AbdelRaouf N, Shebl N, Hafez N, Youssef N, Afdal P, Hozaien R, Menshawey R, Saeed R, Fouda R. A multicenter consensus: A role of furin in the endothelial tropism in obese patients with COVID-19 infection. Obes Med. 2020 Sep;19:100281. doi: 10.1016/j.obmed.2020.100281.

Adkins EA, Brunst KJ. Impacts of Fluoride Neurotoxicity and Mitochondrial Dysfunction on Cognition and Mental Health: A Literature Review. Int J Environ Res Public Health. 2021 Dec 7;18(24):12884. doi: 10.3390/ijerph182412884.

Aggarwal A, Brennan C, Shortal B, Contreras D, Kelz MB, Proekt A. Coherence of Visual-Evoked Gamma Oscillations

Is Disrupted by Propofol but Preserved Under Equipotent Doses of Isoflurane. Front Syst Neurosci. 2019 May 8;13:19. doi: 10.3389/fnsys.2019.00019.

Agnarelli, A., Natali, M., Garcia-Gil, M. et al. The cell-specific pattern of berberine pleiotropic effects on different human cell lines. Sci Rep 8, 10599 (2018). https://doi.org/10.1038/s41598-018-28952-3

Agnati LF, Zunarelli E, Genedani S, Fuxe K. On the existence of a global molecular network enmeshing the whole central nervous system: physiological and pathological implications. Curr Protein Pept Sci. 2006 Feb;7(1):3-15. doi: 10.2174/138920306775474086.

Ahrens AP, Sanchez-Padilla DE, Drew JC, Oli MW, Roesch LFW,Triplett EW. Saliva microbiome, dietary, and genetic markers are associated with suicidal ideation in university students. Sci Rep.2022 Aug 22;12(1):14306. doi: 10.1038/s41598-022-18020-2.

Akbari M, Kirkwood TBL, Bohr VA. Mitochondria in the signaling pathways that control longevity and health span. Ageing Res Rev. 2019 Sep;54:100940. doi: 10.1016/j.arr.2019.100940. Epub 2019 Aug 12. PMID: 31415807; PMCID: PMC7479635.

Al Abed AS, Ducourneau EG, Bouarab C, Sellami A, Marighetto A, Desmedt A. Preventing and treating PTSD-like memory by trauma contextualization. Nat Commun. 2020 Aug 24;11(1):4220. doi: 10.1038/s41467-020-18002-w. PMID: 32839437; PMCID: PMC7445258.

Al-Amin MM, Nasir Uddin MM, Mahmud Reza H. Effects of antipsychotics on the inflammatory response system of patients with schizophrenia in peripheral blood mononuclear cell cultures. Clin Psychopharmacol Neurosci. 2013 Dec;11(3):144-51. doi: 10.9758/cpn.2013.11.3.144. Epub 2013 Dec 24. PMID: 24465251

Alan N Simmons, Estibaliz Arce, Kathryn L Lovero, Murray B Stein, Martin P Paulus, Subchronic SSRI administration reduces insula response during affective anticipation in healthy volunteers, International Journal of Neuropsychopharmacology, Volume 12, Issue 8, September 2009, Pages 1009–1020, https://doi.org/10.1017/S1461145709990149

Albayrak N, Orte Cano C, Karimi S, Dogahe D, Van Praet A, Godefroid A, Del Marmol V, Grimaldi D, Bondue B, Van Vooren JP, Mascart F, Corbière V. Distinct Expression Patterns of Interleukin-22 Receptor 1 on Blood Hematopoietic Cells in SARS-CoV-2 Infection. Front Immunol. 2022 Mar 29;13:769839. doi: 10.3389/fimmu.2022.769839.

Alciati A, Fusi A, D'Arminio Monforte A, Coen M, Ferri A, Mellado C. New-onset delusions and hallucinations in patients infected with HIV. J Psychiatry Neurosci. 2001 May;26(3):229-34. PMID: 11394192; PMCID: PMC1408305.

Aldén M, Olofsson Falla F, Yang D, Barghouth M, Luan C, Rasmussen M, De Marinis Y. Intracellular Reverse Transcription of Pfizer BioNTech COVID-19 mRNA

Vaccine BNT162b2 In Vitro in Human Liver Cell Line. Curr Issues Mol Biol. 2022 Feb 25;44(3):1115-1126. doi: 10.3390/cimb44030073.

Aldosari BN, Alfagih IM, Almurshedi AS. Lipid Nanoparticles as Delivery Systems for RNA-Based Vaccines. Pharmaceutics. 2021 Feb 2;13(2):206. doi: 10.3390/pharmaceutics13020206.

Al-Horani RA, Kar S. Potential Anti-SARS-CoV-2 Therapeutics That Target the Post-Entry Stages of the Viral Life Cycle: A Comprehensive Review. Viruses. 2020;12(10):1092. Published 2020 Sep 26. doi:10.3390/v12101092

Al-Horani RA, Kar S. Potential Anti-SARS-CoV-2 Therapeutics That Target the Post-Entry Stages of the Viral Life Cycle: A Comprehensive Review. Viruses. 2020;12(10):1092. Published 2020 Sep 26. doi:10.3390/v12101092

Ali P, Chen F, Hassan F, Sosa A, Khan S, Badshah M, Shah AA. Bacterial community characterization of Batura Glacier in the Karakoram Range of Pakistan. Int Microbiol. 2021 May;24(2):183-196. doi: 10.1007/s10123-020-00153-x.

Ali Pour P, Hosseinian S, Kheradvar A. Mitochondrial transplantation in cardiomyocytes: foundation, methods, and outcomes. Am J Physiol Cell Physiol. (2021) 321:C489–503. doi: 10.1152/ajpcell.00152.2021

Al-Juhani A, Imran M, Aljaili ZK, Alzhrani MM, Alsalman RA, Ahmed M, Ali DK, Fallatah MI, Yousuf HM, Dajani

LM. Beyond the Pump: A Narrative Study Exploring Heart Memory. Cureus. 2024 Apr 30;16(4):e59385. doi: 10.7759/cureus.59385. PMID: 38694651; PMCID: PMC11061817.

Al-Juhani A, Imran M, Aljaili ZK, Alzhrani MM, Alsalman RA, Ahmed M, Ali DK, Fallatah MI, Yousuf HM, Dajani LM. Beyond the Pump: A Narrative Study Exploring Heart Memory. Cureus. 2024 Apr 30;16(4):e59385. doi: 10.7759/cureus.59385. PMID: 38694651; PMCID: PMC11061817.

Almsherqi ZA. Potential Role of Plasmalogens in the Modulation of Biomembrane Morphology. Front Cell Dev Biol. 2021 Jul 21;9:673917. doi: 10.3389/fcell.2021.673917.

Almulla, A.F.; Thipakorn, Y.; Vasupanrajit, A.; Tunvirachaisakul, C.; Oxenkrug, G.; Al-Hakeim, H.K.; Maes, M. The Tryptophan Catabolite or Kynurenine Pathway in a Major Depressive Episode with Melancholia, Psychotic Features and Suicidal Behaviors: A Systematic Review and Meta-Analysis. Cells 2022, 11, 3112. https://doi.org/10.3390/cells11193112

Alsaleh G, Panse I, Swadling L, Zhang H, Richter FC, Meyer A, Lord J, Barnes E, Klenerman P, Green C, Simon AK. Autophagy in T cells from aged donors is maintained by spermidine and correlates with function and vaccine responses. Elife. 2020 Dec 15;9:e57950. doi: 10.7554/eLife.57950.

Alves I, Staneva G, Tessier C, Salgado GF, Nuss P. The interaction of antipsychotic drugs with lipids and subsequent lipid reorganization investigated using biophysical methods. Biochim Biophys Acta. 2011 Aug;1808(8):2009-18. doi: 10.1016/j.bbamem.2011.02.021

Amir, A., Headley, D. B., Lee, S.-C., Haufler, D., and Paré, D. (2018). Vigilance-Associated Gamma Oscillations Coordinate the Ensemble Activity of Basolateral Amygdala Neurons. Neuron 97, 656–669.e7. doi: 10.1016/j.neuron.2017.12.035

Amritwar AU, Lowry CA, Brenner LA, Hoisington AJ, Hamilton R, Stiller JW, Postolache TT. Mental Health in Allergic Rhinitis: Depression and Suicidal Behavior. Curr Treat Options Allergy. 2017 Mar;4(1):71-97. doi: 10.1007/s40521-017-0110-z

An S, Cho SY, Kang J, Lee S, Kim HS, Min DJ, Son E, Cho KH. Inhibition of 3-phosphoinositide-dependent protein kinase 1 (PDK1) can revert cellular senescence in human dermal fibroblasts. Proc Natl Acad Sci U S A. 2020 Dec 8;117(49):31535-31546. doi: 10.1073/pnas.1920338117. Epub 2020 Nov 23. PMID: 33229519; PMCID: PMC7733858.

Anderson AM, Ma Q, Letendre SL, Iudicello J. Soluble Biomarkers of Cognition and Depression in Adults with HIV Infection in the Combination Therapy Era. Curr HIV/AIDS Rep. 2021 Dec;18(6):558-568. doi: 10.1007/s11904-021-00581-y.

Andries O, Mc Cafferty S, De Smedt SC, Weiss R, Sanders NN, Kitada T. N(1)-methyl pseudouridine-incorporated mRNA outperforms pseudouridine-incorporated mRNA by providing enhanced protein expression and reduced immunogenicity in mammalian cell lines and mice. J Control Release. 2015 Nov 10;217:337-44. doi: 10.1016/j.jconrel.2015.08.051.

Anerillas C, Herman AB, Munk R, Garrido A, Lam KG, Payea MJ, Rossi M, Tsitsipatis D, Martindale JL, Piao Y, Mazan-Mamczarz K, Fan J, Cui CY, De S, Abdelmohsen K, de Cabo R, Gorospe M. A BDNF-TrkB autocrine loop enhances senescent cell viability. Nat Commun. 2022 Oct 20;13(1):6228. doi: 10.1038/s41467-022-33709-8. Erratum in: Nat Commun. 2022 Dec 7;13(1):7540. PMID: 36266274; PMCID: PMC9585019.

Angelucci F, Veverova K, Katonová A, Vyhnalek M, Hort J. Plasminogen activator inhibitor-1 serum levels in frontotemporal lobar degeneration. J Cell Mol Med. 2024 Feb 22;28(5):e18013. doi: 10.1111/jcmm.18013.

Antimisiaris SG, Mourtas S, Marazioti A. Exosomes and Exosome-Inspired Vesicles for Targeted Drug Delivery. Pharmaceutics. 2018 Nov 6;10(4):218. doi: 10.3390/pharmaceutics10040218.

Antonoudiou P, Tan YL, Kontou G, Upton AL, Mann EO. Parvalbumin and Somatostatin Interneurons Contribute to the Generation of Hippocampal Gamma Oscillations. J Neurosci. 2020 Sep 30;40(40):7668-7687. doi: 10.1523/JNEUROSCI.0261-20.2020.

Anzola AM, Trives L, Martínez-Barrio J, Pinilla B, Álvaro-Gracia JM, Molina-Collada J. New-onset giant cell arteritis following COVID-19 mRNA (BioNTech/Pfizer) vaccine: a double-edged sword?. Clin Rheumatol. 2022;41(5):1623-1625. doi:10.1007/s10067-021-06041-7

Arab JP, Sehrawat TS, Simonetto DA, Verma VK, Feng D, Tang T, Dreyer K, Yan X, Daley WL, Sanyal A, Chalasani N, Radaeva S, Yang L, Vargas H, Ibacache M, Gao B, Gores GJ, Malhi H, Kamath PS, Shah VH. An Open-Label, Dose-Escalation Study to Assess the Safety and Efficacy of IL-22 Agonist F-652 in Patients With Alcohol-associated Hepatitis. Hepatology. 2020 Aug;72(2):441-453. doi: 10.1002/hep.31046.

Arai S, Yamamoto H, Itoh K, Kumagai K. Suppressive effect of human natural killer cells on pokeweed mitogen-induced B cell differentiation. J Immunol. 1983 Aug;131(2):651-7. PMID: 6223088.

Arolt V, Weitzsch C, Wilke I, Nolte A, Pinnow M, Rothermundt M, Kirchner H. Production of interferon-gamma in families with multiple occurrence of schizophrenia. Psychiatry Res. 1997 Feb 7;66(2-3):145-52. doi: 10.1016/s0165-1781(96)03023-5

Arraki K, Totoson P, Decendit A, et al. Mammalian Arginase Inhibitory Activity of Methanolic Extracts and Isolated Compounds from Cyperus Species. Molecules. 2021;26(6):1694. Published 2021 Mar 18. doi:10.3390/molecules26061694

Arshad T, Mansur F, Palek R, Manzoor S, Liska V. A Double Edged Sword Role of Interleukin-22 in Wound Healing and Tissue Regeneration. Front Immunol. 2020 Sep 17;11:2148. doi: 10.3389/fimmu.2020.02148.

Artis, D., Spits, H. The biology of innate lymphoid cells. Nature 517, 293–301 (2015). https://doi.org/10.1038/nature14189

Arvola M, Keinänen K. Characterization of the ligand-binding domains of glutamate receptor (GluR)-B and GluR-D subunits expressed in Escherichia coli as periplasmic proteins. J Biol Chem. 1996 Jun 28;271(26):15527-32. doi: 10.1074/jbc.271.26.15527.

Arvola M, Keinänen K. Characterization of the ligand-bindingdomains of glutamate receptor (GluR)-B and GluR-D subunits expressed in Escherichia coli as periplasmic proteins. J Biol Chem.1996 Jun 28;271(26):15527-32. doi: 10.1074/jbc.271.26.15527.PMID: 8663017

Aujla SJ, Chan YR, Zheng M, Fei M, Askew DJ, Pociask DA, Reinhart TA, McAllister F, Edeal J, Gaus K, Husain S, Kreindler JL, Dubin PJ, Pilewski JM, Myerburg MM, Mason CA, Iwakura Y, Kolls JK. IL-22 mediates mucosal host defense against Gram-negative bacterial pneumonia. Nat Med. 2008 Mar;14(3):275-81. doi: 10.1038/nm1710.

Bae, M. - J., Shin, H. S., See, H. - J., Jung, S. Y., Kwon, D. - A., & Shon, D. - H. (2016). Baicalein induces CD4+Foxp3+ T cells and enhances intestinal barrier function in a mouse model of food allergy. Scientific Reports, 6(1), 32225. https://doi.org/10.1038/srep32225

Baharikhoob P, Kolla NJ. Microglial Dysregulation and Suicidality: A Stress-Diathesis Perspective. Front Psychiatry. 2020 Aug 11;11:781. doi: 10.3389/fpsyt.2020.00781.

Baker KE, Coller J. The many routes to regulating mRNA translation. Genome Biol. 2006;7(12):332. doi: 10.1186/gb-2006-7-12-332. PMID: 17176455; PMCID: PMC1794424.

Balasubramanian I, Faheem A, Padhy SK, Menon V. Psychiatric adverse reactions to COVID-19 vaccines: A rapid review of published case reports. Asian J Psychiatr. 2022 May;71:103129. doi: 10.1016/j.ajp.2022.103129.

Bao, C., Tao, X., Cui, W. et al. Natural killer cells associated with SARS-CoV-2 viral RNA shedding, antibody response and mortality in COVID-19 patients. Exp Hematol Oncol 10, 5 (2021). https://doi.org/10.1186/s40164-021-00199-1

Baranov MV, Olea RA, van den Bogaart G. Chasing Uptake: Super-Resolution Microscopy in Endocytosis and Phagocytosis. Trends Cell Biol. 2019 Sep;29(9):727-739. doi: 10.1016/j.tcb.2019.05.006.

Barichello T. The role of innate lymphoid cells (ILCs) in mental health. Discov Ment Health. 2022;2(1):2. doi: 10.1007/s44192-022-00006-1. Epub 2022 Feb 7. PMID: 35224555; PMCID: PMC8855986.

Barichello T. The role of innate lymphoid cells (ILCs) in mental health. Discov Ment Health. 2022;2(1):2. doi: 10.1007/s44192-022-00006-1.

Barrelle A, Luauté JP. Capgras Syndrome and Other Delusional Misidentification Syndromes. Front Neurol Neurosci. 2018;42:35-43. doi: 10.1159/000475680.

Barroso RP, Basso LG, Costa-Filho AJ. Interactions of the antimalarial amodiaquine with lipid model membranes. Chem Phys Lipids. 2015 Feb;186:68-78. doi: 10.1016/j.chemphyslip.2014.12.003.

Bartel L, Mosabbir A. Possible Mechanisms for the Effects of Sound Vibration on Human Health. Healthcare (Basel). 2021 May 18;9(5):597. doi: 10.3390/healthcare9050597. PMID: 34069792; PMCID: PMC8157227.

Bartels C, Wagner M, Wolfsgruber S, Ehrenreich H, Schneider A; Alzheimer's Disease Neuroimaging Initiative. Impact of SSRI Therapy on Risk of Conversion From Mild Cognitive Impairment to Alzheimer's Dementia in Individuals With Previous Depression. Am J Psychiatry. 2018 Mar 1;175(3):232-241. doi: 10.1176/appi.ajp.2017.17040404. Epub 2017 Nov 28. PMID: 29179578.

Barthelemy A, Sencio V, Soulard D, Deruyter L, Faveeuw C, Le Goffic R, Trottein F. Interleukin-22 Immunotherapy during Severe Influenza Enhances Lung Tissue Integrity and Reduces Secondary Bacterial Systemic Invasion. Infect Immun. 2018 Jun 21;86(7):e00706-17. doi: 10.1128/IAI.00706-17.

Başar E. A review of gamma oscillations in healthy subjects and in cognitive impairment. Int J Psychophysiol. 2013 Nov;90(2):99-117. doi: 10.1016/j.ijpsycho.2013.07.005

Batista-Duharte A, Pera A, Aliño SF, Solana R. Regulatory T cells and vaccine effectiveness in older adults. Challenges and prospects. Int Immunopharmacol. 2021 Jul;96:107761. doi: 10.1016/j.intimp.2021.107761

Battistelli M, Falcieri E. Apoptotic Bodies: Particular Extracellular Vesicles Involved in Intercellular Communication. Biology (Basel). 2020 Jan 20;9(1):21. doi: 10.3390/biology9010021. PMID: 31968627; PMCID: PMC7168913.

Baumeister D, Ciufolini S, Mondelli V. Effects of psychotropic drugs on inflammation: consequence or mediator of therapeutic effects in psychiatric treatment? Psychopharmacology (Berl). 2016 May;233(9):1575-89. doi: 10.1007/s00213-015-4044-5.

Bayraktar İ, Yalçın N, Demirkan K. The potential interaction between COVID-19 vaccines and clozapine: A novel approach for clinical trials. Int J Clin Pract. 2021 Aug;75(8):e14441. doi: 10.1111/ijcp.14441. PMID: 34289643; PMCID: PMC8420459.

Bazargani N, Attwell D. Astrocyte calcium signaling: the third wave. Nat Neurosci. 2016 Feb;19(2):182-9. doi: 10.1038/nn.4201. PMID: 26814587.

Beaulieu JM, Zhang X, Rodriguiz RM, Sotnikova TD, Cools MJ, Wetsel WC, Gainetdinov RR, Caron MG. Role of GSK3 beta in behavioral abnormalities induced by serotonin deficiency. Proc Natl Acad Sci U S A. 2008 Jan 29;105(4):1333-8. doi: 10.1073/pnas.0711496105.

Bellavite P, Fazio S, Affuso F. A Descriptive Review of the Action Mechanisms of Berberine, Quercetin and Silymarin on Insulin Resistance/Hyperinsulinemia and Cardiovascular Prevention. Molecules. 2023 Jun 1;28(11):4491. doi: 10.3390/molecules28114491. PMID: 37298967; PMCID: PMC10254920.

Benedetti F, Riccaboni R, Dallaspezia S, Locatelli C, Smeraldi E, Colombo C. Effects of CLOCK gene variants and early stress on hopelessness and suicide in bipolar depression. Chronobiol Int. 2015;32(8):1156-61. doi: 10.3109/07420528.2015.1060603.

Benne N, Leboux RJT, Glandrup M, van Duijn J, Lozano Vigario F, Neustrup MA, Romeijn S, Galli F, Kuiper J, Jiskoot W, Slütter B. Atomic force microscopy measurements of anionic liposomes reveal the effect of liposomal rigidity on antigen-specific regulatory T cell responses. J Control Release. 2020 Feb;318:246-255. doi: 10.1016/j.jconrel.2019.12.003.

Benne N, van Duijn J, Lozano Vigario F, Leboux RJT, van Veelen P, Kuiper J, et al. Anionic 1,2-distearoyl-sn-glycero-3-phosphoglycerol (DSPG) liposomes induce antigen-specific regulatory T cells and prevent atherosclerosis in mice. J Control Release. (2018) 291:135-146. doi: 10.1016/j.jconrel.2018.10.028.

Bergwerk M, Gonen T, Lustig Y, Amit S, Lipsitch M, Cohen C, et al. Covid-19 Breakthrough Infections in Vaccinated Health Care Workers. N Engl J Med. 2021 Oct 14;385(16):1474-1484. doi: 10.1056/NEJMoa2109072.

Beri K. A future perspective for regenerative medicine: understanding the concept of vibrational medicine. Future

Sci OA. 2018 Jan 5;4(3):FSO274. doi: 10.4155/fsoa-2017-0097. PMID: 29568563; PMCID: PMC5859346.

Beristianos MH, Yaffe K, Cohen B, Byers AL. PTSD and Risk of Incident Cardiovascular Disease in Aging Veterans. Am J Geriatr Psychiatry. 2016 Mar;24(3):192-200. doi: 10.1016/j.jagp.2014.12.003. Epub 2014 Dec 9. PMID: 25555625.

Bernot D, Stalin J, Stocker P, Bonardo B, Scroyen I, Alessi MC, Peiretti F. Plasminogen activator inhibitor 1 is an intracellular inhibitor of furin proprotein convertase. J Cell Sci. 2011 Apr 15;124(Pt 8):1224-30. doi: 10.1242/jcs.079889.

Bernstein CN, Hitchon CA, Walld R, Bolton JM, Sareen J, Walker JR, Graff LA, Patten SB, Singer A, Lix LM, El-Gabalawy R, Katz A, Fisk JD, Marrie RA; CIHR Team in Defining the Burden and Managing the Effects of Psychiatric Comorbidity in Chronic Immunoinflammatory Disease. Increased Burden of Psychiatric Disorders in Inflammatory Bowel Disease. Inflamm Bowel Dis. 2019 Jan 10;25(2):360-368. doi: 10.1093/ibd/izy235.

Bernstein CN, Hitchon CA, Walld R, Bolton JM, Sareen J, Walker JR, Graff LA, Patten SB, Singer A, Lix LM, El-Gabalawy R, Katz A, Fisk JD, Marrie RA; CIHR Team in Defining the Burden and Managing the Effects of Psychiatric Comorbidity in Chronic Immunoinflammatory Disease. Increased Burden of Psychiatric Disorders in Inflammatory Bowel Disease. Inflamm Bowel Dis. 2019 Jan 10;25(2):360-368. doi: 10.1093/ibd/izy235.

Beskow LM. Lessons from HeLa Cells: The Ethics and Policy of Biospecimens. Annu Rev Genomics Hum Genet. 2016 Aug 31;17:395-417. doi: 10.1146/annurev-genom-083115-022536. Epub 2016 Mar 3. PMID: 26979405; PMCID: PMC5072843.

Besserve M, Lowe SC, Logothetis NK, Schölkopf B, Panzeri S. Shifts of Gamma Phase across Primary Visual Cortical Sites Reflect Dynamic Stimulus-Modulated Information Transfer. PLOS Biology. 2015;13:e1002257. doi: 10.1371/journal.pbio.1002257.

Beutheu Youmba S, Belmonte L, Galas L, Boukhettala N, Bôle-Feysot C, Déchelotte P, Coëffier M. Methotrexate modulates tight junctions through NF-κB, MEK, and JNK pathways. J Pediatr Gastroenterol Nutr. 2012 Apr;54(4):463-70. doi: 10.1097/MPG.0b013e318247240d.

Bhattacharyya B, Wolff J. Stabilization of microtubules by lithium lithium-ion. Biochem Biophys Res Commun. 1976 Nov 22;73(2):383-90. doi: 10.1016/0006-291x(76)90719-1. PMID: 826253.

Bilinski K, Byth K, Boyages J.Association between Latitude and Breast Cancer Incidence in Mainland Australian Women. Journal of Cancer Research (2014) Volume 2014 | Article ID 149865 | https://doi.org/10.1155/2014/149865

Bindoli A, Rigobello MP, Favel A, Galzigna L. Antioxidant action and photosensitizing effects of three different chlorpromazines. J Neurochem. 1988 Jan;50(1):138-41. doi: 10.1111/j.1471-4159.1988.tb13240.x. PMID: 3335839.

Birge RB, Boeltz S, Kumar S, Carlson J, Wanderley J, Calianese D, et al. Phosphatidylserine is a global immunosuppressive signal in efferocytosis, infectious disease, and cancer. Cell Death Differ. 2016 Jun;23(6):962-78. doi: 10.1038/cdd.2016.11.

Birge, R., Boeltz, S., Kumar, S. et al. Phosphatidylserine is a global immunosuppressive signal in efferocytosis, infectious disease, and cancer. Cell Death Differ 23, 962–978 (2016). https://doi.org/10.1038/cdd.2016.11

Björkstén, K.S., Kripke, D.F. & Bjerregaard, P. Accentuation of suicides but not homicides with rising latitudes of Greenland in the sunny months. BMC Psychiatry 9, 20 (2009). https://doi.org/10.1186/1471-244X-9-20

Blalock, Z.N., Wu, G.W.Y., Lindqvist, D. et al. Circulating cell-free mitochondrial DNA levels and glucocorticoid sensitivity in a cohort of male veterans with and without combat-related PTSD. Transl Psychiatry 14, 22 (2024). https://doi.org/10.1038/s41398-023-02721-x

Blanco-Duque C, Chan D, Kahn MC, Murdock MH, Tsai L-H. Audiovisual gamma stimulation for the treatment of neurodegeneration. J Intern Med. 2024; 295: 146–170.

Bocchetta A. Psychotic mania in glucose-6-phosphate-dehydrogenase-deficient subjects. Ann Gen Hosp Psychiatry. 2003;2(1):6. Published 2003 Jun 13. doi:10.1186/1475-2832-2-6

Boccuto L, Chen CF, Pittman AR, Skinner CD, McCartney HJ, Jones K, Bochner BR, Stevenson RE, Schwartz CE.

Decreased tryptophan metabolism in patients with autism spectrum disorders. Mol Autism. 2013 Jun 3;4(1):16. doi: 10.1186/2040-2392-4-16.

Bohan D, Ert HV, Ruggio N, Rogers KJ, Badreddine M, Aguilar Briseño JA, et al. Phosphatidylserine Receptors Enhance SARS-CoV-2 Infection: AXL as a Therapeutic Target for COVID-19. bioRxiv [Preprint]. 2021 Jun 24:2021.06.15.448419. doi: 10.1101/2021.06.15.448419. Update in: PLoS Pathog. 2021 Nov 19;17(11):e1009743. PMID: 34159331; PMCID: PMC8219095.

Borovcanin MM, Minic Janicijevic S, Jovanovic IP, Gajovic NM, Jurisevic MM, Arsenijevic NN. Type 17 Immune Response Facilitates Progression of Inflammation and Correlates with Cognition in Stable Schizophrenia. Diagnostics (Basel). 2020 Nov 10;10(11):926. doi: 10.3390/diagnostics10110926.

Borovikova, L.V.; Ivanova, S.; Zhang, M.; Yang, H.; Botchkina, G.I.; Watkins, L.R.; Wang, H.; Abumrad, N.; Eaton, J.W.; Tracey, K.J. Vagus nerve stimulation attenuates the systemic inflammatory response to endotoxin. Nature 2000, 405, 458–462. [Google Scholar] [CrossRef]

Bouarab, C., Roullot-Lacarrière, V., Vallée, M. et al. PAI-1 protein is a key molecular effector in the transition from normal to PTSD-like fear memory. Mol Psychiatry 26, 4968–4981 (2021). https://doi.org/10.1038/s41380-021-01024-1

Bouarab, C., Roullot-Lacarrière, V., Vallée, M. et al. PAI-1 protein is a key molecular effector in the transition from normal to PTSD-like fear memory. Mol Psychiatry 26, 4968–4981 (2021). https://doi.org/10.1038/s41380-021-01024-1

Boule, L.A.; Burke, C.G.; Jin, G.-B.; Lawrence, B.P. Aryl hydrocarbon receptor signaling modulates antiviral immune responses: Ligand metabolism rather than chemical source is the stronger predictor of outcome. Sci. Rep. 2018, 8, 1826.

Bourgin M, Derosa L, Silva CAC, Goubet AG, Dubuisson A, et al. Circulating acetylated polyamines correlate with Covid-19 severity in cancer patients. Aging (Albany NY). 2021 Sep 13;13(17):20860-20885. doi: 10.18632/aging.203525

Breier A. 39. VIRUSES AND SCHIZOPHRENIA: IMPLICATIONS FOR PATHOPHYSIOLOGY AND TREATMENT. Schizophr Bull. 2018;44(Suppl 1):S61-S62. doi:10.1093/schbul/sby014.158

Brest P, Mograbi B, Hofman P, Milano G. COVID-19 vaccination and cancer immunotherapy: should they stick together? Br J Cancer. 2022 Jan;126(1):1-3. doi: 10.1038/s41416-021-01618-0.

Brieva JA, Targan S, Stevens RH. NK and T cell subsets regulate antibody production by human in vivo antigen-induced lymphoblastoid B cells. J Immunol. 1984 Feb;132(2):611-5. PMID: 6228592.

Brock DJ, Kondow-McConaghy HM, Hager EC, Pellois JP. Endosomal Escape and Cytosolic Penetration of Macromolecules Mediated by Synthetic Delivery Agents.

Bioconjug Chem. 2019 Feb 20;30(2):293-304. doi: 10.1021/acs.bioconjchem.8b00799.

Brown AS, Begg MD, Gravenstein S, Schaefer CA, Wyatt RJ, Bresnahan M, Babulas VP, Susser ES. Serologic evidence of prenatal influenza in the etiology of schizophrenia. Arch Gen Psychiatry. 2004 Aug;61(8):774-780. doi: 10.1001/archpsyc.61.8.774. PMID: 15289276.

Brundin, L., Bryleva, E. & Thirtamara Rajamani, K. Role of Inflammation in Suicide: From Mechanisms to Treatment. Neuropsychopharmacol 42, 271–283 (2017). https://doi.org/10.1038/npp.2016.116

Buchholz U, Bernard H, Werber D, Böhmer MM, Remschmidt C, Wilking H, Deleré Y, an der Heiden M, Adlhoch C, Dreesman J, Ehlers J, Ethelberg S, Faber M, Frank C, Fricke G, Greiner M, Höhle M, Ivarsson S, Jark U, Kirchner M, Koch J, Krause G, Luber P, Rosner B, Stark K, Kühne M. German outbreak of Escherichia coli O104:H4 associated with sprouts. N Engl J Med. 2011 Nov 10;365(19):1763-70. doi: 10.1056/NEJMoa1106482.

Buchrieser, J.; Dufloo, J.; et al. Syncytia Formation by SARS-CoV-2-infected Cells. EMBO J 2020, 39 (23). https://doi.org/10.15252/embj.2020106267

Bunzel B, Schmidl-Mohl B, Grundböck A, Wollenek G. Does changing the heart mean changing personality? A retrospective inquiry on 47 heart transplant patients. Qual Life Res. 1992 Aug;1(4):251-6. doi: 10.1007/BF00435634. PMID: 1299456.

Burkhardt, C., Kelly, J. P., Lim, Y. H., Filley, C. M. & Parker, W. D. Jr. Neuroleptic medications inhibit complex I of the electron transport chain. Ann. Neurol. 33, 512–517 (1993).

Burton, D. G. A.; Krizhanovsky, V. Physiological and Pathological Consequences of Cellular Senescence. Cellular and Molecular Life Sciences 2014, 71 (22), 4373–4386. https://doi.org/10.1007/s00018-014-1691-3.

Caetano-Silva, M.E., Rund, L., Hutchinson, N.T. et al. Inhibition of inflammatory microglia by dietary fiber and short-chain fatty acids. Sci Rep 13,

Cahn, W.; Pol HE, H.; Lems, E.B.; van Haren, N.E.; Schnack, H.G.; van der Linden, J.A.; Schothorst, P.F.; van Engeland, H.; Kahn, R.S. Brain volume changes in first-episode schizophrenia: A 1-year follow-up study. Arch. Gen. Psychiatry 2002, 59, 1002–1010

Cai LF, Wang SB, Hou CL, Li ZB, Liao YJ, Jia FJ. Association Between Non-Suicidal Self-Injury and Gut Microbial Characteristics in Chinese Adolescents. Neuropsychiatr Dis Treat. 2022 Jul 1;18:1315-1328. doi: 10.2147/NDT.S360588.

Calamassi D, Pomponi GP. Music Tuned to 440 Hz Versus 432 Hz and the Health Effects: A Double-blind Cross-over Pilot Study. Explore (NY). 2019 Jul-Aug;15(4):283-290. doi: 10.1016/j.explore.2019.04.001. Epub 2019 Apr 6. Erratum in: Explore (NY). 2020 Jan - Feb;16(1):8. PMID: 31031095.

Calcutt NA, Smith DR, Frizzi K, Sabbir MG, Chowdhury SK, Mixcoatl-Zecuatl T, et al. Selective antagonism of muscarinic receptors is neuroprotective in peripheral neuropathy. J Clin Invest. 2017 Feb 1;127(2):608-622. doi: 10.1172/JCI88321. Epub 2017 Jan 17. PMID: 28094765; PMCID: PMC5272197.

Caldara M, Marmiroli N. Antimicrobial Properties of Antidepressants and Antipsychotics-Possibilities and Implications. Pharmaceuticals (Basel). 2021 Sep 10;14(9):915. doi: 10.3390/ph14090915. PMID: 34577614; PMCID: PMC8470654.

Canfrán-Duque A, Barrio LC, Lerma M, de la Peña G, Serna J, Pastor O,. First-Generation Antipsychotic Haloperidol Alters the Functionality of the Late Endosomal/Lysosomal Compartment in Vitro. Int J Mol Sci. 2016 Mar 18;17(3):404. doi: 10.3390/ijms17030404.

Cao L, Thut G, Gross J. The role of brain oscillations in predicting self-generated sounds. Neuroimage. 2017 Feb 15;147:895-903. doi: 10.1016/j.neuroimage.2016.11.001. Epub 2016 Nov 3. PMID: 27818209; PMCID: PMC5315057.

Cao Y, Gao GF. mRNA vaccines: A matter of delivery. EClinicalMedicine. 2021 Feb 3;32:100746. doi: 10.1016/j.eclinm.2021.100746. PMID: 33644722

Carbon CC. Wearing Face Masks Strongly Confuses Counterparts in Reading Emotions. Front Psychol. 2020 Sep 25;11:566886. doi: 10.3389/fpsyg.2020.566886.

Cardon I, Grobecker S, Jenne F, Jahner T, Rupprecht R, Milenkovic VM, Wetzel CH. Serotonin effects on human iPSC-derived neural cell functions: from mitochondria to depression. Mol Psychiatry. 2024 Mar 26. doi: 10.1038/s41380-024-02538-0.

Carlberg C, Velleuer E. Vitamin D and the risk for cancer: A molecular analysis. Biochem Pharmacol. 2022 Feb;196:114735. doi: 10.1016/j.bcp.2021.114735.

Carneiro-Filho BA, Lima IP, Araujo DH, Cavalcante MC, Carvalho GH, Brito GA, Lima V, Monteiro SM, Santos FN, Ribeiro RA, Lima AA. Intestinal barrier function and secretion in methotrexate-induced rat intestinal mucositis. Dig Dis Sci. 2004 Jan;49(1):65-72. doi: 10.1023/b:ddas.0000011604.45531.2c. PMID: 14992437.

Carneiro-Filho BA, Lima IP, Araujo DH, Cavalcante MC,Carvalho GH, Brito GA, Lima V, Monteiro SM, Santos FN, RibeiroRA, Lima AA. Intestinal barrier function and secretion in methotrexate-induced rat intestinal mucositis. Dig Dis Sci. 2004Jan;49(1):65-72. doi: 10.1023/b:ddas.0000011604.45531.2c.

Carragher DJ, Hancock PJB. Surgical face masks impair human face matching performance for familiar and unfamiliar faces. Cogn Res Princ Implic. 2020 Nov 19;5(1):59. doi: 10.1186/s41235-020- 00258-x.

Carter, B.; Khoshnaw, L.; Simmons, M.; Hines, L.; Wolfe, B.; Liester, M. Personality Changes Associated with Organ Transplants. Transplantology 2024, 5, 12-26. https://doi.org/10.3390/transplantology5010002

Caspani G, Kennedy S, Foster JA, Swann J. Gut microbial metabolites in depression: understanding the biochemical mechanisms. Microb Cell. 2019 Sep 27;6(10):454-481. doi: 10.15698/mic2019.10.693.

Cavaliere, F., Fornarelli, A., Bertan, F. et al. The tricyclic antidepressant clomipramine inhibits neuronal autophagic flux. Sci Rep 9, 4881 (2019). https://doi.org/10.1038/s41598-019-40887-x

Cefis, M., Chaney, R., Quirié, A. et al. Endothelial cells are an important source of BDNF in rat skeletal muscle. Sci Rep 12, 311 (2022). https://doi.org/10.1038/s41598-021-03740-8.

Cella M, Fuchs A, Vermi W, Facchetti F, Otero K, Lennerz JK, Doherty JM, Mills JC, Colonna M. A human natural killer cell subset provides an innate source of IL-22 for mucosal immunity. Colonna M. Interleukin-22-producing natural killer cells and lymphoid tissue inducer-like cells in mucosal immunity. Immunity. 2009 Jul 17;31(1):15-23. doi: 10.1016/j.immuni.2009.06.008. Nature. 2009 Feb 5;457(7230):722-5. doi: 10.1038/nature07537. Epub 2008 Nov 2.

Cenik B, Cenik C, Snyder MP, Brown ES. Plasma sterols and depressive symptom severity in a population-based cohort. PLoS One. 2017 Sep 8;12(9):e0184382. doi: 10.1371/journal.pone.0184382. PMID: 28886149; PMCID: PMC5590924.

Cham S, Koslik HJ, Golomb BA. Mood, Personality, and Behavior Changes During Treatment with Statins: A Case

Series. Drug Saf Case Rep. 2016 Dec;3(1):1. doi: 10.1007/s40800-015-0024-2. PMID: 27747681; PMCID: PMC5005588.

Chambers ES, Preston T, Frost G, Morrison DJ. Role of gut microbiota-generated short-chain fatty acids in metabolic and cardiovascular health. Curr Nutr Rep. (2018) 7:198–206. 10.1007/s13668-018-0248-8

Chan D, Suk HJ, Jackson BL, Milman NP, Stark D, Klerman EB, Kitchener E, Fernandez Avalos VS, de Weck G, Banerjee A, Beach SD, et al. Gamma frequency sensory stimulation in mild probable Alzheimer's dementia patients: Results of feasibility and pilot studies. PLoS One. 2022 Dec 1;17(12):e0278412. doi: 10.1371/journal.pone.0278412.

Chan ST, McCarthy MJ, Vawter MP. Psychiatric drugs impact mitochondrial function in the brain and other tissues. Schizophr Res. 2020 Mar;217:136-147. doi: 10.1016/j.schres.2019.09.007

Chandrasekaran V, Juszkiewicz S, Choi J, Puglisi JD, Brown A, Shao S, Ramakrishnan V, Hegde RS. Mechanism of ribosome stalling during translation of a poly(A) tail. Nat Struct Mol Biol. 2019 Dec;26(12):1132-1140. doi: 10.1038/s41594-019-0331-x.

Chang CC, Wu M, Yuan F. Role of specific endocytic pathways in electrotransfection of cells. Mol Ther Methods Clin Dev. 2014 Dec 17;1:14058. doi: 10.1038/mtm.2014.58.

Chaurio RA, Janko C, Muñoz LE, Frey B, Herrmann M, Gaipl US. Phospholipids: key players in apoptosis and immune regulation. Molecules. 2009 Nov 30;14(12):4892-914. doi: 10.3390/molecules14124892

Chawla G, Azharuddin M, Ahmad I, Hussain ME. Effect of Whole-body Vibration on Depression, Anxiety, Stress, and Quality of Life in College Students: A Randomized Controlled Trial. Oman Med J. 2022 Jul 31;37(4):e408. doi: 10.5001/omj.2022.72.

Cheemala A, Kimble AL, Tyburski JD, Leclair NK, Zuberi AR, Murphy M, Jellison ER, Reese B, Hu X, Lutz CM, Yan R, Murphy PA. Loss of Endothelial TDP-43 Leads to Blood Brain Barrier Defects in Mouse Models of Amyotrophic Lateral Sclerosis and Frontotemporal Dementia. bioRxiv [Preprint]. 2023 Dec 14:2023.12.13.571184. doi: 10.1101/2023.12.13.571184.

Chen BY, Hsu CC, Chen YZ, Lin JJ, Tseng HH, Jang FL, Chen PS, Chen WN, Chen CS, Lin SH. Profiling antibody signature of schizophrenia by Escherichia coli proteome microarrays. Brain Behav Immun. 2022 Nov;106:11-20. doi: 10.1016/j.bbi.2022.07.162.

Chen CM, Stanford AD, Mao X, Abi-Dargham A, Shungu DC, Lisanby SH, Schroeder CE, Kegeles LS. GABA level, gamma oscillation, and working memory performance in schizophrenia. Neuroimage Clin. 2014 Mar 20;4:531-9. doi: 10.1016/j.nicl.2014.03.007

Chen LY, Qi J, Xu HL, Lin XY, Sun YJ, Ju SQ. The Value of Serum Cell-Free DNA Levels in Patients With Schizophrenia. Front Psychiatry. 2021 Mar 30;12:637789. doi: 10.3389/fpsyt.2021.637789.

Chen S, Aruldass AR, Cardinal RN. Mental health outcomes after SARS-CoV-2 vaccination in the United States: A national cross-sectional study. J Affect Disord. 2022 Feb 1;298(Pt A):396-399. doi: 10.1016/j.jad.2021.10.134.

Chen X, Winstead A, Yu H, Peng J. Taccalonolides: A Novel Class of Microtubule-Stabilizing Anticancer Agents. Cancers (Basel). 2021 Feb 22;13(4):920. doi: 10.3390/cancers13040920. PMID: 33671665; PMCID: PMC7926778.

Chen X, Zhao HX, Bai C, Zhou XY. Blockade of high-mobility group box 1 attenuates intestinal mucosal barrier dysfunction in experimental acute pancreatitis. Sci Rep. 2017 Jul 28;7(1):6799. doi: 10.1038/s41598-017-07094-y.

Chen, Xi, Wang, Z., Zheng, P., Dongol, A., Xie, Y., Ge, X., Zheng, M., Dang, X., Seyhan, Z. B., Nagaratnam, N., Yu, Y., & Huang, X.-F. (2023). Impaired mitophagosome–lysosome fusion mediates olanzapine-induced aging. Aging Cell, 22, e14003. https://doi.org/10.1111/acel.14003

Cheng Y, Wang T, Zhang T, Yi S, Zhao S, Li N, Yang Y, Zhang F, Xu L, Shan B, Xu X, Xu J. Increased Blood-Brain Barrier Permeability of the Thalamus Correlated With Symptom Severity and Brain Volume Alterations in Patients With Schizophrenia. Biol Psychiatry Cogn Neurosci Neuroimaging. 2022 Oct;7(10):1025-1034. doi: 10.1016/j.bpsc.2022.06.006.

Chesnokova V, Zonis S, Apostolou A, Estrada HQ, Knott S, Wawrowsky K, Michelsen K, Ben-Shlomo A, Barrett R, Gorbunova V, Karalis K, Melmed S. Local non-pituitary growth hormone is induced with aging and facilitates epithelial damage. Cell Rep. 2021 Dec 14;37(11):110068. doi: 10.1016/j.celrep.2021.110068. PMID: 34910915

Chester DS, Lynam DR, Milich R, DeWall CN. Physical aggressiveness and gray matter deficits in ventromedial prefrontal cortex. Cortex. 2017 Dec;97:17-22. doi: 10.1016/j.cortex.2017.09.024. Epub 2017 Oct 7. PMID: 29073459; PMCID: PMC5716918.

Chou T. Stochastic entry of enveloped viruses: fusion versus endocytosis. Biophys J. 2007;93(4):1116-1123. doi:10.1529/biophysj.107.106708

Choy O. Nutritional factors associated with aggression. Front Psychiatry. 2023 Jun 21;14:1176061. doi: 10.3389/fpsyt.2023.1176061. PMID: 37415691; PMCID: PMC10320003.

Chuprin, A.; Gal, H.; et al. Cell Fusion Induced by ERVWE1 or Measles Virus Causes Cellular Senescence. Genes Dev 2013, 27 (21), 2356–2366. https://doi.org/10.1101/gad.227512.113.

Clark MA, Shay JW. Mitochondrial transformation of mammalian cells. Nature. (1982) 295:605–7. doi: 10.1038/295605a0

Clemente GS, van Waarde A, F Antunes I, Dömling A, H Elsinga P. Arginase as a Potential Biomarker of Disease Progression: A Molecular Imaging Perspective. Int J Mol Sci. 2020 Jul 25;21(15):5291. doi: 10.3390/ijms21155291. PMID: 32722521; PMCID: PMC7432485.

Colonna M. Interleukin-22-producing natural killer cells and lymphoid tissue inducer-like cells in mucosal immunity. Immunity. 2009 Jul 17;31(1):15-23. doi: 10.1016/j.immuni.2009.06.008. PMID: 19604490.

Congdon, E.E.; Wu, J.W.; Myeku, N.; Figueroa, Y.H.; Herman, M.; Marinec, P.S.; Gestwicki, J.E.; Dickey, C.A.; Yu, W.H.; Duff, K.E. Methylthioninium chloride (methylene blue) induces autophagy and attenuates tauopathy in vitro and in vivo. Autophagy 2012, 8, 609–622.

Coppé JP, Desprez PY, Krtolica A, Campisi J. The senescence-associated secretory phenotype: the dark side of tumor suppression. Annu Rev Pathol. 2010;5:99-118. doi: 10.1146/annurev-pathol-121808-102144.

Correia-Melo C, Marques FDM, Anderson R, Hewitt G, Hewitt R, Cole J, Carroll BM, Miwa S, Birch J, Merz A, Rushton MD, Charles M, Jurk D, Tait SWG, Czapiewski R, Greaves L, Nelson G, Bohlooly-Y M, Rodriguez-Cuenca S, Vidal-Puig A, Mann D, Saretzki G, Quarato G, Green DR, Adams PD, von Zglinicki T, Korolchuk VI & Passos JF (2016) Mitochondria are required for pro-ageing features of the senescent phenotype. EMBO J 35, 724–42

Corsi-Zuelli F, Deakin B, de Lima MHF, Qureshi O, Barnes NM, Upthegrove R, Louzada-Junior P, Del-Ben CM. T regulatory cells as a potential therapeutic target in psychosis? Current challenges and future perspectives. Brain Behav Immun Health. 2021 Aug 19;17:100330. doi: 10.1016/j.bbih.2021.100330.

Coughlin SS. Anxiety and Depression: Linkages with Viral Diseases. Public Health Rev. 2012;34(2):7. doi:10.1007/BF03391675

Craddock TJ, Tuszynski JA, Hameroff S. Cytoskeletal signaling: is memory encoded in microtubule lattices by CaMKII phosphorylation? PLoS Comput Biol. 2012;8(3):e1002421. doi: 10.1371/journal.pcbi.1002421. Epub 2012 Mar 8. PMID: 22412364; PMCID: PMC3297561

Craddock TJ, Tuszynski JA, Hameroff S. Cytoskeletal signaling: is memory encoded in microtubule lattices by CaMKII phosphorylation? PLoS Comput Biol. 2012;8(3):e1002421. doi: 10.1371/journal.pcbi.1002421. Epub 2012 Mar 8. PMID: 22412364; PMCID: PMC3297561.

Critchley, H.D.; Wiens, S.; Rotshtein, P.; Öhman, A.; Dolan, R.J. Neural systems supporting interoceptive awareness. Nat. Neurosci. 2004, 7, 189–195. [Google Scholar] [CrossRef] [Green Version]

Crockett MJ, Clark L, Hauser MD, Robbins TW. Serotonin selectively influences moral judgment and behavior through effects on harm aversion. Proc Natl Acad Sci U S A. 2010 Oct 5;107(40):17433-8. doi: 10.1073/pnas.1009396107.

Cullis PR, Hope MJ. Lipid Nanoparticle Systems for Enabling Gene Therapies. Mol Ther. 2017 Jul 5;25(7):1467-1475. doi: 10.1016/j.ymthe.2017.03.013

d'Adda di Fagagna, F. Living on a break: cellular senescence as a DNA-damage response. Nat Rev Cancer 8, 512–522 (2008). https://doi.org/10.1038/nrc2440

Dagorn A, Chapalain A, Mijouin L, Hillion M, Duclairoir-Poc C, Chevalier S, Taupin L, Orange N, Feuilloley MG. Effect of GABA, a bacterial metabolite, on Pseudomonas fluorescens surface properties and cytotoxicity. Int J Mol Sci. 2013 Jun 6;14(6):12186-204. doi: 10.3390/ijms140612186.

Damasio, A.; Damasio, H.; Tranel, D. Persistence of Feelings and Sentience after Bilateral Damage of the Insula. Cereb. Cortex 2012, 23, 833–846. [Google Scholar] [CrossRef] [Green Version]

D'Ambrosi N, Milani M, Apolloni S. S100A4 in the Physiology and Pathology of the Central and Peripheral Nervous System. Cells. 2021;10(4):798. Published 2021 Apr 2. doi:10.3390/cells10040798

Dang X, Hanson BA, Orban ZS, Jimenez M, Suchy S, Koralnik IJ. Characterization of the brain virome in human immunodeficiency virus infection and substance use disorder. PLoS One. 2024 Apr 17;19(4):e0299891. doi: 10.1371/journal.pone.0299891. PMID: 38630782; PMCID: PMC11023569.

Dang Y, An Y, He J, Huang B, Zhu J, Gao M, Zhang S, Wang X, Yang B, Xie Z. Berberine ameliorates cellular senescence and extends the lifespan of mice via regulating p16 and cyclin protein expression. Aging Cell. 2020 Jan;19(1):e13060. doi: 10.1111/acel.13060.

Daniel WA. Mechanisms of cellular distribution of psychotropic drugs. Significance for drug action and interactions. Prog Neuropsychopharmacol Biol Psychiatry. 2003 Feb;27(1):65-73. doi: 10.1016/s0278-5846(02)00317-2. PMID: 12551728.

Das S, St Croix C, Good M, Chen J, Zhao J, Hu S, Ross M, Myerburg MM, Pilewski JM, Williams J, Wenzel SE, Kolls JK, Ray A, Ray P. Interleukin-22 Inhibits Respiratory Syncytial Virus Production by Blocking Virus-Mediated Subversion of Cellular Autophagy. iScience. 2020 Jul 24;23(7):101256. doi: 10.1016/j.isci.2020.101256.

Davis GE, Lowell WE. Evidence that latitude is directly related to variation in suicide rates. Can J Psychiatry. 2002 Aug;47(6):572-4. doi: 10.1177/070674370204700611.

Davis ZW, Muller L, Martinez-Trujillo J, Sejnowski T, Reynolds JH. Spontaneous travelling cortical waves gate perception in behaving primates. Nature. 2020;587:432–436. doi: 10.1038/s41586-020-2802-y.

de De Souza Cardoso R, Viana RMM, Vitti BC, Coelho ACL, de Jesus BLS, de Paula Souza J, Pontelli MC, Murakami T, Ventura AM, Ono A, Arruda E. Human Respiratory Syncytial Virus Infection in a Human T Cell Line Is Hampered at Multiple Steps. Viruses. 2021 Feb 2;13(2):231. doi: 10.3390/v13020231

de la Monte SM. Triangulated mal-signaling in Alzheimer's disease: roles of neurotoxic ceramides, ER stress, and insulin resistance reviewed. J Alzheimers Dis. 2012;30 Suppl 2(0 2):S231-49. doi: 10.3233/JAD-2012-111727.

De Renzi E, Perani D, Carlesimo GA, Silveri MC, Fazio F. Prosopagnosia can be associated with damage confined to the right hemisphere--an MRI and PET study and a review of the literature. Neuropsychologia. 1994 Aug;32(8):893-902. doi: 10.1016/0028-3932(94)90041-8.

de Ronchi D, Faranca I, Forti P, Ravaglia G, Borderi M, Manfredi R, Volterra V. Development of acute psychotic disorders and HIV-1 infection. Int J Psychiatry Med. 2000;30(2):173-83. doi: 10.2190/PLGX-N48F-RBHJ-UF8K. PMID: 11001280.

Dean B, Laws SM, Hone E, Taddei K, Scarr E, Thomas EA, et al. Increased levels of apolipoprotein E in the frontal cortex of subjects with schizophrenia. Biol Psychiatry. 2003 Sep 15;54(6):616-22. doi: 10.1016/s0006-3223(03)00075-1

Dean MJ, Ochoa JB, Sanchez-Pino MD, Zabaleta J, Garai J, Del Valle L, et al. Severe COVID-19 Is Characterized by an Impaired Type I Interferon Response and Elevated Levels of Arginase Producing Granulocytic Myeloid Derived Suppressor Cells. Front Immunol. 2021 Jul 14;12:695972. doi: 10.3389/fimmu.2021.695972. PMID: 34341659; PMCID: PMC8324422.

Deb S, Arrighi S. Potential Effects of COVID-19 on Cytochrome P450-Mediated Drug Metabolism and Disposition in Infected Patients. Eur J Drug Metab Pharmacokinet. 2021 Mar;46(2):185-203. doi: 10.1007/s13318-020-00668-8.

Dehhaghi M, Kazemi Shariat Panahi H, Guillemin GJ. Microorganisms, Tryptophan Metabolism, and Kynurenine

Pathway: A Complex Interconnected Loop Influencing Human Health Status. Int J Tryptophan Res. 2019 Jun 19;12:1178646919852996. doi: 10.1177/1178646919852996.

Dehhaghi M, Kazemi Shariat Panahi H, Heng B, Guillemin GJ. The Gut Microbiota, Kynurenine Pathway, and Immune System Interaction in the Development of Brain Cancer. Front Cell Dev Biol. 2020 Nov 19;8:562812. doi: 10.3389/fcell.2020.562812.

Della Bella S, Bierti L, Presicce P, Arienti R, Valenti M, Saresella M, Vergani C, Villa ML. Peripheral blood dendritic cells and monocytes are differently regulated in the elderly. Clin Immunol. 2007 Feb;122(2):220-8. doi: 10.1016/j.clim.2006.09.012.

Dempsey, L. Antimicrobial IL-22. Nat Immunol 18, 373 (2017). https://doi.org/10.1038/ni.3722

Den Besten G, van Eunen K, Groen AK, Venema K, Reijngoud D-J, Bakker BM. The role of short-chain fatty acids in the interplay between diet, gut microbiota, and host energy metabolism. J Lipid Res (2013) 54(9):2325–40. 10.1194/jlr.R036012

Derakhshani A, Hemmat N, Asadzadeh Z, Ghaseminia M, Shadbad MA, Jadideslam G, et al. Arginase 1 (Arg1) as an Up-Regulated Gene in COVID-19 Patients: A Promising Marker in COVID-19 Immunopathy. J Clin Med. 2021 Mar 4;10(5):1051. doi: 10.3390/jcm10051051. PMID: 33806290; PMCID: PMC7961773.

Derhovanessian E, Pawelec G. Vaccination in the elderly. Microb Biotechnol. 2012 Mar;5(2):226-32. doi: 10.1111/j.1751-7915.2011.00283.x. Epub 2011 Aug 31. PMID: 21880118; PMCID: PMC3815782.

Deveau CM, Rodriguez E, Schroering A, Yamamoto BK. Serotonin transporter regulation by cholesterol-independent lipid signaling. Biochem Pharmacol. 2021 Jan;183:114349. doi: 10.1016/j.bcp.2020.114349.

Devinsky O, Davachi L, Santchi C, Quinn BT, Staresina BP, Thesen T. Hyperfamiliarity for faces. Neurology. 2010 Mar 23;74(12):970-4. doi: 10.1212/WNL.0b013e3181d5dc22.

Devue, C.; Collette, F.; Balteau, E.; Degueldre, C.; Luxen, A.; Maquet, P.; Brédart, S. Here I am: The cortical correlates of visual self-recognition. Brain Res. 2007, 1143, 169–182.

Di Micco, R.; Krizhanovsky, V.; et al. Cellular Senescence in Ageing: From Mechanisms to Therapeutic Opportunities. Nat Rev Mol Cell Biol 2021, 22 (2), 75–95.https://doi.org/10.1038/s41580-020-00314-w.

Di Micco, R.; Krizhanovsky, V.; et al. Cellular Senescence in Ageing: From Mechanisms to Therapeutic Opportunities. Nat Rev Mol Cell Biol 2021, 22 (2), 75–95.https://doi.org/10.1038/s41580-020-00314-w.

Di Pierro F, Iqtadar S, Khan A, et al. Potential Clinical Benefits of Quercetin in the Early Stage of COVID-19: Results of a Second, Pilot, Randomized, Controlled and Open-Label Clinical Trial. Int J Gen Med. 2021;14:2807-2816. Published 2021 Jun 24. doi:10.2147/IJGM.S318949

Diani-Moore S, Labitzke E, Brown R, Garvin A, Wong L, Rifkind AB. Sunlight generates multiple tryptophan photoproducts eliciting high efficacy CYP1A induction in chick hepatocytes and in vivo. Toxicol Sci. 2006 Mar;90(1):96-110. doi: 10.1093/toxsci/kfj065.

Dickerson F, Jones-Brando L, Ford G, Genovese G, Stallings C, Origoni A, O'Dushlaine C, Katsafanas E, Sweeney K, Khushalani S, Yolken R. Schizophrenia is Associated With an Aberrant Immune Response to Epstein-Barr Virus. Schizophr Bull. 2019 Sep 11;45(5):1112-1119. doi: 10.1093/schbul/sby164.

Dickerson F, Severance E, Yolken R. The microbiome, immunity, and schizophrenia and bipolar disorder. Brain Behav Immun. 2017 May;62:46-52. doi: 10.1016/j.bbi.2016.12.010.6.

Diebold M, Derfuss T. The monoclonal antibody GNbAC1: targeting human endogenous retroviruses in multiple sclerosis. Ther Adv Neurol Disord. 2019;12:1756286419833574. Published 2019 Mar 7. doi:10.1177/1756286419833574

Dietrich C, Kaina B. The aryl hydrocarbon receptor (AhR) in the regulation of cell-cell contact and tumor growth. Carcinogenesis. 2010 Aug;31(8):1319-28. doi: 10.1093/carcin/bgq028. Epub 2010 Jan 27. PMID: 20106901; PMCID: PMC6276890.

Digney A, Keriakous D, Scarr E, Thomas E, Dean B. Differential changes in apolipoprotein E in schizophrenia and bipolar I disorder. Biol Psychiatry. 2005 Apr

1;57(7):711-5. doi: 10.1016/j.biopsych.2004.12.028. PMID: 15820227.

Dikongué E, Ségurel L. Latitude as a co-driver of human gut microbial diversity? Bioessays. 2017 Mar;39(3). doi: 10.1002/bies.201600145. Epub 2017 Jan 13. PMID: 28083908.

Ding F, Zhang H, Cui J, Li Q, Yang C. Boosting ionizable lipid nanoparticle-mediated in vivo mRNA delivery through optimization of lipid amine-head groups. Biomater Sci. 2021 Nov 9;9(22):7534-7546. doi: 10.1039/d1bm00866h. PMID: 34647548.

Ding L, Ren C, Yang L, Wu Z, Li F, Jiang D, Zhu Y, Lu J. OSU-03012 Disrupts Akt Signaling and Prevents Endometrial Carcinoma Progression in vitro and in vivo. Drug Des Devel Ther. 2021 Apr 30;15:1797-1810. doi: 10.2147/DDDT.S304128

Diomede L, Cassata G, Fiordaliso F, Salio M, Ami D, et al. (2010) Tetracycline and its analogueues protect Caenorhabditis elegans from βamyloid-induced toxicity by targeting oligomers. Neurobiol Dis 40: 424-431.

Dipoppa, M., Ranson, A., Krumin, M., Pachitariu, M., Carandini, M., and Harris, K. D. (2018). Vision and Locomotion Shape the Interactions between Neuron Types in Mouse Visual Cortex. Neuron 98, 602–615.e8. doi: 10.1016/j.neuron.2018.03.037

Dominic P, Ahmad J, Bhandari R, Pardue S, Solorzano J, Jaisingh K, et al. Decreased availability of nitric oxide and hydrogen sulfide is a hallmark of COVID-19. Redox Biol. 2021 Jul;43:101982. doi: 10.1016/j.redox.2021.101982. Epub 2021 May 8. PMID: 34020311; PMCID: PMC8106525.

Dompe C, Moncrieff L, Matys J, Grzech-Leśniak K, Kocherova I, Bryja A, Bruska M, Dominiak M, Mozdziak P, Skiba THI, Shibli JA, Angelova Volponi A, Kempisty B, Dyszkiewicz-Konwińska M. Photobiomodulation-Underlying Mechanism and Clinical Applications. J Clin Med. 2020 Jun 3;9(6):1724. doi: 10.3390/jcm9061724. PMID: 32503238; PMCID: PMC7356229.

Dong F, Perdew GH. The aryl hydrocarbon receptor as a mediator of host-microbiota interplay. Gut Microbes. 2020 Nov 9;12(1):1859812. doi: 10.1080/19490976.2020.1859812.

Donley DW, Realing M, Gigley JP, Fox JH. Iron activates microglia and directly stimulates indoleamine-2,3-dioxygenase activity in the N171-82Q mouse model of Huntington's disease. PLoS One. 2021 May 14;16(5):e0250606. doi: 10.1371/journal.pone.0250606.

Doyle GA, Crist RC, Karatas ET, Hammond MJ, Ewing AD, Ferraro TN, Hahn CG, Berrettini WH. Analysis of LINE-1 Elements in DNA from Postmortem Brains of Individuals with Schizophrenia. Neuropsychopharmacology. 2017 Dec;42(13):2602-2611. doi: 10.1038/npp.2017.115.

Du GJ, Zhang Z, Wen XD, et al. Epigallocatechin Gallate (EGCG) is the most effective cancer chemopreventive polyphenol in green tea. Nutrients. 2012;4(11):1679-1691. Published 2012 Nov 8. doi:10.3390/nu4111679

Dudakov JA, Hanash AM, Jenq RR, Young LF, Ghosh A, Singer NV, West ML, Smith OM, Holland AM, Tsai JJ, Boyd RL, van den Brink MR. Interleukin-22 drives endogenous thymic regeneration in mice. Science. 2012 Apr 6;336(6077):91-5. doi: 10.1126/science.1218004. Epub 2012 Mar 1. PMID: 22383805

Ebringer A, Rashid T, Wilson C. The role of Acinetobacter in the pathogenesis of multiple sclerosis examined by using Popper sequences. Med Hypotheses. 2012 Jun;78(6):763-9. doi: 10.1016/j.mehy.2012.02.026

Egbujor MC, Tucci P, Buttari B, Nwobodo DC, Marini P, Saso L. Phenothiazines: Nrf2 activation and antioxidant effects. J Biochem Mol Toxicol. 2024 Mar;38(3):e23661.

Einstein, Albert (1905). "Über die von der molekularkinetischen Theorie der Wärme geforderte Bewegung von in ruhenden Flüssigkeiten suspendierten Teilchen" [On the Movement of Small Particles Suspended in Stationary Liquids Required by the Molecular-Kinetic Theory of Heat] (PDF). Annalen der Physik (in German). 322 (8): 549-560. Bibcode:1905AnP...322..549E. doi:10.1002/andp.19053220806. Archived (PDF) from the original on 9 October 2022.

Ellett L, Schlier B, Kingston JL, Zhu C, So SH, Lincoln TM, Morris EMJ, Gaudiano BA. Pandemic paranoia in the general population: international prevalence and sociodemographic profile. Psychol Med. 2022 Sep 6:1-8. doi: 10.1017/S0033291722002975.

Ellinwood, E.H. Perception of faces: Disorders in organic and psychopathological states. Psych Quar 43, 622–646 (1969). https://doi.org/10.1007/BF01564275

Ellul P, Mariotti-Ferrandiz E, Leboyer M, Klatzmann D. Regulatory T Cells As Supporters of Psychoimmune Resilience: Toward Immunotherapy of Major Depressive Disorder. Front Neurol. 2018 Mar 20;9:167. doi: 10.3389/fneur.2018.00167.

Elmi S, Sahu G, Malavade K, Jacob T. Role of tissue plasminogen activator and plasminogen activator inhibitor as potential biomarkers in psychosis. Asian J Psychiatr. 2019 Jun;43:105-110. doi: 10.1016/j.ajp.2019.05.021.

Elmi S, Sahu G, Malavade K, Jacob T. Role of tissue plasminogen activator and plasminogen activator inhibitor as potential biomarkers in psychosis. Asian J Psychiatr. 2019 Jun;43:105-110. doi: 10.1016/j.ajp.2019.05.021.

Emamian ES. AKT/GSK3 signaling pathway and schizophrenia. Front Mol Neurosci. 2012 Mar 15;5:33. doi: 10.3389/fnmol.2012.00033.

Emamian ES. AKT/GSK3 signaling pathway and schizophrenia. Front Mol Neurosci. 2012 Mar 15;5:33. doi: 10.3389/fnmol.2012.00033.

Engin E, Treit D. Anxiolytic and antidepressant actions of somatostatin: the role of sst2 and sst3 receptors.

Psychopharmacology (Berl). 2009 Oct;206(2):281-9. doi: 10.1007/s00213-009-1605-5.

Engwa G.A., Ayuk E.L., Igbojekwe B.U., Unaegbu M. Potential Antioxidant Activity of New Tetracyclic and Pentacyclic Nonlinear Phenothiazine Derivatives. Biochem. Res. Int. 2016;2016:9896575. doi: 10.1155/2016/9896575.

Erkin Şeker , Bacterial Vibrations.Sci. Transl. Med.5,196ec126-
196ec126(2013).DOI:10.1126/scitranslmed.3007046

Erro R, Buonomo AR, Barone P, Pellecchia MT. Severe Dyskinesia After Administration of SARS-CoV2 mRNA Vaccine in Parkinson's Disease. Mov Disord. 2021 Oct;36(10):2219. doi: 10.1002/mds.28772.

Essali N, Miller BJ. Psychosis as an adverse effect of antibiotics. Brain Behav Immun Health. 2020 Sep 19;9:100148. doi: 10.1016/j.bbih.2020.100148. PMID: 34589893; PMCID: PMC8474525.

Evatt ML, Delong MR, Khazai N, Rosen A, Triche S, Tangpricha V. Prevalence of vitamin d insufficiency in patients with Parkinson disease and Alzheimer disease. Arch Neurol. 2008 Oct;65(10):1348-52. doi: 10.1001/archneur.65.10.1348.

Eygeris Y, Patel S, Jozic A, Sahay G. Deconvoluting Lipid Nanoparticle Structure for Messenger RNA Delivery. Nano Lett. 2020 Jun 10;20(6):4543-4549. doi: 10.1021/acs.nanolett.0c01386.

Ezeonwumelu IJ, Garcia-Vidal E, Ballana E. JAK-STAT Pathway: A Novel Target to Tackle Viral Infections. Viruses. 2021 Nov 27;13(12):2379. doi: 10.3390/v13122379. PMID: 34960648; PMCID: PMC8704679.

Falk W. A ticket to the gut for thymic T cells. Gut. 2006 Jul;55(7):910-2. doi: 10.1136/gut.2005.087288. PMID: 16766746; PMCID: PMC1856347.

Fan H, Wang A, Wang Y, Sun Y, Han J, Chen W, Wang S, Wu Y, Lu Y. Innate Lymphoid Cells: Regulators of Gut Barrier Function and Immune Homeostasis. J Immunol Res. 2019 Dec 20;2019:2525984. doi: 10.1155/2019/2525984.

Fang W, Jiang J, Su L, et al. The role of NO in COVID-19 and potential therapeutic strategies. Free Radic Biol Med. 2021;163:153-162.
doi:10.1016/j.freeradbiomed.2020.12.008

Fang Y, Xue J, Gao S, Lu A, Yang D, Jiang H, He Y, Shi K. Cleavable PEGylation: a strategy for overcoming the "PEG dilemma" in efficient drug delivery. Drug Deliv. 2017 Dec;24(sup1):22-32. doi: 10.1080/10717544.2017.1388451.

Farkas CB, Dudás G, Babinszky GC, Földi L. Analysis of the Virus SARS-CoV-2 as a Potential Bioweapon in Light of International Literature. Mil Med. 2023 Mar 20;188(3-4):531-540. doi: 10.1093/milmed/usac123. PMID: 35569934; PMCID: PMC9384074

Farmer H, Hewstone M, Spiegler O, Morse H, Saifullah A, Pan X, Fell B, Charlesford J, Terbeck S. Positive intergroup contact modulates fusiform gyrus activity to black and white faces. Sci Rep. 2020 Feb 14;10(1):2700. doi: 10.1038/s41598-020-59633-9.

Fehsel K, Schwanke K, Kappel BA, Fahimi E, Meisenzahl-Lechner E, Esser C, Hemmrich K, Haarmann-Stemmann T, Kojda G, Lange-Asschenfeldt C. Activation of the aryl hydrocarbon receptor by clozapine induces preadipocyte differentiation and contributes to endothelial dysfunction. J Psychopharmacol. 2022 Feb;36(2):191-201. doi: 10.1177/02698811211055811

Fehsel K, Schwanke K, Kappel BA, Fahimi E, Meisenzahl-Lechner E, Esser C, Hemmrich K, Haarmann-Stemmann T, Kojda G, Lange-Asschenfeldt C. Activation of the aryl hydrocarbon receptor by clozapine induces preadipocyte differentiation and contributes to endothelial dysfunction. J Psychopharmacol. 2022 Feb;36(2):191-201. doi: 10.1177/02698811211055811.

Fei F, Qu J, Zhang M, Li Y, Zhang S. S100A4 in cancer progression and metastasis: A systematic review. Oncotarget. 2017;8(42):73219-73239. Published 2017 May 19. doi:10.18632/oncotarget.18016

Fernández VC, Alonso N, Melamud L, Villa AM. Psychiatric comorbidities and suicidality among patients with neuromyelitis optica spectrum disorders in Argentina. Mult Scler Relat Disord. 2018 Jan;19:40-43. doi: 10.1016/j.msard.2017.11.002.

Fernández-Arjona MDM, Grondona JM, Fernández-Llebrez P, López-Ávalos MD. Microglial activation by microbial neuraminidase through TLR2 and TLR4 receptors. J Neuroinflammation. 2019 Dec 2;16(1):245. doi: 10.1186/s12974-019-1643-9. PMID: 31791382

Fernandez-Egea E, Vértes PE, Flint SM, Turner L, Mustafa S, Hatton A, Smith KG, Lyons PA, Bullmore ET. Peripheral Immune Cell Populations Associated with Cognitive Deficits and Negative Symptoms of Treatment-Resistant Schizophrenia. PLoS One. 2016 May 31;11(5):e0155631. doi: 10.1371/journal.pone.0155631.

Fernandez-Valenzuela JJ, Sanchez-Varo R, Muñoz-Castro C, De Castro V, Sanchez-Mejias E, Navarro V, et al. Enhancing microtubule stabilization rescues cognitive deficits and ameliorates pathological phenotype in an amyloidogenic Alzheimer's disease model. Sci Rep. 2020 Sep 8;10(1):14776. doi: 10.1038/s41598-020-71767-4. PMID: 32901091; PMCID: PMC7479116.

Ficarra S, Russo A, Barreca D, Giunta E, Galtieri A, Tellone E. Short-Term Effects of Chlorpromazine on Oxidative Stress in Erythrocyte Functionality: Activation of Metabolism and Membrane Perturbation. Oxid Med Cell Longev. 2016;2016:2394130. doi: 10.1155/2016/2394130.

Fiori LM, Turecki G. Implication of the polyamine system in mental disorders. J Psychiatry Neurosci. 2008 Mar;33(2):102-10. PMID: 18330456; PMCID: PMC2265312.

Firpo MR, Mastrodomenico V, Hawkins GM, Prot M, Levillayer L, Gallagher T, Simon-Loriere E, Mounce BC. Targeting Polyamines Inhibits Coronavirus Infection by Reducing Cellular Attachment and Entry. ACS Infect Dis. 2021 Jun 11;7(6):1423-1432. doi: 10.1021/acsinfecdis.0c00491.

Fitzgerald PJ, Watson BO. Gamma oscillations as a biomarker for major depression: an emerging topic. Transl Psychiatry. 2018 Sep 4;8(1):177. doi: 10.1038/s41398-018-0239-y. PMID: 30181587; PMCID: PMC6123432.

Fleshner M, Crane CR. Exosomes, DAMPs, and miRNA: Features of Stress Physiology and Immune Homeostasis. Trends Immunol. 2017 Oct;38(10):768-776. doi: 10.1016/j.it.2017.08.002.

Fond G, Macgregor A, Tamouza R, Hamdani N, Meary A, Leboyer M, Dubremetz JF. Comparative analysis of anti-toxoplasmic activity of antipsychotic drugs and valproate. Eur Arch Psychiatry Clin Neurosci. 2014 Mar;264(2):179-83. doi: 10.1007/s00406-013-0413-4. Epub 2013 Jun 15. PMID: 23771405.

Forloni G, Colombo L, Girola L, Tagliavini F, Salmona M. Anti-amyloidogenic activity of tetracyclines: studies in vitro. FEBS Lett. 2001 Jan 5;487(3):404-7. doi: 10.1016/s0014-5793(00)02380-2. PMID: 11163366.

Formiga FR, Leblanc R, de Souza Rebouças J, Farias LP, de Oliveira RN, Pena L. Ivermectin: an award-winning drug with expected antiviral activity against COVID-19. J

Control Release. 2021 Jan 10;329:758-761. doi: 10.1016/j.jconrel.2020.10.009

Franchi L, Muñoz-Planillo R, Núñez G. Sensing and reacting to microbes through the inflammasomes. Nat Immunol. 2012 Mar 19;13(4):325-32. doi: 10.1038/ni.2231.

Fredrikson S, Cheng Q, Jiang GX, Wasserman D. Elevated suicide risk among patients with multiple sclerosis in Sweden. Neuroepidemiology. 2003 Mar-Apr;22(2):146-52. doi: 10.1159/000068746. PMID: 12629281.

Freud E, Di Giammarino D, Camilleri C. Mask-wearing selectivity alters observers' face perception. Cogn Res Princ Implic. 2022 Nov 16;7(1):97. doi: 10.1186/s41235-022-00444-z.

Friedrich MJ. Depression Is the Leading Cause of Disability Around the World. JAMA. 2017 Apr 18;317(15):1517. doi: 10.1001/jama.2017.3826. PMID: 28418490.

Fromer M, Roussos P, Sieberts SK, Johnson JS, Kavanagh DH, Perumal TM, et al. Gene expression elucidates functional impact of polygenic risk for schizophrenia. Nat Neurosci. 2016;19(11):1442–1453. doi: 10.1038/nn.4399

Fu G, Zhang W, Dai J, Liu J, Li F, Wu D, Xiao Y, Shah C, Sweeney JA, Wu M, Lui S. Increased Peripheral Interleukin 10 Relate to White Matter Integrity in Schizophrenia. Front Neurosci. 2019 Feb 7;13:52. doi: 10.3389/fnins.2019.00052.

Fujimoto H, Matsuoka T, Kato Y, Shibata K, Nakamura K, Yamada K, Narumoto J. Brain regions associated with anosognosia for memory disturbance in Alzheimer's disease: a magnetic resonance imaging study. Neuropsychiatr Dis Treat. 2017 Jul 5;13:1753-1759. doi: 10.2147/NDT.S139177.

Fujino M, Fukuda J, Isogai H, Ogaki T, Mawatari S, Takaki A, Wakana C, Fujino T. Orally Administered Plasmalogens Alleviate Negative Mood States and Enhance Mental Concentration: A Randomized, Double-Blind, Placebo-Controlled Trial. Front Cell Dev Biol. 2022 Jun 2;10:894734. doi: 10.3389/fcell.2022.894734.

Fusco D, Accornero N, Lavoie B, Shenoy SM, Blanchard JM, Singer RH, Bertrand E. Single mRNA molecules demonstrate probabilistic movement in living mammalian cells. Curr Biol. 2003 Jan 21;13(2):161-167. doi: 10.1016/s0960-9822(02)01436-7.

Gal H, Krizhanovsky V. Cell fusion induced senescence. Aging (Albany, NY). 2014;6(5):353-354. doi:10.18632/aging.100670

Gal, H.; Krizhanovsky, V. Cell Fusion Induced Senescence. Aging 2014, 6 (5), 353–354.https://doi.org/10.18632/aging.100670.

Galle, E., Wong, CW., Ghosh, A., et al. H3K18 lactylation marks tissue-specific active enhancers. Genome Biol 23, 207 (2022). https://doi.org/10.1186/s13059-022-02775-y

Gallotto S, Sack AT, Schuhmann T, de Graaf TA. Oscillatory Correlates of Visual Consciousness. Front Psychol. 2017 Jul 7;8:1147. doi: 10.3389/fpsyg.2017.01147.

Galván-Peña S, Leon J, Chowdhary K, Michelson DA, Vijaykumar B, Yang L, et al. MGH COVID-19 Collection & Processing Team, Mathis D, Benoist C. Profound Treg perturbations correlate with COVID-19 severity. Proc Natl Acad Sci U S A. 2021 Sep 14;118(37):e2111315118. doi: 10.1073/pnas.2111315118.

Gamba P, Testa G, Gargiulo S, Staurenghi E, Poli G, Leonarduzzi G. Oxidized cholesterol as the driving force behind the development of Alzheimer's disease. Front Aging Neurosci. 2015 Jun 19;7:119. doi: 10.3389/fnagi.2015.00119.

Gao C, Jiang J, Tan Y, Chen S. Microglia in neurodegenerative diseases: mechanism and potential therapeutic targets. Signal Transduct Target Ther. 2023 Sep 22;8(1):359. doi: 10.1038/s41392-023-01588-0.

Gao X, Huang L. Potentiation of cationic liposome-mediated gene delivery by polycations. Biochemistry. 1996 Jan 23;35(3):1027-36. doi: 10.1021/bi952436a. PMID: 8547238.

Garcia, R., Dati, L., Torres, L. et al. M1 and M3 muscarinic receptors may play a role in the neurotoxicity of anhydroecgonine methyl ester, a cocaine pyrolysis product. Sci Rep 5, 17555 (2015). https://doi.org/10.1038/srep17555

Garcia-Montojo M, Nath A. HERV-W envelope expression in blood leukocytes as a marker of disease severity of COVID-19. EBioMedicine. 2021 May;67:103363. doi: 10.1016/j.ebiom.2021.103363. Epub 2021 May 13. PMID: 33993053; PMCID: PMC8116818.

Gebre, M.S., Rauch, S., Roth, N. et al. Optimization of non-coding regions for a non-modified mRNA COVID-19 vaccine. Nature 601, 410–414 (2022). https://doi.org/10.1038/s41586-021-04231-6

Gersztenkorn D, Lee AG. Palinopsia revamped: a systematic review of the literature. Surv Ophthalmol. 2015 Jan-Feb;60(1):1- 35. doi: 10.1016/j.survophthal.2014.06.003.

Giménez-Orenga, K.; Pierquin, J.; et al. HERV-W ENV Antigenemia and Correlation of Increased Anti-SARS-CoV-2 Immunoglobulin Levels with Post-COVID-19 Symptoms. Front Immunol 2022, 13. https://doi.org/10.3389/fimmu.2022.1020064.

Ginsberg L., Rafique S., Xuereb J.H., Rapoport S.I., Gershfeld N.L. Disease and Anatomic Specificity of Ethanolamine Plasmalogen Deficiency in Alzheimer's Disease Brain. Brain Res. 1995;698:223–226. doi: 10.1016/0006-8993(95)00931-F. [PubMed] [CrossRef] [Google Scholar]

Giovannoni, F., Li, Z., Remes-Lenicov, F. et al. AHR signaling is induced by infection with coronaviruses. Nat Commun 12, 5148 (2021). https://doi.org/10.1038/s41467-021-25412-x

Girard-Thernier C, Pham TN, Demougeot C. The Promise of Plant-Derived Substances as Inhibitors of Arginase. Mini Rev Med Chem. 2015;15(10):798-808. doi: 10.2174/1389557515666150511153852. PMID: 25963565.

Girgis RR, Lieberman JA. Anti-viral properties of antipsychotic medications in the time of COVID-19. Psychiatry Res. 2021 Jan;295:113626. doi: 10.1016/j.psychres.2020.113626. Epub 2020 Nov 30. PMID: 33290940; PMCID: PMC7833567.

Girgis RR, Lieberman JA. Anti-viral properties of antipsychotic medications in the time of COVID-19. Psychiatry Res. 2021 Jan;295:113626. doi: 10.1016/j.psychres.2020.113626.

Gobin V, Van Steendam K, Denys D, Deforce D. Selective serotonin reuptake inhibitors as a novel class of immunosuppressants. Int Immunopharmacol. 2014 May;20(1):148-56. doi: 10.1016/j.intimp.2014.02.030.

Goldman SD, Funk RS, Rajewski RA, Krise JP. Mechanisms of amine accumulation in, and egress from, lysosomes. Bioanalysis. 2009 Nov;1(8):1445-59. doi: 10.4155/bio.09.128.

Goldsmith SK. Haloperidol reduces IgG immunoreactivity in the rat brain. Int J Neuropsychopharmacol. 2002 Dec;5(4):309-13. doi: 10.1017/s146114570200305x. PMID: 14710722.

Golomb BA, Stattin H, Mednick S. Low cholesterol and violent crime. J Psychiatr Res. 2000 Jul-Oct;34(4-5):301-9. doi: 10.1016/s0022-3956(00)00024-8. PMID: 11104842.

Gombash SE, Lee PW, Sawdai E, Lovett-Racke AE. Vitamin D as a Risk Factor for Multiple Sclerosis:

Immunoregulatory or Neuroprotective? Front Neurol. 2022 May 16;13:796933. doi: 10.3389/fneur.2022.796933.

Gomez-Pinedo U, Cuevas JA, Benito-Martín MS, Moreno-Jiménez L, Esteban-Garcia N, Torre-Fuentes L, Matías-Guiu JA, Pytel V, Montero P, Matías-Guiu J. Vitamin D increases remyelination by promoting oligodendrocyte lineage differentiation. Brain Behav. 2020 Jan;10(1):e01498. doi: 10.1002/brb3.1498

Gong Q, Li Q, Zhang X, et al. Pre-COVID resting-state brain activity in the fusiform gyrus prospectively predicts social anxiety alterations during the pandemic. Research Square; 2022. DOI: 10.21203/rs.3.rs-2177845/v1.

Gonzalez-Lima, F, and Barrett, DW. Augmentation of cognitive brain functions with transcranial lasers. Front Syst Neurosci. (2014) 8:36. doi: 10.3389/fnsys.2014.00036

Goodenowe DB, Haroon J, Kling MA, Zielinski M, Mahdavi K, Habelhah B, Shtilkind L, Jordan S. Targeted Plasmalogen Supplementation: Effects on Blood Plasmalogens, Oxidative Stress Biomarkers, Cognition, and Mobility in Cognitively Impaired Persons. Front Cell Dev Biol. 2022 Jul 6;10:864842. doi: 10.3389/fcell.2022.864842.

Gozes I. The ADNP Syndrome and CP201 (NAP) Potential and Hope. Front Neurol. 2020 Nov 24;11:608444. doi: 10.3389/fneur.2020.608444. PMID: 33329371; PMCID: PMC7732499.

Graham KL, Carson CM, Ezeoke A, Buckley PF, Miller BJ. Urinary tract infections in acute psychosis. J Clin Psychiatry. 2014 Apr;75(4):379-85. doi: 10.4088/JCP.13m08469

Green MJ, Matheson SL, Shepherd A, Weickert CS, Carr VJ. Brain-derived neurotrophic factor levels in schizophrenia: a systematic review with meta-analysis. Mol Psychiatry. 2011 Sep;16(9):960-72. doi: 10.1038/mp.2010.88. Epub 2010 Aug 24. PMID: 20733577.

Greene C, Hanley N, Campbell M. Blood-brain barrier associated tight junction disruption is a hallmark feature of major psychiatric disorders. Transl Psychiatry. 2020 Nov 2;10(1):373. doi: 10.1038/s41398-020-01054-3.

Gregory J Anderson, David M Frazer, Lactate as a regulator of iron homeostasis, Life Metabolism, Volume 2, Issue 5, October 2023, load033, https://doi.org/10.1093/lifemeta/load033

Grimes JM, Khan S, Badeaux M, Rao RM, Rowlinson SW, Carvajal RD. Arginine depletion as a therapeutic approach for patients with COVID-19. Int J Infect Dis. 2021;102:566-570. doi:10.1016/j.ijid.2020.10.100

Griskova-Bulanova I, Dapsys K, Melynyte S, Voicikas A, Maciulis V, Andruskevicius S, Korostenskaja M. 40Hz auditory steady-state response in schizophrenia: Sensitivity to stimulation type (clicks versus flutter amplitude-modulated tones). Neurosci Lett. 2018 Jan 1;662:152-157. doi: 10.1016/j.neulet.2017.10.025.

Gropman AL. Neuroimaging in mitochondrial disorders. Neurotherapeutics. 2013 Apr;10(2):273-85. doi: 10.1007/s13311-012-0161-6. PMID: 23208728; PMCID: PMC3625392.

Gross CG. Genealogy of the "grandmother cell". Neuroscientist. 2002 Oct;8(5):512-8. doi: 10.1177/107385802237175.

Gross JA, Turecki G. Suicide and the polyamine system. CNS Neurol Disord Drug Targets. 2013 Nov;12(7):980-8. doi: 10.2174/18715273113129990095.

Grossberg, S. (2013). Adaptive Resonance Theory: how a brain learns to consciously attend, learn, and recognize a changing world. Neural. Netw. 37, 1–47. doi: 10.1016/j.neunet.2012.09.017

Grosse L et al. Defined p16(High) Senescent Cell Types Are Indispensable for Mouse Healthspan. Cell Metab 32, 87–99.e86 (2020). 10.1016/j.cmet.2020.05.002

Grosse, L. et al. Deficiencies of the T and natural killer cell system in major depressive disorder: T regulatory cell defects are associated with inflammatory monocyte activation. Brain Behav. Immun. 54, 38–44 (2016).

Grube M. Violent behavior in cancer patients--a rarely addressed phenomenon in oncological treatment. J Interpers Violence. 2012 Jul;27(11):2163-82. doi: 10.1177/0886260511431434. PMID: 22767207.

Guadagna S, Esiri MM, Williams RJ, Francis PT. Tau phosphorylation in human brain: relationship to behavioral disturbance in dementia. Neurobiol Aging. 2012 Dec;33(12):2798-806. doi: 10.1016/j.neurobiolaging.2012.01.015.

Guerra B., Issinger O.G. Natural Compounds and Derivatives as Ser/Thr Protein Kinase Modulators and Inhibitors. Pharmaceuticals. 2019;12:4. doi: 10.3390/ph12010004. [PMC free article] [PubMed] [CrossRef] [Google Scholar]i

Gulbins, A., Schumacher, F., Becker, K.A. et al. Antidepressants act by inducing autophagy controlled by sphingomyelin–ceramide. Mol Psychiatry 23, 2324–2346 (2018). https://doi.org/10.1038/s41380-018-0090-9

Guo J, Hu H, Chen Z, Xu J, Nie J, Lu J, Ma L, Ji H, Yuan J, Xu B. Cold Exposure Induces Intestinal Barrier Damage and Endoplasmic Reticulum Stress in the Colon via the SIRT1/Nrf2 Signaling Pathway. Front Physiol. 2022 Apr 20;13:822348. doi: 10.3389/fphys.2022.822348.

Guo SJ, Ma CG, Hu YY, Bai G, Song ZJ, Cao XQ. Solid lipid nanoparticles for phytosterols delivery: The acyl chain number of the glyceride matrix affects the arrangement, stability, and release. Food Chem. 2022 Jun 7;394:133412. doi: 10.1016/j.foodchem.2022.133412.

Gurguis, G., Antai-Otong, D., Vo, S. et al. Adrenergic Receptor Function in Panic Disorder: I. Platelet α2 Receptors Gi Protein Coupling, Effects of Imipramine, and Relationship to Treatment Outcome.

Neuropsychopharmacol 20, 162–176 (1999). https://doi.org/10.1016/S0893-133X(98)00062-1

Gurung, S., Perocheau, D., Touramanidou, L. et al. The exosome journey: from biogenesis to uptake and intracellular signalling. Cell Commun Signal 19, 47 (2021). https://doi.org/10.1186/s12964-021-00730-1

Hagihara H, Shoji H, Otabi H, Toyoda A, Katoh K, Namihira M, Miyakawa T. Protein lactylation induced by neural excitation. Cell Rep. 2021 Oct 12;37(2):109820. doi: 10.1016/j.celrep.2021.109820. PMID: 34644564.

Hallett M. Volitional control of movement: the physiology of free will. Clin Neurophysiol. 2007 Jun;118(6):1179-92. doi: 10.1016/j.clinph.2007.03.019.

Hamsanathan, S.; Gurkar, A.U. Lipids as Regulators of Cellular Senescence. Front. Physiol. 2022, 13, 796850.

Han CH, Chung JH. Asthma and other allergic diseases in relation to suicidal behavior among South Korean adolescents. J Psychosom Res. 2018 Dec;115:94-100. doi: 10.1016/j.jpsychores.2018.10.015.

Han, X., Zhang, H., Butowska, K. et al. An ionizable lipid toolbox for RNA delivery. Nat Commun 12, 7233 (2021). https://doi.org/10.1038/s41467-021-27493-0

Handono K, Sidarta YO, Pradana BA, Nugroho RA, Hartono IA, Kalim H, Endharti AT. Vitamin D prevents endothelial damage induced by increased neutrophil extracellular traps formation in patients with systemic lupus erythematosus. Acta Med Indones. 2014 Jul;46(3):189

Harrington A, Oepen G, Spitzer M. Disordered recognition and perception of human faces in acute schizophrenia and experimental psychosis. Compr Psychiatry. 1989 Sep-Oct;30(5):376-84. doi: 10.1016/0010-440x(89)9000

Harris MJ, Jeste DV, Gleghorn A, Sewell DD. New-onset psychosis in HIV-infected patients. J Clin Psychiatry. 1991 Sep;52(9):369-76. PMID: 1894589.

Harrison, G.; Hopper, K.; Craig, T.; Laska, E.; Siegel, C.; Wanderling, J.; Dube, K.C.; Ganev, K.; Giel, R.; Der Heiden, W.A.; et al. Recovery from psychotic illness: A 15- and 25-year international follow-up study. Br. J. Psychiatry 2001, 178, 506–517.

Hayakawa K, Esposito E, Wang X, Terasaki Y, Liu Y, Xing C, et al. Transfer of mitochondria from astrocytes to neurons after stroke. Nature. (2016) 535:551–5. doi: 10.1038/nature18928

He B, Sheng C, Yu X, Zhang L, Chen F, Han Y. Alterations of gut microbiota are associated with brain structural changes in the spectrum of Alzheimer's disease: the SILCODE study in Hainan cohort. Front Aging Neurosci. 2023 Jul 14;15:1216509. doi: 10.3389/fnagi.2023.1216509.

He J, Kong J, Tan QR, Li XM. Neuroprotective effect of atypical antipsychotics in cognitive and non-cognitive behavioral impairment in animal models. Cell Adh Migr. 2009 Jan-Mar;3(1):129-37. doi: 10.4161/cam.3.1.7401.

Epub 2009 Jan 13. PMID: 19372744; PMCID: PMC2675159.

Hecht D. Cerebral lateralization of pro- and anti-social tendencies. Exp Neurobiol. 2014 Mar;23(1):1-27. doi: 10.5607/en.2014.23.1.1. Epub 2014 Mar 27. PMID: 24737936; PMCID: PMC3984952.

Heiczman A, Tóth M. Effect of chlorpromazine on the synthesis of neutral lipids and phospholipids from [3H]glycerol in the primordial human placenta. Placenta. 1995 Jun;16(4):347-58. doi: 10.1016/0143-4004(95)90092-6. PMID: 7567797.

Hein S, Benz NI, Eisert J, Herrlein ML, Oberle D, Dreher M, Stingl JC, Hildt C, Hildt E. Comirnaty-Elicited and Convalescent Sera Recognize Different Spike Epitopes. Vaccines (Basel). 2021 Dec 1;9(12):1419. doi: 10.3390/vaccines9121419.

Heltberg MS, Lucchetti A, Hsieh FS, Minh Nguyen DP, Chen SH, Jensen MH. Enhanced DNA repair through droplet formation and p53 oscillations. Cell. 2022 Nov 10;185(23):4394-4408.c10. doi: 10.1016/j.cell.2022.10.004

Herceg D, Mimica N, Herceg M, Puljić K. Aggression in Women with Schizophrenia Is Associated with Lower HDL Cholesterol Levels. Int J Mol Sci. 2022 Oct 6;23(19):11858. doi: 10.3390/ijms231911858.

Herda LR, Felix SB, Boege F. Drug-like actions of autoantibodies against receptors of the autonomous nervous system and their impact on human heart function. Br J

Pharmacol. 2012 Jun;166(3):847-57. doi: 10.1111/j.1476-5381.2012.01828.x.

Hering H, Lin CC, Sheng M. Lipid rafts in the maintenance of synapses, dendritic spines, and surface AMPA receptor stability. J Neurosci. 2003 Apr 15;23(8):3262-71. doi: 10.1523/JNEUROSCI.23-08-03262.2003.

Hilliard M, Giordano-Santini R, Li Z et al. Fusogen-mediated neuron–neuron fusion disrupts neural circuit connectivity and alters animal behavior. PNAS. 2020. doi: 10.1073/pnas.1919063117

Himmerich H, Milenović S, Fulda S, Plümäkers B, Sheldrick AJ, Michel TM, Kircher T, Rink L. Regulatory T cells increased while IL-1β decreased during antidepressant therapy. J Psychiatr Res. 2010 Nov;44(15):1052-7. doi: 10.1016/j.jpsychires.2010.03.005

Ho, B.C.; Andreasen, N.C.; Ziebell, S.; Pierson, R.; Magnotta, V. Long-term antipsychotic treatment and brain volumes: A longitudinal study of first-episode schizophrenia. Arch. Gen. Psychiatry 2011, 68, 128–137.

Hofhansel, L., Weidler, C., Votinov, M. et al. Morphology of the criminal brain: gray matter reductions are linked to antisocial behavior in offenders. Brain Struct Funct 225, 2017–2028 (2020). https://doi.org/10.1007/s00429-020-02106-6

Holm, M.; Taipale, H.; Tanskanen, A.; Tiihonen, J.; Mitterdorfer-Rutz, E. Employment among people with schizophrenia or bipolar disorder: A population-based study using nationwide registers. Acta Psychiatr. Scand. 2020, 143, 61–71.

Horn, A.; Jaiswal, J.K. Structural and signaling role of lipids in plasma membrane repair. Curr. Top. Membr. 2019, 84, 67–98.172.

Hörnich BF, Großkopf AK, Schlagowski S, Tenbusch M, Kleine-Weber H, Neipel F, et al. SARS-CoV-2 and SARS-CoV Spike-Mediated Cell-Cell Fusion Differ in Their Requirements for Receptor Expression and Proteolytic Activation. J Virol. 2021 Apr 12;95(9):e00002-21. doi: 10.1128/JVI.00002-21.

Hou, X., Zaks, T., Langer, R. et al. Lipid nanoparticles for mRNA delivery. Nat Rev Mater 6, 1078–1094 (2021). https://doi.org/10.1038/s41578-021-00358-0

Houtepen LC, van Bergen AH, Vinkers CH, Boks MP. DNA methylation signatures of mood stabilizers and antipsychotics in bipolar disorder. Epigenomics. 2016 Feb;8(2):197-208. doi: 10.2217/epi.15.98.

Howes, O.D.; Cummings, C.; Chapman, G.E.; Shatalina, E. Neuroimaging in schizophrenia: An overview of findings and their implications for synaptic changes. Neuropsychopharmacology 2022, 48, 151–167

Hu S, Chen Y, Chen Y, Wang C. Depression and Anxiety Disorders in Patients With Inflammatory Bowel Disease. Front Psychiatry. 2021 Oct 8;12:714057. doi: 10.3389/fpsyt.2021.714057. PMID: 34690829; PMCID: PMC8531580.

Hu Y, Fryatt GL, Ghorbani M, Obst J, Menassa DA, Martin-Estebane M, Muntslag TAO, Olmos-Alonso A, Guerrero-Carrasco M, Thomas D, Cragg MS, Gomez-Nicola D. Replicative senescence dictates the emergence of disease-associated microglia and contributes to Aβ pathology. Cell Rep. 2021 Jun 8;35(10):109228. doi: 10.1016/j.celrep.2021.109228.

Hu, J., Chen, X., Lu, X. et al. A spike protein S2 antibody efficiently neutralizes the Omicron variant. Cell Mol Immunol 19, 644–646 (2022). https://doi.org/10.1038/s41423-022-00847-4

Hu, J., Ding, Y., Liu, W. et al. When AHR signaling pathways meet viral infections. Cell Commun Signal 21, 42 (2023). https://doi.org/10.1186/s12964-023-01058-8

Hugdahl K, Løberg EM, Jørgensen HA, Lundervold A, Lund A, Green MF, Rund B. Left hemisphere lateralisation of auditory hallucinations in schizophrenia: a dichotic listening study. Cogn Neuropsychiatry. 2008 Mar;13(2):166-79. doi: 10.1080/13546800801906808.

Hughes LE, Smith PA, Bonell S, Natt RS, Wilson C, Rashid T, Amor S, Thompson EJ, Croker J, Ebringer A. Cross-reactivity between related sequences found in Acinetobacter sp., Pseudomonas aeruginosa, myelin basic protein and myelin oligodendrocyte glycoprotein in multiple sclerosis. J Neuroimmunol. 2003 Nov;144(1-2):105-15. doi: 10.1016/s0165-5728(03)00274-1.

Hung SY, Fu WM. Drug candidates in clinical trials for Alzheimer's disease. J Biomed Sci. 2017;24(1):47. Published 2017 Jul 19. doi:10.1186/s12929-017-0355-7

Hussain T, Murtaza G, Kalhoro DH, Kalhoro MS, Metwally E, Chughtai MI, Mazhar MU, Khan SA. Relationship between gut microbiota and host-metabolism: Emphasis on hormones related to reproductive function. Anim Nutr. 2021 Mar;7(1):1-10. doi: 10.1016/j.aninu.2020.11.005.

Hussar AE, Cradle JL, Beiser SM. A study of the immunologic and allergic responsiveness of chronic schizophrenics. Br J Psychiatry. 1971 Jan;118(542):91-2. doi: 10.1192/bjp.118.542.91. PMID: 5576273.

Hutton J. Does Rubella Cause Autism: A 2015 Reappraisal? Front Hum Neurosci. 2016;10:25. Published 2016 Feb 1. doi:10.3389/fnhum.2016.00025

Hwang KA, Kim HR, Kang I. Aging and human CD4(+) regulatory T cells. Mech Ageing Dev. 2009 Aug;130(8):509-17. doi: 10.1016/j.mad.2009.06.003.

Iida T, Onodera K, Nakase H. Role of autophagy in the pathogenesis of inflammatory bowel disease. World J Gastroenterol. 2017 Mar 21;23(11):1944-1953. doi: 10.3748/wjg.v23.i11.1944.

Ingersoll MA, Starkey MR. Interleukin-22 in urinary tract disease - new experimental directions. Clin Transl Immunology. 2020 Jun 7;9(6):e1143. doi: 10.1002/cti2.1143.

Inoue Y, Tanaka N, Tanaka Y, Inoue S, Morita K, Zhuang M, Hattori T, Sugamura K. Clathrin-dependent entry of severe acute respiratory syndrome coronavirus into target cells expressing ACE2 with the cytoplasmic tail deleted. J Virol. 2007 Aug;81(16):8722-9. doi: 10.1128/JVI.00253-07.

Islam MS, Quispe C, Hossain R, et al. Neuropharmacological Effects of Quercetin: A Literature-Based Review. Front Pharmacol. 2021;12:665031. Published 2021 Jun 17. doi:10.3389/fphar.2021.665031

Issinger O.G., Guerra B. Phytochemicals in cancer and their effect on the PI3K/AKT-mediated cellular signalling. Biomed. Pharmacother. 2021;139:111650. doi: 10.1016/j.biopha.2021.111650. [PubMed] [CrossRef] [Google Scholar]

J. R. Evans, Quantitative EEG findings in a group of death row inmates, Archives of Clinical Neuropsychology, Volume 12, Issue 4, 1997, Pages 315–316, https://doi.org/10.1093/arclin/12.4.315a

Jääskeläinen, E.; Juola, P.; Hirvonen, N.; McGrath, J.J.; Saha, S.; Isohanni, M.; Veijola, J.; Miettunen, J. A Systematic Review and Meta-Analysis of Recovery in Schizophrenia. Schizophr. Bull. 2012, 39, 1296–1306.

James R. Evans, Ph.D. & Nan-Sook Park M.A. (1997) Quantitative EEG Findings Among Men Convicted of Murder, Journal of Neurotherapy: Investigations in Neuromodulation, Neurofeedback and Applied Neuroscience, 2:2, 31-39, DOI: 10.1300/J184v02n02_05

Jang HJ, Chung H, Rowland JM, Richards BA, Kohl MM, Kwag J. Distinct roles of parvalbumin and somatostatin interneurons in gating the synchronization of spike times in the neocortex. Sci Adv. 2020 Apr 22;6(17):eaay5333. doi: 10.1126/sciadv.aay5333.

Jaworski T, Banach-Kasper E, Gralec K. GSK-3β at the Intersection of Neuronal Plasticity and Neurodegeneration. Neural Plast. 2019 May 2;2019:4209475. doi: 10.1155/2019/4209475. PMID: 31191636; PMCID: PMC6525914.

Jeeva S, Kim KH, Shin CH, Wang BZ, Kang SM. An Update on mRNA-Based Viral Vaccines. Vaccines (Basel). 2021;9(9):965. Published 2021 Aug 29. doi:10.3390/vaccines9090965

Jiang Y, Lu Q, Wang Y, Xu E, Ho A, Singh P, et al. Quantitating Endosomal Escape of a Library of Polymers for mRNA Delivery. Nano Lett. 2020 Feb 12;20(2):1117-1123. doi: 10.1021/acs.nanolett.9b04426

Jiang, H., Li, X., Chen, S. et al. Plasminogen Activator Inhibitor-1 in depression: Results from Animal and Clinical Studies. Sci Rep 6, 30464 (2016). https://doi.org/10.1038/srep30464

Jin WN, Shi K, He W, Sun JH, Van Kaer L, Shi FD, Liu Q. Neuroblast senescence in the aged brain augments natural killer cell cytotoxicity leading to impaired neurogenesis and cognition. Nat Neurosci. 2021 Jan;24(1):61-73. doi: 10.1038/s41593-020-00745-w.

Johnson, E.L., Heaver, S.L., Waters, J.L. et al. Sphingolipids produced by gut bacteria enter host metabolic pathways, impacting ceramide levels. Nat Commun 11, 2471 (2020). https://doi.org/10.1038/s41467-020-16274-w

Jones KT, Zhen J, Reith ME. Importance of cholesterol in dopamine transporter function. J Neurochem. 2012 Dec;123(5):700-15. doi: 10.1111/jnc.12007.

Juanola O, Piñero P, Gómez-Hurtado I, Caparrós E, García-Villalba R, Marín A, Zapater P, Tarín F, González-Navajas JM, Tomás-Barberán FA, Francés R. Regulatory T Cells Restrict Permeability to Bacterial Antigen Translocation and Preserve Short-Chain Fatty Acids in Experimental Cirrhosis. Hepatol Commun. 2018 Oct 22;2(12):1610-1623. doi: 10.1002/hep4.1268.

Juengst, S.; Skidmore, E.; Pramuka, M.; McCue, M.; Becker, J. Factors contributing to impaired self-awareness of cognitive functioning in an HIV positive and at-risk population. Disabil. Rehabil. 2011, 34, 19–25

Jutila A, Söderlund T, Pakkanen AL, Huttunen M, Kinnunen PK. Comparison of the effects of clozapine, chlorpromazine, and haloperidol on membrane lateral heterogeneity. Chem Phys Lipids. 2001 Aug;112(2):151-63. doi: 10.1016/s0009-3084(01)00175-x.

Kaddurah-Daouk R, McEvoy J, Baillie R, Zhu H, K Yao J, Nimgaonkar VL, Buckley PF, Keshavan MS, Georgiades A, Nasrallah HA. Impaired plasmalogens in patients with schizophrenia. Psychiatry Res. 2012 Aug 15;198(3):347-52.

doi: 10.1016/j.psychres.2012.02.019. Epub 2012 Apr 16. PMID: 22513041.

Kanayama M, Hayashida M, Hashioka S, Miyaoka T, Inagaki M. Decreased Clostridium Abundance after Electroconvulsive Therapy in the Gut Microbiota of a Patient with Schizophrenia. Case Rep Psychiatry. 2019 Feb 25;2019:4576842. doi: 10.1155/2019/4576842.

Kapelski P, Skibinska M, Maciukiewicz M, Pawlak J, Zaremba D, Twarowska-Hauser J. Family-based association study of interleukin 10 (IL10) and interleukin 10 receptor alpha (IL10RA) functional polymorphisms in schizophrenia in Polish population. J Neuroimmunol. 2016 Aug 15;297:92-7. doi: 10.1016/j.jneuroim.2016.05.010.

Kar M, Ghosh D, Sengupta J. Molecular correlates of syncytialization in muscle and placenta. Indian J Physiol Pharmacol. 2007 Oct-Dec;51(4):311-25. PMID: 18476385.

Karamyshev AL, Karamysheva ZN. Lost in Translation: Ribosome-Associated mRNA and Protein Quality Controls. Front Genet. 2018 Oct 4;9:431. doi: 10.3389/fgene.2018.00431.

Karczewski P, Pohlmann A, Wagenhaus B, Wisbrun N, Hempel P, Lemke B, Kunze R, Niendorf T, Bimmler M. Antibodies to the α1-adrenergic receptor cause vascular impairments in rat brain as demonstrated by magnetic resonance angiography. PLoS One. 2012;7(7):e41602. doi: 10.1371/journal.pone.0041602.

Karczmar, A.G. Cholinergic Behaviors, Emotions, and the "Self". J. Mol. Neurosci. 2013, 53, 291–297. [Google Scholar] [CrossRef]

Katharina Kunzelmann, Matthias Grieder, Claudia van Swam, Philipp Homan, Stephanie Winkelbeiner, Daniela Hubl, Thomas Dierks. Am I hallucinating or is my fusiform cortex activated? Functional activation differences in schizophrenia patients with and without hallucinations, The European Journal of Psychiatry, Volume 33, Issue 1, 2019, Pages 1-7, https://doi.org/10.1016/j.ejpsy.2018.06.002.

Kato T, Mizoguchi Y, Monji A, Horikawa H, Suzuki SO, Seki Y, Iwaki T, Hashioka S, Kanba S. Inhibitory effects of aripiprazole on interferon-gamma-induced microglial activation via intracellular Ca2+ regulation in vitro. J Neurochem. 2008 Jul;106(2):815-25. doi: 10.1111/j.1471-4159.2008.05435.x

Kato T, Monji A, Hashioka S, Kanba S. Risperidone significantly inhibits interferon-gamma-induced microglial activation in vitro. Schizophr Res. 2007 May;92(1-3):108-15. doi: 10.1016/j.schres.2007.01.019.

Katoozi S, Skauli N, Zahl S, Deshpande T, Ezan P, Palazzo C, Steinhäuser C, Frigeri A, Cohen-Salmon M, Ottersen OP, Amiry-Moghaddam M. Uncoupling of the Astrocyte Syncytium Differentially Affects AQP4 Isoforms. Cells. 2020 Feb 7;9(2):382. doi: 10.3390/cells9020382.

Katrangi E, D'Souza G, Boddapati SV, Kulawiec M, Singh KK, Bigger B, et al. Xenogenic transfer of isolated murine mitochondria into human rho0 cells can improve respiratory function. Rejuvenation Res. (2007) 10:561–70. doi: 10.1089/rej.2007.0575

Kavanagh, E. Long Covid Brain Fog: A Neuroinflammation Phenomenon? Oxf Open Immunol 2022, 3 (1). https://doi.org/10.1093/oxfimm/iqac007.

Kawamoto S, Hara E. Crosstalk between gut microbiota and cellular senescence: a vicious cycle leading to aging gut. Trends Cell Biol. 2024 Jan 13:S0962-8924(23)00254-4. doi: 10.1016/j.tcb.2023.12.004. Epub ahead of print. PMID: 38220548.

Keir M, Yi Y, Lu T, Ghilardi N. The role of IL-22 in intestinal health and disease. J Exp Med. 2020 Feb 13;217(3):e20192195. doi: 10.1084/jem.20192195.

Kelly DL, Kane MA, Fraser CM, Sayer MA, Grant-Beurmann S, Liu T, Gold JM, Notarangelo FM, Vyas GR, Richardson CM, August SM, Kotnana B, Miller J, Liu F, Buchanan RW. Prebiotic Treatment Increases Serum Butyrate in People With Schizophrenia: Results of an Open-Label Inpatient Pilot Clinical Trial. J Clin Psychopharmacol. 2021 Mar-Apr 01;41(2):200-202. doi: 10.1097/JCP.0000000000001364.

Kelly DL, Li X, Kilday C, Feldman S, Clark S, Liu F, Buchanan RW, Tonelli LH. Increased circulating regulatory T cells in medicated people with schizophrenia. Psychiatry Res. 2018 Nov;269:517-523. doi: 10.1016/j.psychres.2018.09.006

Kelly DL, Li X, Kilday C, Feldman S, Clark S, Liu F, Buchanan RW, Tonelli LH. Increased circulating regulatory T cells in medicated people with schizophrenia. Psychiatry Res. 2018 Nov;269:517-523. doi: 10.1016/j.psychres.2018.09.006.

Kelly DL, Li X, Kilday C, Feldman S, Clark S, Liu F, Buchanan RW, Tonelli LH. Increased circulating regulatory T cells in medicated people with schizophrenia. Psychiatry Res. 2018 Nov;269:517-523. doi: 10.1016/j.psychres.2018.09.006.

Kępińska AP, Iyegbe CO, Vernon AC, Yolken R, Murray RM, Pollak TA. Schizophrenia and Influenza at the Centenary of the 1918-1919 Spanish Influenza Pandemic: Mechanisms of Psychosis Risk. Front Psychiatry. 2020;11:72. Published 2020 Feb 26. doi:10.3389/fpsyt.2020.00072

Khalefah MM, Khalifah AM. Determining the relationship between SARS-CoV-2 infection, dopamine, and COVID-19 complications. J Taibah Univ Med Sci. 2020 Dec;15(6):550-553. doi: 10.1016/j.jtumed.2020.10.006.

Khan H, Ullah H, Aschner M, Cheang WS, Akkol EK. Neuroprotective Effects of Quercetin in Alzheimer's Disease. Biomolecules. 2019;10(1):59. Published 2019 Dec 30. doi:10.3390/biom10010059

Khan MF, Murphy CD. Bacterial degradation of the anti-depressant drug fluoxetine produces trifluoroacetic acid and fluoride ion. Appl Microbiol Biotechnol. 2021 Dec;105(24):9359-9369. doi: 10.1007/s00253-021-11675-3

Khan MF, Murphy CD. Bacterial degradation of the antidepressant drug fluoxetine produces trifluoroacetic acid and fluoride ion. Appl Microbiol Biotechnol. 2021 Dec;105(24):9359-9369. doi: 10.1007/s00253-021-11675-3

Khan, M.; Baussan, Y.; Hebert-Chatelain, E. Connecting Dots between Mitochondrial Dysfunction and Depression. Biomolecules 2023, 13, 695. https://doi.org/10.3390/biom13040695

Kidson C, Moreau MC, Asher DM, et al. Cell fusion induced by scrapie and Creutzfeldt-Jakob virus-infected brain preparations. Proc Natl Acad Sci U S A. 1978;75(6):2969-2971. doi:10.1073/pnas.75.6.2969

Kim CJ, Nazli A, Rojas OL, Chege D, Alidina Z, Huibner S, Mujib S, Benko E, Kovacs C, Shin LY, Grin A, Kandel G, Loutfy M, Ostrowski M, Gommerman JL, Kaushic C, Kaul R. A role for mucosal IL-22 production and Th22 cells in HIV-associated mucosal immunopathogenesis. Mucosal Immunol. 2012 Nov;5(6):670-80. doi: 10.1038/mi.2012.72.

Kim GW, Park SY, Kim IS. Novel function of stabilin-2 in myoblast fusion: the recognition of extracellular phosphatidylserine as a "fuse-me" signal. BMB Rep. 2016 Jun;49(6):303-4. doi: 10.5483/bmbrep.2016.49.6.078.

Kim SH, Park S, Yu HS, Ko KH, Park HG, Kim YS. The antipsychotic agent clozapine induces autophagy via the AMPK-ULK1-Beclin1 signaling pathway in the rat frontal cortex. Prog Neuropsychopharmacol Biol Psychiatry. 2018 Feb 2;81:96-104. doi: 10.1016/j.pnpbp.2017.10.012.

Kim YK, Suh IB, Kim H, Han CS, Lim CS, Choi SH, Licinio J. The plasma levels of interleukin-12 in schizophrenia, major depression, and bipolar mania: effects of psychotropic drugs. Mol Psychiatry. 2002;7(10):1107-14. doi: 10.1038/sj.mp.4001084. PMID: 12476326.

Kim, H.s., Kim, S., Shin, S.J. et al. Gram-negative bacteria and their lipopolysaccharides in Alzheimer's disease: pathologic roles and therapeutic implications. Transl Neurodegener 10, 49 (2021). https://doi.org/10.1186/s40035-021-00273-y

Kim, H.S.; Kim, S.; Shin, S.J.; Park, Y.H.; Nam, Y.; Kim, C.W.; Lee, K.W.; Kim, S.-M.; Jung, I.D.; Yang, H.D.; et al. Gram-negative bacteria and their lipopolysaccharides in Alzheimer's disease: Pathologic roles and therapeutic implications. Transl. Neurodegener. 2021, 10, 49. [Google Scholar] [CrossRef]

Kim, H.S.; Kim, S.; Shin, S.J.; Park, Y.H.; Nam, Y.; Kim, C.W.; Lee, K.W.; Kim, S.-M.; Jung, I.D.; Yang, H.D.; et al. Gram-negative bacteria and their lipopolysaccharides in Alzheimer's disease: Pathologic roles and therapeutic implications. Transl. Neurodegener. 2021, 10, 49. [Google Scholar] [CrossRef]

Kindred R, Bates GW. The Influence of the COVID-19 Pandemic on Social Anxiety: A Systematic Review. Int J Environ Res Public Health. 2023 Jan 29;20(3):2362. doi: 10.3390/ijerph20032362.

Kinney DK, Teixeira P, Hsu D, Napoleon SC, Crowley DJ, Miller A, Hyman W, Huang E. Relation of schizophrenia prevalence to latitude, climate, fish consumption, infant mortality, and skin color: a role for prenatal vitamin d deficiency and infections? Schizophr Bull. 2009 May;35(3):582-95. doi: 10.1093/schbul/sbp023.

Kleimann A, Toto S, Eberlein CK, Kielstein JT, Bleich S, Frieling H, Sieberer M. Psychiatric symptoms in patients with Shiga toxin-producing E. coli O104:H4 induced haemolytic-uraemic syndrome. PLoS One. 2014 Jul 9;9(7):e101839. doi: 10.1371/journal.pone.0101839.

Kleimann A, Toto S, Eberlein CK, Kielstein JT, Bleich S, Frieling H, Sieberer M. Psychiatric symptoms in patients with Shiga toxin-producing E. coli O104:H4 induced haemolytic-uraemic syndrome. PLoS One. 2014 Jul 9;9(7):e101839. doi: 10.1371/journal.pone.0101839.

Kobayashi T, Motomura Y, Moro K. The discovery of group 2 innate lymphoid cells has changed the concept of type 2 immune diseases. Int Immunol. 2021 Nov 25;33(12):705-709. doi: 10.1093/intimm/dxab063

Kopf A, Kiermaier E. Dynamic Microtubule Arrays in Leukocytes and Their Role in Cell Migration and Immune Synapse Formation. Front Cell Dev Biol. 2021 Feb 9;9:635511. doi: 10.3389/fcell.2021.635511. PMID: 33634136; PMCID: PMC7900162.

Korade Ž, Liu W, Warren EB, Armstrong K, Porter NA, Konradi C. Effect of psychotropic drug treatment on sterol metabolism. Schizophr Res. 2017 Sep;187:74-81. doi: 10.1016/j.schres.2017.02.001. Epub 2017 Feb 12. PMID: 28202290; PMCID: PMC555446

Koren T, Yifa R, Amer M, Krot M, Boshnak N, Ben-Shaanan TL, Azulay-Debby H, Zalayat I, Avishai E, Hajjo H, Schiller M, Haykin H, Korin B, Farfara D, Hakim F, Kobiler O, Rosenblum K, Rolls A. Insular cortex neurons encode and retrieve specific immune responses. Cell. 2021 Nov 24;184(24):5902-5915.e17. doi: 10.1016/j.cell.2021.10.013.

Koshiyama, D. et al. Auditory gamma oscillations predict global symptomatic outcome in the early stages of psychosis: a longitudinal investigation. Clin. Neurophysiol. 129, 2268–2275 (2018).

Kovalevich, J., Cornec, A. S., Yao, Y., James, M., Crowe, A., Lee, V. M., et al. (2016). Characterization of the brain–penetrant pyrimidine–containing molecules with differential microtubule–-stabilizing activities developed as potential therapeutic agents for Alzheimer's disease and related tauopathies. J. Pharmacol. Exp. Ther. 357, 432–450. doi: 10.1124/jpet.115.231175

Kovtun O, Dickson VK, Kelly BT, Owen DJ, Briggs JAG. Architecture of the AP2/clathrin coat on the membranes of clathrin-coated vesicles. Sci Adv. 2020 Jul 22;6(30):eaba8381. doi: 10.1126/sciadv.aba8381.

Kow CS, Hasan SS. Potential interactions between COVID-19 vaccines and antiepileptic drugs. Seizure. 2021 Mar;86:80-81. doi: 10.1016/j.seizure.2021.01.021.

Kozloff N, Mulsant BH, Stergiopoulos V, Voineskos AN. The COVID-19 Global Pandemic: Implications for People With Schizophrenia and Related Disorders. Schizophr Bull.

2020 Jul 8;46(4):752-757. doi: 10.1093/schbul/sbaa051. PMID: 32343342; PMCID: PMC7197583

Krstić G. Asthma prevalence associated with geographical latitude and regional insolation in the United States of America and Australia. PLoS One. 2011 Apr 8;6(4):e18492. doi: 10.1371/journal.pone.0018492. PMID: 21494627; PMCID: PMC3072993.

Kucharz EJ, Sierakowski S, Staite ND, Goodwin JS. Mechanism of lithium-induced augmentation of T-cell proliferation. Int J Immunopharmacol. 1988;10(3):253-9. doi: 10.1016/0192-0561(88)90056-2. PMID: 3263331.

Kulkarni JA, Cullis PR, van der Meel R. Lipid Nanoparticles Enabling Gene Therapies: From Concepts to Clinical Utility. Nucleic Acid Ther. 2018 Jun;28(3):146-157. doi: 10.1089/nat.2018.0721

Kumar CS, Dey D, Ghosh S, Banerjee M. Breach: Host Membrane Penetration and Entry by Nonenveloped Viruses. Trends Microbiol. 2018 Jun;26(6):525-537. doi: 10.1016/j.tim.2017.09.010. Epub 2017 Oct 25. PMID: 29079499.

Kumar P, Thakar MS, Ouyang W, Malarkannan S. IL-22 from conventional NK cells is epithelial regenerative and inflammation protective during influenza infection. Mucosal Immunol. 2013 Jan;6(1):69-82. doi: 10.1038/mi.2012.49.

Lai SW, Kuo YH, Liao KF. Chronic hydroxychloroquine exposure and the risk of Alzheimer's disease. Ann Rheum

Dis. 2021 Jul;80(7):e105. doi: 10.1136/annrheumdis-2019-216173. Epub 2019 Aug 21. PMID: 31434638.

Langer V, Vivi E, Regensburger D, Winkler TH, Waldner MJ, Rath T, Schmid B, Skottke L, Lee S, Jeon NL, Wohlfahrt T, Kramer V, Tripal P, Schumann M, Kersting S, Handtrack C, Geppert CI, Suchowski K, Adams RH, Becker C, Ramming A, Naschberger E, Britzen-Laurent N, Stürzl M. IFN-γ drives inflammatory bowel disease pathogenesis through VE-cadherin-directed vascular barrier disruption. J Clin Invest. 2019 Nov 1;129(11):4691-4707. doi: 10.1172/JCI124884.

Lau, D.H.W., Hartopp, N., Welsh, N.J. et al. Disruption of ER−mitochondria signalling in frontotemporal dementia and related amyotrophic lateral sclerosis. Cell Death Dis 9, 327 (2018). https://doi.org/10.1038/s41419-017-0022-7

Laursen TM. Life expectancy among persons with schizophrenia or bipolar affective disorder. Schizophr Res. 2011 Sep;131(1-3):101-4. doi: 10.1016/j.schres.2011.06.008.

Lavazza A. Free Will and Neuroscience: From Explaining Freedom Away to New Ways of Operationalizing and Measuring It. Front Hum Neurosci. 2016 Jun 1;10:262. doi: 10.3389/fnhum.2016.00262.

Lazebnik Y. Cell fusion as a link between the SARS-CoV-2 spike protein, COVID-19 complications, and vaccine side effects. Oncotarget. 2021;12(25):2476-2488. Published 2021 Dec 7. doi:10.18632/oncotarget.28088

Le Dréan, G., Blottière, H.M. Glutamate from the microbiome controls host metabolism. Nat Metab (2024). https://doi.org/10.1038/s42255-024-01050-7

Le PT, Pearce MM, Zhang S, Campbell EM, Fok CS, Mueller ER, Brincat CA, Wolfe AJ, Brubaker L. IL22 regulates human urothelial cell sensory and innate functions through modulation of the acetylcholine response, immunoregulatory cytokines and antimicrobial peptides: assessment of an in vitro model. PLoS One. 2014 Oct 29;9(10):e111375. doi: 10.1371/journal.pone.0111375.

Le T, Le SC, Zhang Y, Liang P, Yang H. Evidence that polyphenols do not inhibit the phospholipid scramblase TMEM16F. J Biol Chem. 2020 Aug 28;295(35):12537-12544. doi: 10.1074/jbc.AC120.014872. Epub 2020 Jul 24. PMID: 32709749; PMCID: PMC7458812.

Le TH, Oh JM, Rami FZ, Li L, Chun SK, Chung YC. Effects of Social Defeat Stress on Microtubule Regulating Proteins and Tubulin Polymerization. Clin Psychopharmacol Neurosci. 2024 Feb 29;22(1):129-138. doi: 10.9758/cpn.23.1077. Epub 2023 Aug 10. PMID: 38247419; PMCID: PMC10811395.

Lee B, Shim I, Lee H, Hahm DH. Berberine alleviates symptoms of anxiety by enhancing dopamine expression in rats with post-traumatic stress disorder. Korean J Physiol Pharmacol. 2018 Mar;22(2):183-192. doi: 10.4196/kjpp.2018.22.2.183.

Lee J, Patel DS, Ståhle J, Park SJ, Kern NR, Kim S, Lee J, et al. CHARMM-GUI Membrane Builder for Complex

Biological Membrane Simulations with Glycolipids and Lipoglycans. J Chem Theory Comput. 2019 Jan 8;15(1):775-786. doi: 10.1021/acs.jctc.8b01066.

Lee S, Yu Y, Trimpert J, Benthani F, Mairhofer M, Richter-Pechanska P, Wyler E, et al. Virus-induced senescence is a driver and therapeutic target in COVID-19. Nature. 2021 Nov;599(7884):283-289. doi: 10.1038/s41586-021-03995-1.

Lefèvre PL, Palin MF, Murphy BD. Polyamines on the reproductive landscape. Endocr Rev. 2011 Oct;32(5):694-712. doi: 10.1210/er.2011-0012. Epub 2011 Jul 26. PMID: 21791568.

Lehmann ML, Poffenberger CN, Elkahloun AG, Herkenham M. Analysis of cerebrovascular dysfunction caused by chronic social defeat in mice. Brain Behav Immun. 2020 Aug;88:735-747. doi: 10.1016/j.bbi.2020.05.030.

Lenz P, Søgaard-Andersen L. Temporal and spatial oscillations in bacteria. Nat Rev Microbiol. 2011 Aug 15;9(8):565-77. doi: 10.1038/nrmicro2612.

Leppien E, Mulcahy K, Demler TL, Trigoboff E, Opler L. Effects of Statins and Cholesterol on Patient Aggression: Is There a Connection? Innov Clin Neurosci. 2018 Apr 1;15(3-4):24-27. PMID: 29707423; PMCID: PMC5906086.

Leung, M.; Cheung, C.; Yu, K.; Yip, B.; Sham, P.; Li, Q.; Chua, S.; McAlonan, G. Gray Matter in First-Episode Schizophrenia Before and After Antipsychotic Drug Treatment. Anatomical Likelihood Estimation Meta-analyses With Sample Size Weighting. Schizophr. Bull. 2009, 37, 199–211

Lévesque, I.S.; Abdel-Baki, A. Homeless youth with first-episode psychosis: A 2-year outcome study. Schizophr. Res. 2019, 216, 460–469.

Leykin I, Mayer R, Shinitzky M. Short and long-term immunosuppressive effects of clozapine and haloperidol. Immunopharmacology. 1997 Aug;37(1):75-86. doi: 10.1016/s0162-3109(97)00037-4. PMID: 9285246.

Li D, Zhang H, Lyons TW, Lu M, Achab A, Pu Q, Childers M, et al. Comprehensive Strategies to Bicyclic Prolines: Applications in the Synthesis of Potent Arginase Inhibitors. ACS Med Chem Lett. 2021 Oct 13;12(11):1678-1688. doi: 10.1021/acsmedchemlett.1c00258. PMID: 34795856; PMCID: PMC8591728.

Li J, He Y, Wang W, Wu C, Hong C, Hammond PT. Polyamine-Mediated Stoichiometric Assembly of Ribonucleoproteins for Enhanced mRNA Delivery. Angew Chem Int Ed Engl. 2017 Oct 23;56(44):13709-13712. doi: 10.1002/anie.201707466.

Li J, Song D, Wang S, Dai Y, Zhou J, Gu J. Antiviral Effect of Epigallocatechin Gallate via Impairing Porcine Circovirus Type 2 Attachment to Host Cell Receptor. Viruses. 2020;12(2):176. Published 2020 Feb 4. doi:10.3390/v12020176

Li LJ, Gong C, Zhao MH, Feng BS. Role of interleukin-22 in inflammatory bowel disease. World J Gastroenterol. 2014 Dec 28;20(48):18177-88. doi: 10.3748/wjg.v20.i48.18177

Li X, Fan X, Yuan X, Pang L, Hu S, Wang Y, Huang X, Song X. The Role of Butyric Acid in Treatment Response in Drug-Naïve First Episode Schizophrenia. Front Psychiatry. 2021 Aug 23;12:724664. doi: 10.3389/fpsyt.2021.724664.

Li Y, Kröger M, Liu WK. Endocytosis of PEGylated nanoparticles accompanied by structural and free energy changes of the grafted polyethylene glycol. Biomaterials. 2014 Oct;35(30):8467-78. doi: 10.1016/j.biomaterials.2014.06.032

Li Y, Wang J, Li Y, Wu H, Zhao S, Yu Q. Protecting intestinal epithelial cells against deoxynivalenol and E. coli damage by recombinant porcine IL-22. Vet Microbiol. 2019 Apr;231:154-159. doi: 10.1016/j.vetmic.2019.02.027.

Li, S., Song, J., Ke, P. et al. The gut microbiome is associated with brain structure and function in schizophrenia. Sci Rep 11, 9743 (2021). https://doi.org/10.1038/s41598-021-89166-8

Li, W., Zhu, L., Chen, Y. et al. Association between mitochondrial DNA levels and depression: a systematic review and meta-analysis. BMC Psychiatry 23, 866 (2023). https://doi.org/10.1186/s12888-023-05358-8

Liang H, Luo D, Liao H, Li S. Coronavirus Usurps the Autophagy-Lysosome Pathway and Induces Membranes Rearrangement for Infection and Pathogenesis. Front

Microbiol. 2022 Mar 2;13:846543. doi: 10.3389/fmicb.2022.846543.

Liester MB. Personality changes following heart transplantation: The role of cellular memory. Med Hypotheses. 2020 Feb;135:109468. doi: 10.1016/j.mehy.2019.109468. Epub 2019 Oct 31. PMID: 31739081.

Liguz-Lecznar M, Urban-Ciecko J, Kossut M. Somatostatin and Somatostatin-Containing Neurons in Shaping Neuronal Activity and Plasticity. Front Neural Circuits. 2016 Jun 30;10:48. doi: 10.3389/fncir.2016.00048.

Lim ICZY, Tam WWS, Chudzicka-Czupała A, McIntyre RS, Teopiz KM, Ho RC, Ho CSH. Prevalence of depression, anxiety and post-traumatic stress in war- and conflict-afflicted areas: A meta-analysis. Front Psychiatry. 2022 Sep 16;13:978703. doi: 10.3389/fpsyt.2022.978703.

Lin DY, Gu Y, Wheeler B, Young H, Holloway S, Sunny SK, Moore Z, Zeng D. Effectiveness of Covid-19 Vaccines over a 9-Month Period in North Carolina. N Engl J Med. 2022 Mar 10;386(10):933-941. doi: 10.1056/NEJMoa2117128.

Lin L, Zhou XF, Bobrovskaya L. Blockage of p75NTR ameliorates depressive-like behaviours of mice under chronic unpredictable mild stress. Behav Brain Res. 2021 Jan 1;396:112905. doi: 10.1016/j.bbr.2020.112905. Epub 2020 Sep 11. PMID: 32926907.

Lin WC, Blanchette CD, Ratto TV, Longo ML. Lipid asymmetry in DLPC/DSPC-supported lipid bilayers: a combined AFM and fluorescence microscopy study. Biophys J. 2006 Jan 1;90(1):228-37. doi: 10.1529/biophysj.105.067066.

Lin, C.-H., Chen, C.-C., Chou, C.-M., Wang, C.-Y., Hung, C.-C., Chen, J.Y., Chang, H.-W., Chen, Y.-C., Yeh, G.C. and Lee, Y.-H. (2009), Knockdown of the aryl hydrocarbon receptor attenuates excitotoxicity and enhances NMDA-induced BDNF expression in cortical neurons. Journal of Neurochemistry, 111: 777-789. https://doi.org/10.1111/j.1471-4159.2009.06364.x

Lin, H. R., Wang, C. H., Deng, Q. L., Xu, C., Deng, Z. K., and Zhou, C. (2021). Review on chaotic dynamics of memristive neuron and neural network. Nonlinear Dyn. 106, 959–973. doi: 10.1007/s11071-021-06853-x

Lin, L., Li, Q., Wang, Y. et al. Syncytia formation during SARS-CoV-2 lung infection: a disastrous unity to eliminate lymphocytes. Cell Death Differ 28, 2019–2021 (2021). https://doi.org/10.1038/s41418-021-00795-y

Lindqvist D, Fernström J, Grudet C, Ljunggren L, Träskman-Bendz L, Ohlsson L, Westrin Å. Increased plasma levels of circulating cell-free mitochondrial DNA in suicide attempters: associations with HPA-axis hyperactivity. Transl Psychiatry. 2016 Dec 6;6(12):e971. doi: 10.1038/tp.2016.236.

Lindqvist, D.; Epel, E.S.; Mellon, S.H.; Penninx, B.W.; Révész, D.; Verhoeven, J.E.; Reus, V.I.; Lin, J.; Mahan, L.;

Hough, C.M.; et al. Psychiatric disorders and leukocyte telomere length: Underlying mechanisms linking mental illness with cellular aging. Neurosci. Biobehav. Rev. 2015, 55, 333–364.

Link CD. Is There a Brain Microbiome? Neurosci Insights. 2021 May 27;16:26331055211018709. doi: 10.1177/26331055211018709.

Liu J, Conboy JC. Phase Behavior of Planar Supported Lipid Membranes Composed of Cholesterol and 1,2-Distearoyl-sn-Glycerol-3-Phosphocholine Examined by Sum-Frequency Vibrational Spectroscopy. Vib Spectrosc. 2009 May 26;50(1):106-115. doi: 10.1016/j.vibspec.2008.09.004

Liu J, Prindle A, Humphries J, Gabalda-Sagarra M, Asally M, Lee DY, Ly S, Garcia-Ojalvo J, Süel GM. Metabolic co-dependence gives rise to collective oscillations within biofilms. Nature. 2015 Jul 30;523(7562):550-4. doi: 10.1038/nature14660.

Liu J, Prindle A, Humphries J, Gabalda-Sagarra M, Asally M, Lee DY, Ly S, Garcia-Ojalvo J, Süel GM. Metabolic co-dependence gives rise to collective oscillations within biofilms. Nature. 2015 Jul 30;523(7562):550-4. doi: 10.1038/nature14660.

Liu M, Chu Y, Liu H, Su Y, Zhang Q, Jiao J, et al. Accelerated Blood Clearance of Nanoemulsions Modified with PEG-Cholesterol and PEG-Phospholipid Derivatives in Rats: The Effect of PEG-Lipid Linkages and PEG Molecular Weights. Mol Pharm. 2020 Apr 6;17(4):1059-1070. doi: 10.1021/acs.molpharmaceut.9b00770.

Liu Q, He H, Yang J, Feng X, Zhao F, Lyu J. Changes in the global burden of depression from 1990 to 2017: Findings from the Global Burden of Disease study. J Psychiatr Res. 2020 Jul;126:134-140. doi: 10.1016/j.jpsychires.2019.08.002

Liu X., Yao Z. Chronic over-nutrition and dysregulation of GSK3 in diseases. Nutr. Metab. 2016;13:49. doi: 10.1186/s12986-016-0108-8. [PMC free article] [PubMed] [CrossRef] [Google Scholar]

Liu Y, Dai M. Trimethylamine N-Oxide Generated by the Gut Microbiota Is Associated with Vascular Inflammation: New Insights into Atherosclerosis. Mediators Inflamm. 2020 Feb 17;2020:4634172. doi: 10.1155/2020/4634172.

Liu ZSJ, Truong TTT, Bortolasci CC, Spolding B, Panizzutti B, Swinton C, et al. Effects of Psychotropic Drugs on Ribosomal Genes and Protein Synthesis. Int J Mol Sci. 2022 Jun 28;23(13):7180. doi: 10.3390/ijms23137180.

Lotter C, Alter CL, Bolten JS, Detampel P, Palivan CG, Einfalt T, Huwyler J. Incorporation of phosphatidylserine improves the efficiency of lipid lipid-based gene delivery systems. Eur J Pharm Biopharm. 2022 Mar;172:134-143. doi: 10.1016/j.ejpb.2022.02.007.

Lotz C, Muellenbach RM, Meybohm P, Mutlak H, Lepper PM, Rolfes CB, et all. Effects of inhaled nitric oxide in COVID-19-induced ARDS - Is it worthwhile? Acta Anaesthesiol Scand. 2021 May;65(5):629-632. doi: 10.1111/aas.13757. Epub 2020 Dec 20. PMID: 33296498.

Lovero KL, Simmons AN, Aron JL, Paulus MP. Anterior insular cortex anticipates impending stimulus significance. Neuroimage. 2009 Apr 15;45(3):976-83. doi: 10.1016/j.neuroimage.2008.12.070.

Lozano R, Marin R, Santacruz MJ, Pascual A. Selective Immunoglobulin M Deficiency Among Clozapine-Treated Patients: A Nested Case-Control Study. Prim Care Companion CNS Disord. 2015 Jul 2;17(4):10.4088/PCC.15m01782. doi: 10.4088/PCC.15m01782.

Lu F, Zhang Y, Trivedi A, Jiang X, Chandra D, Zheng J, Nakano Y, Abduweli Uyghurturk D, Jalai R, Onur SG, Mentes A, DenBesten PK. Fluoride related changes in behavioral outcomes may relate to increased serotonin. Physiol Behav. 2019 Jul 1;206:76-83. doi: 10.1016/j.physbeh.2019.02.017.

Lu F, Zhang Y, Trivedi A, Jiang X, Chandra D, Zheng J, Nakano Y, Abduweli Uyghurturk D, Jalai R, Onur SG, Mentes A, DenBesten PK. Fluoride related changes in behavioral outcomes may relate to increased serotonin. Physiol Behav. 2019 Jul 1;206:76-83. doi: 10.1016/j.physbeh.2019.02.017.

Lucas, N.; Saj, A.; Schwartz, S.; Ptak, R.; Schnider, A.; Thomas, C.; Conne, P.; Leroy, R.; Pavin, S.; Diserens, K.; et al. Effects of Pro-Cholinergic Treatment in Patients Suffering from Spatial Neglect. Front. Hum. Neurosci. 2013, 7, 574. [Google Scholar] [CrossRef] [Green Version]

Ludvigsson JF, Olén O, Larsson H, Halfvarson J, Almqvist C, Lichtenstein P, Butwicka A. Association Between Inflammatory Bowel Disease and Psychiatric Morbidity and Suicide: A Swedish Nationwide Population-Based Cohort Study With Sibling Comparisons. J Crohns Colitis. 2021 Nov 8;15(11):1824-1836. doi: 10.1093/ecco-jcc/jjab039.

Luisetto M, Tarro G, Edbey K, Khan FA, Ilman A, et al. Coronavirus COVID-19 surface properties: Electrical charges status. Int J Clin Microbiol Biochem Technol. 2021; 4: 016-027.

Luo G, Ambati A, Lin L, Bonvalet M, Partinen M, Ji X, Maecker HT, Mignot EJ. Autoimmunity to hypocretin and molecular mimicry to flu in type 1 narcolepsy. Proc Natl Acad Sci USA. 2018 Dec 26;115(52): E12323-E12332. doi: 10.1073/pnas.1818150116. Epub 2018 Dec 12. PMID: 30541895; PMCID: PMC6310865.

Luquain-Costaz C, Kockx M, Anastasius M, Chow V, Kontush A, Jessup W, Kritharides L. Increased ABCA1 (ATP-Binding Cassette Transporter A1)-Specific Cholesterol Efflux Capacity in Schizophrenia. Arterioscler Thromb Vasc Biol. 2020 Nov;40(11):2728-2737. doi: 10.1161/ATVBAHA.120.314847.

Luu, M., and Visekruna, A. (2019). Short-chain fatty acids: bacterial messengers modulating the immunometabolism of T cells. Eur. J. Immunol. 49, 842–848. doi: 10.1002/eji.201848009

Lyons M, Bootes E, Brewer G, Stratton K, Centifanti L. "COVID-19 spreads round the planet, and so do paranoid thoughts". A qualitative investigation into personal experiences of psychosis during the COVID-19 pandemic. Curr Psychol. 2021 Oct 12:1-10. doi: 10.1007/s12144-021-02369-0.

Maazi H, Akbari O. Type two innate lymphoid cells: the Janus cells in health and disease. Immunol Rev. 2017 Jul;278(1):192-206. doi: 10.1111/imr.12554. PMID: 28658553; PMCID: PMC5492968.

Madison CA, Hillbrick L, Kuempel J, Albrecht GL, Landrock KK, Safe S, Chapkin RS, Eitan S. Intestinal epithelium aryl hydrocarbon receptor is involved in stress sensitivity and maintaining depressive symptoms. Behav Brain Res. 2023 Feb 25;440:114256. doi: 10.1016/j.bbr.2022.114256.

Maes M, Kanchanatawan B, Sirivichayakul S, Carvalho AF. In Schizophrenia, Increased Plasma IgM/IgA Responses to Gut Commensal Bacteria Are Associated with Negative Symptoms, Neurocognitive Impairments, and the Deficit Phenotype. Neurotox Res. 2019 Apr;35(3):684-698. doi: 10.1007/s12640-018-9987-y.

Maes M, Kubera M, Leunis JC. The gut-brain barrier in major depression: intestinal mucosal dysfunction with an increased translocation of LPS from gram negative enterobacteria (leaky gut) plays a role in the inflammatory pathophysiology of depression. Neuro Endocrinol Lett. 2008 Feb;29(1):117-24.

Maes M, Vojdani A, Geffard M, Moreira EG, Barbosa DS, Michelin AP, Semeão LO, Sirivichayakul S,

Kanchanatawan B. Schizophrenia phenomenology comprises a bifactorial general severity and a single-group factor, which are differently associated with neurotoxic immune and immune-regulatory pathways. Biomol Concepts. 2019 Nov 17;10(1):209-225. doi: 10.1515/bmc-2019-0023.

Mahadik SP, Mukherjee S, Laev H, Reddy R, Schnur DB. Abnormal growth of skin fibroblasts from schizophrenic patients. Psychiatry Res. 1991 Jun;37(3):309-20. doi: 10.1016/0165-1781(91)90066-x. PMID: 1891511.

Mahin Ghorbani, Unveiling the Human Brain Virome in Brodmann Area 46: Novel Insights Into Dysbiosis and Its Association With Schizophrenia, Schizophrenia Bulletin Open, Volume 4, Issue 1, January 2023, sgad029, https://doi.org/10.1093/schizbullopen/sgad029

Malashkevich VN, Dulyaninova NG, Ramagopal UA, Liriano MA, Varney KM, Knight D, et al. Phenothiazines inhibit S100A4 function by inducing protein oligomerization. Proc Natl Acad Sci U S A. 2010 May 11;107(19):8605-10. doi: 10.1073/pnas.0913660107. Epub 2010 Apr 26. PMID: 20421509; PMCID: PMC2889333.

Malebari AM, Wang S, Greene TF, O'Boyle NM, Fayne D, Khan MF. Synthesis and Antiproliferative Evaluation of 3-Chloroazetidin-2-ones with Antimitotic Activity: Heterocyclic Bridged Analogues of Combretastatin A-4. Pharmaceuticals (Basel). 2021 Oct 31;14(11):1119. doi: 10.3390/ph14111119. PMID: 34832901; PMCID: PMC8624998.

Malekan M, Nezamabadi SS, Samami E, Mohebalizadeh M, Saghazadeh A, Rezaei N. BDNF and its signaling in cancer. J Cancer Res Clin Oncol. 2023 Jun;149(6):2621-2636. doi: 10.1007/s00432-022-04365-8.

Manjunath K, Reddy JS, Venkateswarlu V. Solid lipid nanoparticles as drug delivery systems. Methods Find Exp Clin Pharmacol. 2005 Mar;27(2):127-44. doi: 10.1358/mf.2005.27.2.876286.

Mankidy R., Ahiahonu P. W., Ma H., Jayasinghe D., Ritchie S. A., Khan M. A., et al. (2010). Membrane Plasmalogen Composition and Cellular Cholesterol Regulation: A Structure Activity Study. Lipids Health Dis. 9 (1), 1–17. 10.1186/1476-511X-9-62

Manzella CR, Ackerman M, Singhal M, Ticho AL, Ceh J, Alrefai WA, Saksena S, Dudeja PK, Gill RK. Serotonin Modulates AhR Activation by Interfering with CYP1A1-Mediated Clearance of AhR Ligands. Cell Physiol Biochem. 2020 Feb 5;54(1):126-141. doi: 10.33594/000000209.

Mar, J.S., Ota, N., Pokorzynski, N.D. et al. IL-22 alters gut microbiota composition and function to increase aryl hydrocarbon receptor activity in mice and humans. Microbiome 11, 47 (2023). https://doi.org/10.1186/s40168-023-01486-1

Mariani N, Everson J, Pariante CM, Borsini A. Modulation of microglial activation by antidepressants. Journal of Psychopharmacology. 2022;36(2):131-150. doi:10.1177/02698811211069110

Marie-Luise Kieseler, Brad Duchaine; Persisting Prosopagnosia due to COVID-19. Journal of Vision 2021;21(9):2408. doi: https://doi.org/10.1167/jov.21.9.2408.

Marrie RA, Walld R, Bolton JM, Sareen J, Walker JR, Patten SB, Singer A, Lix LM, Hitchon CA, El-Gabalawy R, Katz A, Fisk JD, Bernstein CN; CIHR Team in Defining the Burden and Managing the Effects of Psychiatric Comorbidity in Chronic Immunoinflammatory Disease. Increased incidence of psychiatric disorders in immune-mediated inflammatory disease. J Psychosom Res. 2017 Oct;101:17-23. doi: 10.1016/j.jpsychores.2017.07.015

Martin N, Zhu K, Czarnecka-Herok J, Vernier M, Bernard D. Regulation and role of calcium in cellular senescence. Cell Calcium. 2023 Mar;110:102701. doi: 10.1016/j.ceca.2023.102701.

Martin, N.; Bernard, D. Calcium Signaling and Cellular Senescence. Cell Calcium 2018,70, 16–23. https://doi.org/10.1016/j.ceca.2017.04.001

Martinez-Corral R, Liu J, Prindle A, Süel GM, Garcia-Ojalvo J. Metabolic basis of brain-like electrical signalling in bacterial communities. Philos Trans R Soc Lond B Biol Sci. 2019 Jun 10;374(1774):20180382. doi: 10.1098/rstb.2018.0382.

Martinez-Corral R, Liu J, Süel GM, Garcia-Ojalvo J. Bistable emergence of oscillations in growing Bacillus subtilis biofilms. Proc Natl Acad Sci U S SA. 2018 Sep 4;115(36): E8333-E8340. doi: 10.1073/pnas.1805004115.

Martin-Rodriguez, O.; Gauthier, T.; et al. Pro-Resolving Factors Released by Macrophages After Efferocytosis Promote Mucosal Wound Healing in Inflammatory Bowel Disease. Front Immunol 2021, 12. https://doi.org/10.3389/fimmu.2021.754475.

Masaldan, S.; Clatworthy, S. A. S.; et al. Iron Accumulation in Senescent Cells Is Coupled with Impaired Ferritinophagy and Inhibition of Ferroptosis. Redox Biol 2018,14, 100–115. https://doi.org/10.1016/j.redox.2017.08.015

Masaldan, S.; Clatworthy, S. A. S.; et al. Iron Accumulation in Senescent Cells Is Coupled with Impaired Ferritinophagy and Inhibition of Ferroptosis. Redox Biol 2018,14, 100–115. https://doi.org/10.1016/j.redox.2017.08.015

Mascitelli L, Pezzetta F, Goldstein MR. Low cholesterol, delinquency, and suicidality. Prim Care Companion J Clin Psychiatry. 2008;10(5):413-4. doi: 10.4088/pcc.v10n0511c.

Masdrakis VG, Markianos M, Baldwin DS. Apathy associated with antidepressant drugs: a systematic review. Acta Neuropsychiatr. 2023 Aug;35(4):189-204. doi: 10.1017/neu.2023.6.

Mash C, Bornstein MH, Arterberry ME. Brain dynamics in young infants' recognition of faces: EEG oscillatory activity in response to mother and stranger. Neuroreport. 2013 May 8;24(7):359-63. doi: 10.1097/WNR.0b013e32835f6828

Mason PD, Weetman AP, Sissons JG, Borysiewicz LK. Suppressive role of NK cells in pokeweed mitogen-induced immunoglobulin synthesis: effect of depletion/enrichment of

Leu 11b+ cells. Immunology. 1988 Sep;65(1):113-8. PMID: 3053423; PMCID: PMC1385028.

Matsunaga S, Kishi T, Annas P, Basun H, Hampel H, Iwata N. Lithium as a Treatment for Alzheimer's Disease: A Systematic Review and Meta-Analysis. J Alzheimers Dis. 2015;48(2):403-10. doi: 10.3233/JAD-150437. PMID: 26402004.

Mattapallil MJ, Kielczewski JL, Zárate-Bladés CR, St Leger AJ, Raychaudhuri K, Silver PB, Jittayasothorn Y, Chan CC, Caspi RR. Interleukin 22 ameliorates neuropathology and protects from central nervous system autoimmunity. J Autoimmun. 2019 Aug;102:65-76. doi: 10.1016/j.jaut.2019.04.017. Epub 2019 May 9. PMID: 31080013; PMCID: PMC6667188

Matteoni, S.; Matarrese, P.; Ascione, B.; Ricci-Vitiani, L.; Pallini, R.; Villani, V.; Pace, A.; Paggi, M.G.; Abbruzzese, C. Chlorpromazine induces cytotoxic autophagy in glioblastoma cells via endoplasmic reticulum stress and unfolded protein response. J. Exp. Clin. Cancer Res. 2021, 40, 347.

Maugeri, M., Nawaz, M., Papadimitriou, A. et al. Linkage between endosomal escape of LNP-mRNA and loading into EVs for transport to other cells. Nat Commun 10, 4333 (2019). https://doi.org/10.1038/s41467-019-12275-6

Maurya A.K., Vinayak M. PI-103 and Quercetin Attenuate PI3K-AKT Signaling Pathway in T-Cell Lymphoma Exposed to Hydrogen Peroxide. PLoS ONE.

2016;11:e0160686. doi: 10.1371/journal.pone.0160686. [PMC free article] [PubMed] [CrossRef] [Google Scholar]

May M, Beauchemin M, Vary C, Barlow D, Houseknecht KL. The antipsychotic medication, risperidone, causes global immunosuppression in healthy mice. PLoS One. 2019 Jun 26;14(6):e0218937. doi: 10.1371/journal.pone.0218937.

May M, Beauchemin M, Vary C, Barlow D, Houseknecht KL. The antipsychotic medication, risperidone, causes global immunosuppression in healthy mice. PLoS One. 2019 Jun 26;14(6):e0218937. doi: 10.1371/journal.pone.0218937.

Mazereel V, Van Assche K, Detraux J, De Hert M. COVID-19 vaccination for people with severe mental illness: why, what, and how? Lancet Psychiatry. 2021 May;8(5):444-450. doi: 10.1016/S2215-0366(20)30564-2.

McGrath JJ, Pemberton MR, Welham JL, Murray RM. Schizophrenia and the influenza epidemics of 1954, 1957 and 1959: a southern hemisphere study. Schizophr Res. 1994 Dec;14(1):1-8. doi: 10.1016/0920-9964(94)90002-7. PMID: 7893616.

McKone E, Wan L, Pidcock M, Crookes K, Reynolds K, Dawel A, Kidd E, Fiorentini C. A critical period for faces: Other-race face recognition is improved by childhood but not adult social contact. Sci Rep. 2019 Sep 6;9(1):12820. doi: 10.1038/s41598-019-49202- 0. PMID: 31492907

McLaren RA Jr, Trejo FE, Blitz MJ, Bianco A, Limaye M, Brustman L, et al. COVID-related "lockdowns" and birth rates in New York. Am J Obstet Gynecol MFM. 2021 Nov;3(6):100476. doi: 10.1016/j.ajogmf.2021.100476

Melbourne, J.K.; Rosen, C.; Chase, K.A.; Feiner, B.; Sharma, R.P. Monocyte Transcriptional Profiling Highlights a Shift in Immune Signatures Over the Course of Illness in Schizophrenia. Front. Psychiatry 2021, 12, 649494.

Mendez MF. The neurobiology of moral behavior: review and neuropsychiatric implications. CNS Spectr. 2009 Nov;14(11):608-20. doi: 10.1017/s1092852900023853.

Merenlender-Wagner A, Malishkevich A, Shemer Z, Udawela M, Gibbons A, Scarr E, Dean B, Levine J, Agam G, Gozes I. Autophagy has a key role in the pathophysiology of schizophrenia. Mol Psychiatry. 2015 Feb;20(1):126-32. doi: 10.1038/mp.2013.174.

Merenlender-Wagner, A., Malishkevich, A., Shemer, Z. et al. Autophagy has a key role in the pathophysiology of schizophrenia. Mol Psychiatry 20, 126–132 (2015). https://doi.org/10.1038/mp.2013.174

Merkley SD, Chock CJ, Yang XO, Harris J, Castillo EF. Modulating T Cell Responses via Autophagy: The Intrinsic Influence Controlling the Function of Both Antigen-Presenting Cells and T Cells. Front Immunol. 2018 Dec 14;9:2914. doi: 10.3389/fimmu.2018.02914

Meselson M, Guillemin J, Hugh-Jones M, Langmuir A, Popova I, Shelokov A, Yampolskaya O. The Sverdlovsk anthrax outbreak of 1979. Science. 1994; 266:1202–1208.

Messaoud A, Mensi R, Douki W, Neffati F, Najjar MF, Gobbi G, Valtorta F, Gaha L, Comai S. Reduced peripheral availability of tryptophan and increased activation of the kynurenine pathway and cortisol correlate with major depression and suicide. World J Biol Psychiatry. 2019 Nov;20(9):703-711. doi: 10.1080/15622975.2018.1468031.

Meyer N, Henkel L, Linder B, Zielke S, Tascher G, Trautmann S, et al. Autophagy activation, lipotoxicity and lysosomal membrane permeabilization synergize to promote pimozide- and loperamide-induced glioma cell death. Autophagy. 2021 Nov;17(11):3424-3443. doi: 10.1080/15548627.2021.1874208.

Miatmoko A, Nurjannah I, Nehru NF, Rosita N, Hendradi E, Sari R, Ekowati J. Interactions of primaquine and chloroquine with PEGylated phosphatidylcholine liposomes. Sci Rep. 2021 Jun 14;11(1):12420. doi: 10.1038/s41598-021-91866-0.

Michael Gold. A Conspiracy of Cells; One Woman's Immortal Legacy and the Medical Scandal it Caused. State University of New York Press (1986). ISBN:9780887060991, 0887060994

Migliorelli, R.; Tesón, A.; Sabe, L.; Petracca, G.; Petracchi, M.; Leiguarda, R.; E Starkstein, S. Anosognosia in Alzheimer's disease: A study of associated factors. J. Neuropsychiatry 1995, 7, 338–344

Mikkelsen JD, Woldbye DP. Accumulated increase in neuropeptide Y and somatostatin gene expression of the rat in response to repeated electroconvulsive stimulation. J

Psychiatr Res. 2006 Mar;40(2):153-9. doi: 10.1016/j.jpsychires.2005.02.005.

Miller CJ, Nichol RC, Batuski DJ. Acoustic oscillations in the early universe and today. Science. 2001 Jun 22;292(5525):2302-3. doi: 10.1126/science.1060440. Epub 2001 May 24. PMID: 11375481.

Millington-Burgess, S.L., Harper, M.T. Epigallocatechin gallate inhibits the release of extracellular vesicles from platelets without inhibiting phosphatidylserine exposure. Sci Rep 11, 17678 (2021). https://doi.org/10.1038/s41598-021-97212-8

Minozzo BR, Fernandes D, Beltrame FL. Phenolic Compounds as Arginase Inhibitors: New Insights Regarding Endothelial Dysfunction Treatment. Planta Med. 2018 Mar;84(5):277-295. doi: 10.1055/s-0044-100398. Epub 2018 Jan 17. PMID: 29342480.

Minozzo BR, Fernandes D, Beltrame FL. Phenolic Compounds as Arginase Inhibitors: New Insights Regarding Endothelial Dysfunction Treatment. Planta Med. 2018 Mar;84(5):277-295. doi: 10.1055/s-0044-100398. Epub 2018 Jan 17. PMID: 29342480.

Mirzakhani H, Al-Garawi A, Weiss ST, Litonjua AA. Vitamin D and the development of allergic disease: how important is it? Clin Exp Allergy. 2015 Jan;45(1):114-25. doi: 10.1111/cea.12430.

Mirzayans, R.; Andrais, B.; et al. Multinucleated Giant Cancer Cells Produced in Response to Ionizing Radiation

Retain Viability and Replicate Their Genome. Int J Mol Sci 2017, 18 (2), 360. https://doi.org/10.3390/ijms18020360.

Misrani A, Tabassum S, Wang T, Huang H, Jiang J, Diao H, Zhao Y, Huang Z, Tan S, Long C, Yang L. Vibration-reduced anxiety-like behavior relies on ameliorating abnormalities of the somatosensory cortex and medial prefrontal cortex. Neural Regen Res. 2024 Jun 1;19(6):1351-1359. doi: 10.4103/1673-5374.385840.

Miu AC, Balteş FR. Empathy manipulation impacts music-induced emotions: a psychophysiological study on opera. PLoS One. 2012;7(1):e30618. doi: 10.1371/journal.pone.0030618. Epub 2012 Jan 24. PMID: 22292000; PMCID: PMC3265492.

Miyajima H, Adachi J, Kohno S, Takahashi Y, Ueno Y, Naito T. Increased oxysterols associated with iron accumulation in the brains and visceral organs of acaeruloplasminaemia patients. QJM. 2001 Aug;94(8):417-22. doi: 10.1093/qjmed/94.8.417.

Mizuno Y, Muraoka M, Shimabukuro K, Toda K, Miyagawa K, Yoshimatsu H, Tsuchiya M. Inflammatory bowel diseases and thymus disorder: reactivity of thymocytes with monoclonal antibodies. Bull Tokyo Dent Coll. 1990 May;31(2):137-41. PMID: 2131166

Mo R, Lai R, Lu J, Zhuang Y, Zhou T, Jiang S, Ren P, Li Z, Cao Z, Liu Y, Chen L, Xiong L, Wang P, Wang H, Cai W, Xiang X, Bao S, Xie Q. Enhanced autophagy contributes to protective effects of IL-22 against acetaminophen-induced liver injury. Theranostics. 2018 Jul 30;8(15):4170-4180. doi: 10.7150/thno.25798.

Moan J, Porojnicu A, Lagunova Z, Berg JP, Dahlback A. Colon cancer: prognosis for different latitudes, age groups and seasons in Norway. J Photochem Photobiol B. 2007 Dec 14;89(2-3):148-55. doi: 10.1016/j.jphotobiol.2007.09.003.

Mochizuki-Oda, N, Kataoka, Y, Cui, Y, Yamada, H, Heya, M, and Awazu, K. Effects of near-infra-red laser irradiation on adenosine triphosphate and adenosine diphosphate contents of rat brain tissue. Neurosci Lett. (2002) 323:207–10. doi: 10.1016/s0304-3940(02)00159-3

Mogilevski T, Rosella S, Aziz Q, Gibson PR. Transcutaneous vagal nerve stimulation protects against stress-induced intestinal barrier dysfunction in healthy adults. Neurogastroenterol Motil. 2022 Apr 28:e14382. doi: 10.1111/nmo.14382

Mojica-Benavides M, van Niekerk DD, Mijalkov M, Snoep JL, Mehlig B, Volpe G, Goksör M, Adiels CB. Intercellular communication induces glycolytic synchronization waves between individually oscillating cells. Proc Natl Acad Sci U S SA. 2021 Feb 9;118(6):e2010075118. doi: 10.1073/pnas.2010075118.

Mojtabavi H, Saghazadeh A, van den Heuvel L, Bucker J, Rezaei N. Peripheral blood levels of brain-derived neurotrophic factor in patients with post-traumatic stress disorder (PTSD): A systematic review and meta-analysis. PLoS One. 2020 Nov 5;15(11):e0241928. doi:

10.1371/journal.pone.0241928. PMID: 33152026; PMCID: PMC7644072.

Möller M, Du Preez JL, Viljoen FP, Berk M, Emsley R, Harvey BH. Social isolation rearing induces mitochondrial, immunological, neurochemical, and behavioural deficits in rats and is reversed by clozapine or N-acetyl cysteine. Brain Behav Immun. 2013 May;30:156-67. doi: 10.1016/j.bbi.2012.12.011.

Molloy SS, Bresnahan PA, Leppla SH, Klimpel KR, Thomas G. Human furin is a calcium-dependent serine endoprotease that recognizes the sequence Arg-X-X-Arg and efficiently cleaves anthrax toxin protective antigen. J Biol Chem. 1992 Aug 15;267(23):16396-402. PMID: 1644824.

Moncrieff J, Cooper RE, Stockmann T, Amendola S, Hengartner MP, Horowitz MA. The serotonin theory of depression: a systematic umbrella review of the evidence. Mol Psychiatry. 2023;28:3243–56.

Moreira CG, Russell R, Mishra AA, Narayanan S, Ritchie JM, Waldor MK, Curtis MM, Winter SE, Weinshenker D, Sperandio V. Bacterial Adrenergic Sensors Regulate Virulence of Enteric Pathogens in the Gut. mBio. 2016 Jun 7;7(3):e00826-16. doi: 10.1128/mBio.00826-16.

Morozova A, Zorkina Y, Pavlov K, Pavlova O, Abramova O, Ushakova V, Mudrak AV, Zozulya S, Otman I, Sarmanova Z, Klyushnik T, Reznik A, Kostyuk G, Chekhonin V. Associations of Genetic Polymorphisms and Neuroimmune Markers With Some Parameters of Frontal

Lobe Dysfunction in Schizophrenia. Front Psychiatry. 2021 May 7;12:655178. doi: 10.3389/fpsyt.2021.655178.

Moskaliuk VS, Kozhemyakina RV, Khomenko TM, Volcho KP, Salakhutdinov NF, Kulikov AV, Naumenko VS, Kulikova EA. On Associations between Fear-Induced Aggression, Bdnf Transcripts, and Serotonin Receptors in the Brains of Norway Rats: An Influence of Antiaggressive Drug TC-2153. Int J Mol Sci. 2023 Jan 4;24(2):983. doi: 10.3390/ijms24020983.

Mostafa S, Miller BJ. Antibiotic-associated psychosis during treatment of urinary tract infections: a systematic review. J Clin Psychopharmacol. 2014 Aug;34(4):483-90. doi: 10.1097/JCP.0000000000000150.

Mount MP, Lira A, Grimes D, Smith PD, Faucher S, Slack R, Anisman H, Hayley S, Park DS. Involvement of interferon-gamma in microglial-mediated loss of dopaminergic neurons. J Neurosci. 2007 Mar 21;27(12):3328-37. doi: 10.1523/JNEUROSCI.5321-06.2007.

Moyer BJ, Rojas IY, Kerley-Hamilton JS, Hazlett HF, Nemani KV, Trask HW, West RJ, Lupien LE, Collins AJ, Ringelberg CS, Gimi B, Kinlaw WB 3rd, Tomlinson CR. Inhibition of the aryl hydrocarbon receptor prevents Western diet-induced obesity. Model for AHR activation by kynurenine via oxidized-LDL, TLR2/4, TGFβ, and IDO1. Toxicol Appl Pharmacol. 2016 Jun 1;300:13-24. doi: 10.1016/j.taap.2016.03.011. Epub 2016 Mar 25. PMID: 27020609; PMCID

Mufti RM, Balon R, Arfken CL. Low cholesterol and violence. Psychiatr Serv. 1998 Feb;49(2):221-4. doi: 10.1176/ps.49.2.221. PMID: 9575009.

Munawara, U.; Catanzaro, M.; Xu, W.; Tan, C.; Hirokawa, K.; Bosco, N.; Dumoulin, D.; Khalil, A.; Larbi, A.; Lévesque, S.; et al. Hyperactivation of monocytes and macrophages in MCI patients contributes to the progression of Alzheimer's disease. Immun. Aging 2021, 18, 29. [Google Scholar] [CrossRef]

Murru A, Manchia M, Hajek T, et al. Lithium's antiviral effects: a potential drug for CoViD-19 disease? Int J Bipolar Disorder. 2020;8(1):21. Published 2020 May 20. doi:10.1186/s40345-020-00191-4

Murty DVPS, Manikandan K, Kumar WS, Ramesh RG, Purokayastha S, Javali M, Rao NP, Ray S. Gamma oscillations weaken with age in healthy elderly in human EEG. Neuroimage. 2020 Jul 15;215:116826. doi: 10.1016/j.neuroimage.2020.116826

Murueta-Goyena, A., Ortuzar, N., Lafuente, J.V. et al. Enriched Environment Reverts Somatostatin Interneuron Loss in MK-801 Model of Schizophrenia. Mol Neurobiol 57, 125–134 (2020). https://doi.org/10.1007/s12035-019-01762-y

Myrov, V., Siebenhühner, F., Juvonen, J.J. et al. The rhythmicity of neuronal oscillations delineates their cortical and spectral architecture. Commun Biol 7, 405 (2024). https://doi.org/10.1038/s42003-024-06083-y

N'Guessan, K.F., Patel, P.H. & Qi, X. SapC-DOPS – a Phosphatidylserine-targeted Nanovesicle for selective Cancer therapy. Cell Commun Signal 18, 6 (2020). https://doi.org/10.1186/s12964-019-0476-6

Najjar S, Pahlajani S, De Sanctis V, Stern JNH, Najjar A, Chong D. Neurovascular Unit Dysfunction and Blood-Brain Barrier Hyperpermeability Contribute to Schizophrenia Neurobiology: A Theoretical Integration of Clinical and Experimental Evidence. Front Psychiatry. 2017 May 23;8:83. doi: 10.3389/fpsyt.2017.00083.

Nance KD, Meier JL. Modifications in an Emergency: The Role of N1-Methylpseudouridine in COVID-19 Vaccines. ACS Cent Sci. 2021 May 26;7(5):748-756. doi: 10.1021/acscentsci.1c00197.

Nässberger L, Träskman-Bendz L. Increased soluble interleukin-2 receptor concentrations in suicide attempters. Acta PsychiatrScand. 1993 Jul;88(1):48-52. doi: 10.1111/j.1600-

Natah SS, Mouihate A, Pittman QJ, Sharkey KA. Disruption of the blood-brain barrier during TNBS colitis. Neurogastroenterol Motil. 2005 Jun;17(3):433-46. doi: 10.1111/j.1365-2982.2005.00654.x. PMID: 15916631.

Nehme H, Saulnier P, Ramadan AA, Cassisa V, Guillet C, Eveillard M, Umerska A. Antibacterial activity of antipsychotic agents, their association with lipid nanocapsules and its impact on the properties of the nanocarriers and antibacterial activity. PLoS One. 2018 Jan 3;13(1):e0189950. doi: 10.1371/journal.pone.0189950

Nelson Espinosa, Alejandra Alonso, Cristian Morales, Pedro Espinosa, Andrés E Chávez, Pablo Fuentealba, Basal Forebrain Gating by Somatostatin Neurons Drives Prefrontal Cortical Activity, Cerebral Cortex, Volume 29, Issue 1, January 2019, Pages 42–53, https://doi.org/10.1093/cercor/bhx302

Nemani K, Williams SZ, Olfson M, Leckman-Westin E, Finnerty M, Kammer J, et al. Association Between the Use of Psychotropic Medications and the Risk of COVID-19 Infection Among Long-term Inpatients With Serious Mental Illness in a New York State-wide Psychiatric Hospital System. JAMA Netw Open. 2022 May 2;5(5):e2210743. doi: 10.1001/jamanetworkopen.2022.10743.

Neugebauer R, Betz H, Kuhse J. Expression of a soluble glycine binding domain of the NMDA receptor in Escherichia coli. Biochem Biophys Res Commun. 2003 Jun 6;305(3):476-83. doi: 10.1016/s0006-291x(03)00768-x. PMID: 12763017.

Ng PY, McNeely TL, Baker DJ. Untangling senescent and damage-associated microglia in the aging and diseased brain. FEBS J. 2023 Mar;290(5):1326-1339. doi: 10.1111/febs.16315.

Nguyen MC, Park JT, Jeon YG, Jeon BH, Hoe KL, Kim YM, et al. Arginase Inhibition Restores Peroxynitrite-Induced Endothelial Dysfunction via L-Arginine-Dependent Endothelial Nitric Oxide Synthase Phosphorylation. Yonsei Med J. 2016 Nov;57(6):1329-38. doi:

10.3349/ymj.2016.57.6.1329. PMID: 27593859; PMCID: PMC5011263.

Nguyen TT, Kosciolek T, Daly RE, Vázquez-Baeza Y, Swafford A, Knight R, Jeste DV. Gut microbiome in Schizophrenia: Altered functional pathways related to immune modulation and atherosclerotic risk. Brain Behav Immun. 2021 Jan;91:245-256. doi: 10.1016/j.bbi.2020.10.003.

Nicolson G. Continuing research into Gulf War illness. Science. 2001 May 4;292(5518):853. PMID: 11341275.

Nicolson GL, Ferreira de Mattos G, Ash M, Settineri R, Escribá PV. Fundamentals of Membrane Lipid Replacement: A Natural Medicine Approach to Repairing Cellular Membranes and Reducing Fatigue, Pain, and Other Symptoms While Restoring Function in Chronic Illnesses and Aging. Membranes (Basel). 2021 Nov 29;11(12):944. doi: 10.3390/membranes11120944.

Nicolson, G.L.; Ash, M.E. Lipid Replacement Therapy: A natural medicine approach to replacing damaged lipids in cellular membranes and organelles and restoring function. Biochim. Biophys. Acta 2014, 1838, 1657–1679. [CrossRef] [PubMed]170.

Nimmrich V, Eckert A. Calcium channel blockers and dementia. Br J Pharmacol. 2013;169(6):1203-1210. doi:10.1111/bph.12240

Nirisha PL, Bhaskaran AS, Yedavally NA, Suchandra HH, Manjunatha N, Kumar CN, Math SB. First episode psychosis and COVID-19: A case series and mini review. Asian J Psychiatr. 2022 Jul;73:103123. doi: 10.1016/j.ajp.2022.103123.

Nishimi K, Neylan TC, Bertenthal D, Seal KH, O'Donovan A. Association of Psychiatric Disorders With Incidence of SARS-CoV-2 Breakthrough Infection Among Vaccinated Adults. JAMA Netw Open. 2022 Apr 1;5(4):e227287. doi: 10.1001/jamanetworkopen.2022.7287. PMID: 35420660; PMCID: PMC9011123.

Niu R, Xue X, Zhao Y, Sun Z, Yan X, Li X, Feng C, Wang J. Effects of fluoride on microtubule ultrastructure and expression of Tubα1a and Tubβ2a in mouse hippocampus. Chemosphere. 2015 Nov;139:422-7. doi: 10.1016/j.chemosphere.2015.07.011. Epub 2015 Jul 30. PMID: 26232646.

Noh SE, Lee SJ, Lee TG, Park KS, Kim JH. Inhibition of cellular senescence hallmarks by mitochondrial transplantation in senescence-induced ARPE-19 cells. Neurobiol Aging. 2023 Jan;121:157-165. doi: 10.1016/j.neurobiolaging.2022.11.003.

Noll R. Kraepelin's 'lost biological psychiatry'? Autointoxication, organotherapy and surgery for dementia praecox. Hist Psychiatry. 2007 Sep;18(71 Pt 3):301-20. doi: 10.1177/0957154X07078705.

Oberg M, Bergander L, Håkansson H, Rannug U, Rannug A. Identification of the tryptophan photoproduct 6-formylindolo[3,2-b]carbazole, in cell culture medium, as a factor that controls the background aryl hydrocarbon receptor activity. Toxicol Sci. 2005 Jun;85(2):935-43. doi: 10.1093/toxsci/kfi154.

Ohlsson L, Gustafsson A, Lavant E, Suneson K, Brundin L, Westrin Å, Ljunggren L, Lindqvist D. Leaky gut biomarkers in depression and suicidal behavior. Acta Psychiatr Scand. 2019 Feb;139(2):185-193. doi: 10.1111/acps.12978. Epub 2018 Nov 1. Erratum in: Acta Psychiatr Scand. 2020 Nov;142(5):423. PMID: 30347427; PMCID: PMC6587489.

Olanow C.W., Stern M.B., Sethi K. The Scientific and Clinical Basis for the Treatment of Parkinson Disease (2009) Neurology. 2009;72:S1–S136. doi: 10.1212/WNL.0b013e3181a1d44c.

Olfson M, Marcus SC, Druss B, Elinson L, Tanielian T, Pincus HA. National Trends in the Outpatient Treatment of Depression. Journal of the American Medical Association. 2002;287:203–9

Olfson M, Marcus SC, Druss B, Elinson L, Tanielian T, Pincus HA. National trends in the outpatient treatment of depression. JAMA. 2002 Jan 9;287(2):203-9. doi: 10.1001/jama.287.2.203. PMID: 11779262.

Olivier JL, Chachaty C, Wolf C, Daveloose D, Bereziat G. Binding of two spin-labelled derivatives of chlorpromazine to human erythrocytes. Biochem J. 1989 Dec 15;264(3):633-41. doi: 10.1042/bj2640633.

Olson A, Hussong SA, Kayed R, Galvan V. TAU-INDUCED ASTROCYTE SENESCENCE: A NOVEL MECHANISM FOR NEURONAL DYSFUNCTION IN

ALZHEIMER'S DISEASE. Innov Aging. 2019;3(Suppl 1):S91-S92. Published 2019 Nov 8. doi:10.1093/geroni/igz038.348

Onaolapo OJ, Onaolapo AY. Nutrition, nutritional deficiencies, and schizophrenia: An association worthy of constant reassessment. World J Clin Cases. 2021 Oct 6;9(28):8295-8311. doi: 10.12998/wjcc.v9.i28.8295.

Osborne NJ, Ukoumunne OC, Wake M, Allen KJ. Prevalence of eczema and food allergy is associated with latitude in Australia. J Allergy Clin Immunol. 2012 Mar;129(3):865-7. doi: 10.1016/j.jaci.2012.01.037..

Osorio C, Kanukuntla T, Diaz E, Jafri N, Cummings M, Sfera A. The Post-amyloid Era in Alzheimer's Disease: Trust Your Gut Feeling. Front Aging Neurosci. 2019 Jun 26;11:143. doi: 10.3389/fnagi.2019.00143. PMID: 31297054; PMCID: PMC6608545.

Ousingsawat, J., Wanitchakool, P., Schreiber, R. et al. Contribution of TMEM16F to pyroptotic cell death. Cell Death Dis 9, 300 (2018). https://doi.org/10.1038/s41419-018-0373-8

Ovejero-Sánchez M, Rubio-Heras J, Vicente de la Peña MDC, San-Segundo L, Pérez-Losada J, González-Sarmiento R, Herrero AB. Chloroquine-Induced DNA Damage Synergizes with Nonhomologous End Joining Inhibition to Cause Ovarian Cancer Cell Cytotoxicity. Int J Mol Sci. 2022 Jul 7;23(14):7518. doi: 10.3390/ijms23147518.

Ozsvari B, Nuttall JR, Sotgia F, Lisanti MP. Azithromycin and Roxithromycin define a new family of "senolytic" drugs that target senescent human fibroblasts. Aging (Albany, NY). 2018 Nov 14;10(11):3294-3307. doi: 10.18632/aging.101633. PMID: 30428454; PMCID: PMC6286845.

Pacak AP, Preble JM, Kondo H, Seibel P, Levitsky S, del Nido PJ, et al. Actin-dependent mitochondrial internalization in cardiomyocytes: evidence for rescue of mitochondrial function. Biol Open. (2015) 4:622–6. doi: 10.1242/bio.20151147818.

Paliwal SR, Paliwal R, Vyas SP. A review of mechanistic insight and application of pH-sensitive liposomes in drug delivery. Drug Deliv. 2015 May;22(3):231-42. doi: 10.3109/10717544.2014.882469.

Palmos, A.B., Duarte, R.R.R., Smeeth, D.M. et al. Telomere length and human hippocampal neurogenesis. Neuropsychopharmacol. 45, 2239–2247 (2020). https://doi.org/10.1038/s41386-020-00863-w

Paloncýová M, Čechová P, Šrejber M, Kührová P, Otyepka M. Role of Ionizable Lipids in SARS-CoV-2 Vaccines As Revealed by Molecular Dynamics Simulations: From Membrane Structure to Interaction with mRNA Fragments. J Phys Chem Lett. 2021 Nov 18;12(45):11199-11205. doi: 10.1021/acs.jpclett.1c03109.

Pan B, Wang D, Li L, Shang L, Xia F, Zhang F, Zhang Y, Gale RP, Xu M, Li Z, Xu K. IL-22 Accelerates Thymus Regeneration via Stat3/Mcl-1 and Decreases Chronic Graft-versus-Host Disease in Mice after Allotransplants. Biol Blood Marrow Transplant. 2019 Oct;25(10):1911-1919. doi: 10.1016/j.bbmt.2019.06.002.

Panagiotaropoulos TI, Deco G, Kapoor V, Logothetis NK. Neuronal discharges and gamma oscillations explicitly reflect visual consciousness in the lateral prefrontal cortex. Neuron. 2012 Jun;74(5):924-935. DOI: 10.1016/j.neuron.2012.04.013. PMID: 22681695.

Pandurangi AK, Buckley PF. Inflammation, Antipsychotic Drugs, and Evidence for Effectiveness of Anti-inflammatory Agents in Schizophrenia. Curr Top Behav Neurosci. 2020;44:227-244. doi: 10.1007/7854_2019_91.

Papanastasiou E, Gaughran F, Smith S. Schizophrenia as segmental progeria. J R Soc Med. 2011 Nov;104(11):475-84. doi: 10.1258/jrsm.2011.110051. PMID: 22048679; PMCID: PMC3206717.

Papanastasiou E, Gaughran F, Smith S. Schizophrenia as segmental progeria. J R Soc Med. 2011 Nov;104(11):475-84. doi: 10.1258/jrsm.2011.110051.

Pardi N., Hogan M.J., Porter F.W., Weissman D. mRNA vaccines - a new era in vaccinology. Nat Rev Drug Discov. 2018;17:261–279. doi: 10.1038/nrd.2017.243

Paris D, Parker TA, Town T, Suo Z, Fang C, Humphrey J, Crawford F, Mullan M. Role of peroxynitrite in the vasoactive and cytotoxic effects of Alzheimer's beta-amyloid1-40 peptide. Exp Neurol. 1998 Jul;152(1):116-22. doi: 10.1006/exnr.1998.6828. PMID: 9682018.

Park S, Choi YK, Kim S, Lee J, Im W. CHARMM-GUI Membrane Builder for Lipid Nanoparticles with Ionizable Cationic Lipids and PEGylated Lipids. J Chem Inf Model. 2021 Oct 25;61(10):5192-5202. doi: 10.1021/acs.jcim.1c00770.

Party H, Dujarrier C, Hébert M, Lenoir S, Martinez de Lizarrondo S, Delépée R, Fauchon C, Bouton MC, Obiang P, Godefroy O, Save E, Lecardeur L, Chabry J, Vivien D, Agin V. Plasminogen Activator Inhibitor-1 (PAI-1) deficiency predisposes to depression and resistance to treatments. Acta Neuropathol Commun. 2019 Oct 14;7(1):153. doi: 10.1186/s40478-019-0807-2.

Pascalis O, de Haan M, Nelson CA. Is face processing species- specific during the first year of life? Science. 2002 May 17;296(5571):1321-3. doi: 10.1126/science.1070223.

Pastuzyn ED, Day CE, Kearns RB, Kyrke-Smith M, Taibi AV, McCormick J, Yoder N, Belnap DM, Erlendsson S, Morado DR, Briggs JAG, Feschotte C, Shepherd JD. The Neuronal Gene Arc Encodes a Repurposed Retrotransposon Gag Protein that Mediates Intercellular RNA Transfer. Cell. 2018 Jan 11;172(1-2):275-288.e18. doi: 10.1016/j.cell.2017.12.024.

Patel, S. Ashwanikumar N. Robinson E. et al. Naturally-occurring cholesterol analogues in lipid nanoparticles induce polymorphic shape and enhance intracellular delivery of mRNA. Nat Commun 11, 983 (2020). https://doi.org/10.1038/s41467-020-14527-2

Pathak H, Sreeraj VS, Venkatasubramanian G. Transcranial Alternating Current Stimulation (tACS) and Its Role in Schizophrenia: A Scoping Review. Clin Psychopharmacol Neurosci. 2023 Nov 30;21(4):634-649. doi: 10.9758/cpn.22.1042.

Pelkey, K. A., Chittajallu, R., Craig, M. T., Tricoire, L., Wester, J. C., and McBain, C. J. (2017). Hippocampal GABAergic Inhibitory Interneurons. Physiol. Rev. 97, 1619–1747. doi: 10.1152/physrev.00007.2017

Peng XC, Zhang M, Meng YY, Liang YF, Wang YY, Liu XQ, et al. Cell-cell fusion as an important mechanism of tumor metastasis (Review). Oncol Rep. 2021 Jul;46(1):145. doi: 10.3892/or.2021.8096. Epub 2021 Jun 3. PMID: 34080662.

Pennino D, Bhavsar PK, Effner R, Avitabile S, Venn P, Quaranta M, Marzaioli V, Cifuentes L, Durham SR, Cavani A, Eyerich K, Chung KF, Schmidt-Weber CB, Eyerich S. IL-22 suppresses IFN-γ-mediated lung inflammation in asthmatic patients. J Allergy Clin Immunol. 2013 Feb;131(2):562-70. doi: 10.1016/j.jaci.2012.09.036.

Perez JC, Moret-Chalmin C, Montagnier L. Towards the emergence of a new form of the neurodegenerative Creutzfeldt-Jakob disease: Twenty six cases of CJD declared a few days after a COVID-19 "vaccine" Jab. Preprint May 2022 DOI: 10.13140/RG.2.2.14427.03366

Pérez-Cervera, A., Seara, T. M., and Huguet, G. (2020). Phase-locked states in oscillating neural networks and their role in neural communication. Commun. Nonlinear. Sci.

Numer. Simul. 80, 104992. doi: 10.1016/j.cnsns.2019.104992

Perusina Lanfranca M, Lin Y, Fang J, Zou W, Frankel T. Biological and pathological activities of interleukin-22. J Mol Med (Berl). 2016 May;94(5):523-34. doi: 10.1007/s00109-016-1391-6.

Petrie KA, Schmidt D, Bubser M, Fadel J, Carraway RE, Deutch AY. Neurotensin activates GABAergic interneurons in the prefrontal cortex. J Neurosci. 2005 Feb 16;25(7):1629-36. doi: 10.1523/JNEUROSCI.3579-04.2005.

Pham TD. Identifying critical transitions in major depression with fuzzy recurrence entropy. ALL LIFE2022, VOL. 15, NO. 1, 1086–1100https://doi.org/10.1080/26895293.2022.2132017

Piao L, Zhao G, Zhu E, Inoue A, Shibata R, Lei Y, Hu L, Yu C, Yang G, Wu H, Xu W, Okumura K, Ouchi N, Murohara T, Kuzuya M, Cheng XW. Chronic Psychological Stress Accelerates Vascular Senescence and Impairs Ischemia-Induced Neovascularization: The Role of Dipeptidyl Peptidase-4/Glucagon-Like Peptide-1-Adiponectin Axis. J Am Heart Assoc. 2017 Sep 28;6(10):e006421. doi: 10.1161/JAHA.117.006421.

Poblocka, M., Bassey, A.L., Smith, V.M. et al. Targeted clearance of senescent cells using an antibody-drug conjugate against a specific membrane marker. Sci Rep 11, 20358 (2021). https://doi.org/10.1038/s41598-021-99852-2

Pompili M, Forte A, Palermo M, Stefani H, Lamis DA, Serafini G, Amore M, Girardi P. Suicide risk in multiple sclerosis: a systematic review of current literature. J Psychosom Res. 2012 Dec;73(6):411-7. doi: 10.1016/j.jpsychores.2012.09.011.

Ponsford MJ, Pecoraro A, Jolles S. Clozapine-associated secondary antibody deficiency. Curr Opin Allergy Clin Immunol. 2019 Dec;19(6):553-562. doi: 10.1097/ACI.0000000000000592. PMID: 31567398.

Popova, N.V.; Deyev, I.E.; Petrenko, A.G. Clathrin-mediated endocytosis and adaptor proteins. Acta Nat. 2013, 5, 62–73.

Postolache, T.T., Komarow, H. & Tonelli, L.H. Allergy: A risk factor for suicide?. Curr Treat Options Neurol 10, 363–376 (2008). https://doi.org/10.1007/s11940-008-0039-4

Pousa, P.; Souza, R.; Melo, P.; Correa, B.; Mendonça, T.; Simões-E-Silva, A.; Miranda, D. Telomere Shortening and Psychiatric Disorders: A Systematic Review. Cells 2021, 10, 1423.

Powell JB, Goode GD, Eltom SE. The Aryl Hydrocarbon Receptor: A Target for Breast Cancer Therapy. J Cancer Ther. 2013 Sep;4(7):1177-1186. doi: 10.4236/jct.2013.47137.

Pretorius L, Kell DB, Pretorius E. Iron Dysregulation and Dormant Microbes as Causative Agents for Impaired Blood Rheology and Pathological Clotting in Alzheimer's Type

Dementia. Front Neurosci. 2018 Nov 16;12:851. doi: 10.3389/fnins.2018.00851.

Prindle A, Liu J, Asally M, Ly S, Garcia-Ojalvo J, Süel GM. Ion channels enable electrical communication in bacterial communities. Nature. 2015 Nov 5;527(7576):59-63. doi: 10.1038/nature15709.

Prior TI, Baker GB. Interactions between the cytochrome P450 system and the second-generation antipsychotics. J Psychiatry Neurosci. (2003) 28:99–112

Proal AD, Albert PJ, Marshall TG. The human microbiome and autoimmunity. Curr Opin Rheumatol. 2013 Mar;25(2):234-40. doi: 10.1097/BOR.0b013e32835cedbf. PMID: 23370376.

Puvogel, S., Alsema, A., Kracht, L. et al. Single-nucleus RNA sequencing of midbrain blood-brain barrier cells in schizophrenia reveals subtle transcriptional changes with overall preservation of cellular proportions and phenotypes. Mol Psychiatry 27, 4731–4740 (2022). https://doi.org/10.1038/s41380-022-01796-0

Qattan M.Y., Khan M.I., Alharbi S.H., Verma A.K., Al-Saeed F.A., Abduallah A.M., Al Areefy A.A. Therapeutic Importance of Kaempferol in the Treatment of Cancer through the Modulation of Cell Signalling Pathways. Molecules. 2022;27:8864. doi: 10.3390/molecules27248864. [PMC free article] [PubMed] [CrossRef] [Google Scholar]

Qiao G, Li S, Yang B, Li B. Inhibitory effects of artemisinin on voltage-gated ion channels in intact nodose ganglion neurones of adult rats. Basic Clin Pharmacol Toxicol. 2007 Apr;100(4):217-24. doi: 10.1111/j.1742-7843.2006.00009.x. PMID: 17371525.

Qie, S.; Ran, Y.; et al. Candesartan Modulates Microglia Activation and Polarization via NF-KB Signaling Pathway. Int J Immunopathol Pharmacol 2020, 34, 205873842097490.
https://doi.org/10.1177/2058738420974900

Qin J., Fu M., Wang J., Huang F., Liu H., Huangfu M., Yu D., Liu H., Li X., Guan X., et al. PTEN/AKT/mTOR signaling med ates anticancer effects of epigallocatechin-3-gallate in ovarian cancer. Oncol. Rep. 2020;43:1885–1896. doi: 10.3892/or.2020.7571. [PMC free article] [PubMed] [CrossRef] [Google Scholar]

Quiroga RQ. Concept cells: the building blocks of declarative memory functions. Nat Rev Neurosci. 2012 Jul 4;13(8):587-97. doi: 10.1038/nrn3251.

Rachel Caspi, Mary Mattapallil, Rachael Rigden, Carlos Zarate-Blades, Phyllis Silver, Dror Luger, Chi Chao Chan; Neuroprotective effects of IL-22 during CNS inflammation (CCR4P.203). J Immunol 1 May 2015; 194 (1_Supplement): 118.3.

Rachel Kaufman, Prozac Killing E. coli in the Great Lakes. National Geographic (2011).

Raine A, Meloy JR, Bihrle S, Stoddard J, LaCasse L, Buchsbaum MS. Reduced prefrontal and increased subcortical brain functioning assessed using positron emission tomography in predatory and affective murderers. Behav Sci Law. 1998 Summer;16(3):319-32. doi: 10.1002/(sici)1099-0798(199822)16:3<319::aid-bsl311>3.0.co;2-g.

Rannug A, Rannug U, Rosenkranz HS, Winqvist L, Westerholm R, Agurell E, Grafström AK. Certain photooxidized derivatives of tryptophan bind with very high affinity to the Ah receptor and are likely to be endogenous signal substances. J Biol Chem. 1987 Nov 15;262(32):15422-7.

Raskin DM, de Boer PA. Rapid pole-to-pole oscillation of a protein required for directing division to the middle of Escherichia coli. Proc Natl Acad Sci U S A. 1999 Apr 27;96(9):4971-6. doi: 10.1073/pnas.96.9.4971.

Razzoli M, Nyuyki-Dufe K, Gurney A, et al. Social stress shortens lifespan in mice. Aging Cell. 2018;17(4):e12778. doi: 10.1111/acel.12778

Refaeli R, Doron A, Benmelech-Chovav A, Groysman M, Kreisel T, Loewenstein Y, Goshen I. Features of hippocampal astrocytic domains and their spatial relation to excitatory and inhibitory neurons. Glia. 2021 Oct;69(10):2378-2390. doi: 10.1002/glia.24044.

Ren J, Lu Y, Qian Y, Chen B, Wu T, Ji G. Recent progress regarding kaempferol for the treatment of various diseases.

Exp Ther Med. 2019 Oct;18(4):2759-2776. doi: 10.3892/etm.2019.7886.

Ren, F., Zhang, N., Zhang, L. et al. Alternative Polyadenylation: a new frontier in post post-transcriptional regulation. Biomark Res 8, 67 (2020). https://doi.org/10.1186/s40364-020-00249-6

Rentscher KE, Carroll JE, Repetti RL, Cole SW, Reynolds BM, Robles TF. Chronic stress exposure and daily stress appraisals relate to biological aging marker p16 INK4a. Psychoneuroendocrinology. 2019;102:139–148. doi: 10.1016/j.psyneuen.2018.12.006

Rhodes JM, Subramanian S, Laird E, Kenny RA. Editorial: low population mortality from COVID-19 in countries south of latitude 35 degrees North supports vitamin D as a factor determining severity. Aliment Pharmacol Ther. 2020 Jun;51(12):1434-1437. doi: 10.1111/apt.15777.

Richardson, K., Petukhova, R., Hughes, S. et al. The acceptability of lifestyle medicine for the treatment of mental illness: perspectives of people with and without lived experience of mental illness. BMC Public Health 24, 171 (2024). https://doi.org/10.1186/s12889-024-17683-y

Rijkers GT, Weterings N, Obregon-Henao A, Lepolder M, Dutt TS, van Overveld FJ, Henao-Tamayo M. Antigen Presentation of mRNA-Based and Virus-Vectored SARS-CoV-2 Vaccines. Vaccines (Basel). 2021 Aug 3;9(8):848. doi: 10.3390/vaccines9080848.

Rodrigues FR, Papanikolaou A, Holeniewska J, Phillips KG, Saleem AB, Solomon SG. Altered low-frequency brain rhythms precede changes in gamma power during tauopathy. iScience. 2022 Sep 28;25(10):105232. doi: 10.1016/j.isci.2022.105232.

Rodrigues, L. S.; da Silva Nali, L. H.; et al. HERV-K and HERV-W Transcriptional Activity in Myalgic Encephalomyelitis/Chronic Fatigue Syndrome. Autoimmunity Highlights 2019, 10 (1), 12. https://doi.org/10.1186/s13317-019-0122-8.

Rolf L, Sikkema T, Krudde J, van Harten B. Wittestofafwijkingen na een zelfmoordpoging [White matter abnormalities following attempted suicide]. Ned Tijdschr Geneeskd. 2013;157(41):A6526. Dutch. PMID: 24103138.

Ronald A. The etiology of urinary tract infection: traditional and emerging pathogens. Am J Med. 2002 Jul 8;113 Suppl 1A:14S-19S. doi: 10.1016/s0002-9343(02)01055-0

Rose MF, Ahmad KA, Thaller C, Zoghbi HY. Excitatory neurons of the proprioceptive, interoceptive, and arousal hindbrain networks share a developmental requirement for Math1. Proc Natl Acad Sci U S A. 2009 Dec 29;106(52):22462-7. doi: 10.1073/pnas.0911579106.

Rosłoń, I.E., Japaridze, A., Steeneken, P.G. et al. Probing nano motion of single bacteria with graphene drums. Nat. Nanotechnol. 17, 637–642 (2022). https://doi.org/10.1038/s41565-022-01111-6

Rudzki L, Szulc A. "Immune Gate" of Psychopathology-The Role of Gut Derived Immune Activation in Major Psychiatric Disorders. Front Psychiatry. 2018 May 29;9:205. doi: 10.3389/fpsyt.2018.00205

Rulands S, Lee HJ, Clark SJ, Angermueller C, Smallwood SA, Krueger F, Mohammed H, Dean W, Nichols J, Rugg-Gunn P, Kelsey G, Stegle O, Simons BD, Reik W. Genome-Scale Oscillations in DNA Methylation during Exit from Pluripotency. Cell Syst. 2018 Jul 25;7(1):63-76.e12. doi: 10.1016/j.cels.2018.06.012.

Rus, C.P., de Vries, B.E.K., de Vries, I.E.J. et al. Treatment of 95 post-Covid patients with SSRIs. Sci Rep 13, 18599 (2023). https://doi.org/10.1038/s41598-023-45072-9

Russ TC, Murianni L, Icaza G, Slachevsky A, Starr JM. Geographical Variation in Dementia Mortality in Italy, New Zealand, and Chile: The Impact of Latitude, Vitamin D, and Air Pollution. Dement Geriatr Cogn Disord. 2016;42(1-2):31-41. doi: 10.1159/000447449.

Sadeghi Hassanabadi N, Broux B, Marinović S, Gotthardt D. Innate Lymphoid Cells - Neglected Players in Multiple Sclerosis. Front Immunol. 2022 Jun 17;13:909275. doi: 10.3389/fimmu.2022.909275.

Sahay G, Querbes W, Alabi C, Eltoukhy A, Sarkar S, Zurenko C, et al. Efficiency of siRNA delivery by lipid nanoparticles is limited by endocytic recycling. Nat Biotechnol. 2013 Jul;31(7):653-8. doi: 10.1038/nbt.2614

Sahbaz, C., Zibandey, N., Kurtulmus, A. et al. Reduced regulatory T cells with increased proinflammatory response in patients with schizophrenia. Psychopharmacology 237, 1861–1871 (2020). https://doi.org/10.1007/s00213-020-05504-0

Saheki A, Terasaki T, Tamai I, Tsuji A. In vivo and in vitro blood-brain barrier transport of 3-hydroxy-3-methylglutaryl coenzyme A (HMG-CoA) reductase inhibitors. Pharm Res. 1994;11:305–11.

Sakai-Kato K, Yoshida K, Takechi-Haraya Y, Izutsu KI. Physicochemical Characterization of Liposomes That Mimic the Lipid Composition of Exosomes for Effective Intracellular Trafficking. Langmuir. 2020 Oct 27;36(42):12735-12744. doi: 10.1021/acs.langmuir.0c02491.

Salminen A. Aryl hydrocarbon receptor (AhR) reveals evidence of antagonistic pleiotropy in the regulation of the aging process. Cell Mol Life Sci. 2022 Aug 20;79(9):489. doi: 10.1007/s00018-022-04520-x. PMID: 35987825; PMCID: PMC9392714.

Sandler NG, Douek DC. Microbial translocation in HIV infection: causes, consequences and treatment opportunities. Nat Rev Microbiol. 2012 Sep;10(9):655-66. doi: 10.1038/nrmicro2848.

Sansone RA, Sansone LA. SSRI-Induced Indifference. Psychiatry (Edgmont). 2010 Oct;7(10):14-8. PMID: 21103140; PMCID: PMC2989833.

Santiago-Mujika E, Luthi-Carter R, Giorgini F, Kalaria RN, Mukaetova-Ladinska EB. Tubulin and Tubulin Posttranslational Modifications in Alzheimer's Disease and Vascular Dementia. Front Aging Neurosci. 2021;13:730107. Published 2021 Oct 29. doi:10.3389/fnagi.2021.730107

Sargiacomo C, Sotgia F, Lisanti MP. COVID-19 and chronological aging: senolytics and other anti-aging drugs for the treatment or prevention of corona virus infection? Aging (Albany NY). 2020 Mar 30;12(8):6511-6517. doi: 10.18632/aging.103001. Epub 2020 Mar 30. PMID: 32229706; PMCID: PMC7202514.

Sasaki, D., Abe, J., Takeda, A. et al. Transplantation of MITO cells, mitochondria activated cardiac progenitor cells, to the ischemic myocardium of mouse enhances the therapeutic effect. Sci Rep 12, 4344 (2022). https://doi.org/10.1038/s41598-022-08583-521.

Sato, T.; Shapiro, J. S.; et al. Aging Is Associated with Increased Brain Iron through Cortex-Derived Hepcidin Expression. Elife 2022, 11. https://doi.org/10.7554/eLife.73456.

Sato, T.; Shapiro, J. S.; et al. Aging Is Associated with Increased Brain Iron through Cortex-Derived Hepcidin Expression. Elife 2022, 11. https://doi.org/10.7554/eLife.73456.

Schleuning MJ, Duggan A, Reem GH. Inhibition by chlorpromazine of lymphokine-specific mRNA expression in human thymocytes. Eur J Immunol. 1989

Aug;19(8):1491-5. doi: 10.1002/eji.1830190822. PMID: 2550248.

Schoenmaker L, Witzigmann D, Kulkarni JA, et al. mRNA-lipid nanoparticle COVID-19 vaccines: Structure and stability. Int J Pharm. 2021;601:120586. doi:10.1016/j.ijpharm.2021.120586

Schubert KO, Föcking M, Cotter DR. Proteomic pathway analysis of the hippocampus in schizophrenia and bipolar affective disorder implicates 14-3-3 signaling, aryl hydrocarbon receptor signaling, and glucose metabolism: potential roles in GABAergic interneuron pathology. Schizophr Res. 2015 Sep;167(1-3):64-72. doi: 10.1016/j.schres.2015.02.002

Schug RA, Yang Y, Raine A, Han C, Liu J, Li L. Resting EEG deficits in accused murderers with schizophrenia. Psychiatry Res. 2011 Oct 31;194(1):85-94. doi: 10.1016/j.pscychresns.2010.12.017.

Schwarz E., Prabakaran S., Whitfield P., Major H., Leweke F. M., Keothe D., et al.. (2008). High troughput lipidomic profiling of schizophrenia and bipolar disorder brain tissue reveals alterations of free fatty acids, phosphatidylcolines and ceramides. J. Proteome Res. 7, 4266–4277. 10.1021/pr800188y

Sebastiani F, Yanez Arteta M, Lerche M, Porcar L, Lang C, Bragg RA, et al. Apolipoprotein E Binding Drives Structural and Compositional Rearrangement of mRNA-Containing Lipid Nanoparticles. ACS Nano. 2021 Apr 27;15(4):6709-6722. doi: 10.1021/acsnano.0c10064.

Secher T, Samba-Louaka A, Oswald E, Nougayrède JP. Escherichia coli producing colibactin triggers premature and transmissible senescence in mammalian cells. PLoS One. 2013 Oct 8;8(10):e77157. doi: 10.1371/journal.pone.0077157.

Secher T, Samba-Louaka A, Oswald E, Nougayrède JP. Escherichia coli producing colibactin triggers premature and transmissible senescence in mammalian cells. PLoS One. 2013 Oct 8;8(10):e77157. doi: 10.1371/journal.pone.0077157.

Sedgwick AJ, Ghazanfari N, Constantinescu P, Mantamadiotis T, Barrow AD. The Role of NK Cells and Innate Lymphoid Cells in Brain Cancer. Front Immunol. 2020 Jul 31;11:1549. doi: 10.3389/fimmu.2020.01549.

Seoane R, Vidal S, Bouzaher YH, El Motiam A, Rivas C. The Interaction of Viruses with the Cellular Senescence Response. Biology (Basel). 2020 Dec 9;9(12):455. doi: 10.3390/biology9120455.

Settanni G, Brill W, Haas H, Schmid F. pH-Dependent Behavior of Ionizable Cationic Lipids in mRNA-Carrying Lipoplexes Investigated by Molecular Dynamics Simulations. Macromol Rapid Commun. 2022 Jun;43(12):e2100683. doi: 10.1002/marc.202100683.

Severance EG, Gressitt KL, Stallings CR, Origoni AE, Khushalani S, Leweke FM, Dickerson FB, Yolken RH. Discordant patterns of bacterial translocation markers and implications for innate immune imbalances in schizophrenia. Schizophr Res. 2013 Aug;148(1-3):130-7. doi: 10.1016/j.schres.2013.05.018.

Severance EG, Gressitt KL, Stallings CR, Origoni AE, Khushalani S, Leweke FM, Dickerson FB, Yolken RH. Discordant patterns of bacterial translocation markers and implications for innate immune imbalances in schizophrenia. Schizophr Res. 2013 Aug;148(1-3):130-7. doi: 10.1016/j.schres.2013.05.018.

Severance EG, Gressitt KL, Stallings CR, Origoni AE, Khushalani S, Leweke FM, Dickerson FB, Yolken RH. Discordant patterns of bacterial translocation markers and implications for innate immune imbalances in schizophrenia. Schizophr Res. 2013 Aug;148(1-3):130-7. doi: 10.1016/j.schres.2013.05.018.

Severance EG, Yolken RH. From Infection to the Microbiome: An Evolving Role of Microbes in Schizophrenia. Curr Top Behav Neurosci. 2020;44:67-84. doi: 10.1007/7854_2018_84.

Sewell DD. Schizophrenia and HIV. Schizophr Bull. 1996;22(3):465-73. doi: 10.1093/schbul/22.3.465. PMID: 8873297.

Sfera A, Osorio C, Afzaal J, Del Campo, Z-M, Kozlakidis Z. COVID-19: A Catalyst for Novel Psychiatric Paradigms May 2021 DOI: 10.5772/intechopen.96940. In book: Biotechnology to Combat COVID-19

Sfera A, Osorio C, Rahman L, Zapata-Martín Del Campo CM, Maldonado JC, Jafri N, Cummings MA, Maurer S,

Kozlakidis Z. PTSD as an Endothelial Disease: Insights From COVID-19. Front Cell Neurosci. 2021 Oct 29;15:770387. doi: 10.3389/fncel.2021.770387. PMID: 34776871; PMCID: PMC8586713.

Sfera A. Targeted intermittent treatment in chronic schizophrenia. Front Psychiatry. 2013 Mar 14;4:13. doi: 10.3389/fpsyt.2013.00013. PMID: 23505392; PMCID: PMC3596804.

Sfera, A.; Anton, J.J.; Imran, H.; Kozlakidis, Z.; Klein, C.; Osorio, C. Of Soldiers and Their Ghosts: Are We Ready for a Review of PTSD Evidence? BioMed 2023, 3, 484-506. https://doi.org/10.3390/biomed3040039

Sfera, A.; Hazan, S.; Klein, C.; del Campo, C.M.Z.-M.; Sasannia, S.; Anton, J.J.; Rahman, L.; Andronescu, C.V.; Sfera, D.O.; Kozlakidis, Z.; Nicolson, G.L. Microbial Translocation Disorders: Assigning an Etiology to Idiopathic Illnesses. Appl. Microbiol. 2023, 3, 212-240. https://doi.org/10.3390/applmicrobiol3010015

Sha Paciorek, A.; Skora, L. Vagus Nerve Stimulation as a Gateway to Interoception. Front. Psychol. 2020, 11, 1659.

Shang L, Duah M, Xu Y, Liang Y, Wang D, Xia F, Li L, Sun Z, Yan Z, Xu K, Pan B. Dynamic of plasma IL-22 level is an indicator of thymic output after allogeneic hematopoietic cell transplantation. Life Sci. 2021 Jan 15;265:118849. doi: 10.1016/j.lfs.2020.118849.

Shantakumari N, Ahmed M. Whole body vibration therapy and cognitive functions: a systematic review. AIMS

Neurosci. 2023 May 18;10(2):130-143. doi: 10.3934/Neuroscience.2023010.

Shao, L., Xiong, X., Zhang, Y. et al. IL-22 ameliorates LPS-induced acute liver injury by autophagy activation through ATF4-ATG7 signaling. Cell Death Dis 11, 970 (2020). https://doi.org/10.1038/s41419-020-03176-4

Sharma N, Tan MA, An SSA. Phytosterols: Potential Metabolic Modulators in Neurodegenerative Diseases. Int J Mol Sci. 2021 Nov 12;22(22):12255. doi: 10.3390/ijms222212255. PMID: 34830148; PMCID: PMC8618769.

Sharma R. Emerging Interrelationship Between the Gut Microbiome and Cellular Senescence in the Context of Aging and Disease: Perspectives and Therapeutic Opportunities. Probiotics Antimicrob Proteins. 2022 Aug;14(4):648-663. doi: 10.1007/s12602-021-09903-3.

Sherman MA, Linthicum DS, Bolger MB. Haloperidol binding to monoclonal antibodies: conformational analysis and relationships to D-2 receptor binding. Mol Pharmacol. 1986 Jun;29(6):589-98. PMID: 2423865.

Sibony M, Abdullah M, Greenfield L, Raju D, Wu T, Rodrigues DM, Galindo-Mata E, Mascarenhas H, Philpott DJ, Silverberg MS, Jones NL. Microbial Disruption of Autophagy Alters Expression of the RISC Component AGO2, a Critical Regulator of the miRNA Silencing Pathway. Inflamm Bowel Dis. 2015 Dec;21(12):2778-86. doi: 10.1097/MIB.0000000000000553.

Siegel JZ, Crockett MJ. How serotonin shapes moral judgment and behavior. Ann N Y Acad Sci. 2013 Sep;1299(1):42-51. doi: 10.1111/nyas.12229. PMID: 25627116; PMCID: PMC3817523.

Simpson HL, Campbell BJ. Review article: dietary fibre-microbiota interactions. Aliment Pharmacol Ther (2015) 42(2):158–79. 10.1111/apt.13248

Singh RK, Dai Y, Staudinger JL, Muma NA. Activation of the JAK-STAT pathway is necessary for desensitization of 5-HT2A receptor-stimulated phospholipase C signalling by olanzapine, clozapine and MDL 100907. Int J Neuropsychopharmacol. 2009 Jun;12(5):651-65. doi: 10.1017/S1461145708009590.

Singh S., Srivastava P. Molecular Docking Studies of Myricetin and Its Analogues against Human PDK-1 Kinase as Candidate Drugs for Cancer. Comput. Mol. Biosci. 2015;5:20. doi: 10.4236/cmb.2015.52004. [CrossRef] [Google Scholar]

Sirakanyan S, Arabyan E, Hakobyan A, Hakobyan T, Chilingaryan G, Sahakyan H, et al. A new microtubule-stabilizing agent shows potent antiviral effects against African swine fever virus with no cytotoxicity. Emerg Microbes Infect. 2021 Dec;10(1):783-796. doi: 10.1080/22221751.2021.1902751. PMID: 33706677; PMCID: PMC8079068.

Sirtori CR. The pharmacology of statins. Pharmacol Res. 2014 Oct;88:3-11. doi: 10.1016/j.phrs.2014.03.002. Epub 2014 Mar 20. PMID: 24657242.

Siwaszek A, Ukleja M, Dziembowski A. Proteins involved in the degradation of cytoplasmic mRNA in the major eukaryotic model systems. RNA Biol. 2014;11(9):1122-36. doi: 10.4161/rna.34406. PMID: 25483043; PMCID: PMC4615280.

Skloot R. The Immortal Life of Henrietta Lacks. New York: Crown; 2010.

Slavin J. Fiber and prebiotics: mechanisms and health benefits. Nutrients. (2013) 5:1417–35. 10.3390/nu5041417

Slavin J. Fiber and prebiotics: mechanisms and health benefits. Nutrients (2013) 5(4):1417–35. 10.3390/nu5041417

Solaimanzadeh I. Nifedipine and Amlodipine Are Associated With Improved Mortality and Decreased Risk for Intubation and Mechanical Ventilation in Elderly Patients Hospitalized for COVID-19. Cureus. 2020 May 12;12(5):e8069. doi: 10.7759/cureus.8069. PMID: 32411566; PMCID: PMC7219014.

Solana C, Pereira D, Tarazona R. Early Senescence and Leukocyte Telomere Shortening in SCHIZOPHRENIA: A Role for Cytomegalovirus Infection? Brain Sci. 2018 Oct 18;8(10):188. doi: 10.3390/brainsci8100188.

Solmi, M., Seitidis, G., Mavridis, D. et al. Incidence, prevalence, and global burden of schizophrenia - data, with critical appraisal, from the Global Burden of Disease (GBD) 2019. Mol Psychiatry 28, 5319–5327 (2023). https://doi.org/10.1038/s41380-023-02138-4

Solomon GF, Rubbo SD, Batchelder E. Secondary immune response to tetanus toxoid in psychiatric patients. J Psychiatr Res. 1970 Feb;7(3):201-7. doi: 10.1016/0022-3956(70)90007-5. PMID: 5440860.

Sommer A, Kordowski F, Büch J, Maretzky T, Evers A, Andrä J, et al. Phosphatidylserine exposure is required for ADAM17 sheddase function. Nat Commun. 2016 May 10;7:11523. doi: 10.1038/ncomms11523

Song Y, Slominski RM, Qayyum S, Kim TK, Janjetovic Z, Raman C, Tuckey RC, Song Y, Slominski AT. Molecular and structural basis of interactions of vitamin D3 hydroxyderivatives with aryl hydrocarbon receptor (AhR): An integrated experimental and computational study. Int J Biol Macromol. 2022 Jun 1;209(Pt A):1111-1123. doi: 10.1016/j.ijbiomac.2022.04.048.

Soulet D, Gagnon B, Rivest S, Audette M, Poulin R. A fluorescent probe of polyamine transport accumulates into intracellular acidic vesicles via a two-step mechanism. J Biol Chem. 2004 Nov 19;279(47):49355-66. doi: 10.1074/jbc.M401287200.

Spagna A, Hajhajate D, Liu J, Bartolomeo P. Visual mental imagery engages the left fusiform gyrus, but not the early visual cortex: A meta-analysis of neuroimaging evidence. Neurosci Biobehav Rev. 2021 Mar;122:201-217. doi: 10.1016/j.neubiorev.2020.12.029.

Squassina A, Manchia M, Chillotti C, Deiana V, Congiu D, Paribello F, et al. Differential effect of lithium on spermidine/spermine N1-acetyltransferase expression in suicidal behaviour. Int J Neuropsychopharmacol. 2013 Nov;16(10):2209-18. doi: 10.1017/S1461145713000655.

Srivastava, V., Buzas, B., Momenan, R. et al. Association of SOD2, a Mitochondrial Antioxidant Enzyme, with Gray Matter Volume Shrinkage in Alcoholics. Neuropsychopharmacol 35, 1120–1128 (2010). https://doi.org/10.1038/npp.2009.217

Stadlmann, S.; Hein-Kuhnt, R.; et al. Viropathic Multinuclear Syncytial Giant Cells in Bronchial Fluid from a Patient with COVID-19. J Clin Pathol 2020, 73 (9), 607–608. https://doi.org/10.1136/jclinpath-2020-206657.

Stanbouly D, Chuang SK. What are the Psychosocial Consequences of Chronic Mask-Wearing in the COVID-19 Pandemic? J Oral Maxillofac Surg. 2021 Sep;79(9):1815-1816. doi: 10.1016/j.joms.2021.04.014.

Stankovic I, Notaras M, Wolujewicz P, Lu T, Lis R, Ross ME, Colak D. Schizophrenia endothelial cells exhibit higher permeability and altered angiogenesis patterns in patient-derived organoids. Transl Psychiatry. 2024 Jan 23;14(1):53. doi: 10.1038/s41398-024-02740-2. PMID: 38263175; PMCID: PMC10806043.

Stapel B, Sieve I, Falk CS, Bleich S, Hilfiker-Kleiner D, Kahl KG. Second generation atypical antipsychotics olanzapine and aripiprazole reduce expression and secretion of inflammatory cytokines in human immune cells. J Psychiatr Res. 2018 Oct;105:95-102. doi: 10.1016/j.jpsychires.2018.08.017.

Steel AW, Mela CM, Lindsay JO, Gazzard BG, Goodier MR. Increased proportion of CD16(+) NK cells in the colonic lamina propria of inflammatory bowel disease patients, but not after azathioprine treatment. Aliment Pharmacol Ther. 2011 Jan;33(1):115-26. doi: 10.1111/j.1365-2036.2010.04499.x.

Stehle JR Jr, Leng X, Kitzman DW, Nicklas BJ, Kritchevsky SB, High KP. Lipopolysaccharide-binding protein, a surrogate marker of microbial translocation, is associated with physical function in healthy older adults. J Gerontol A Biol Sci Med Sci. 2012 Nov;67(11):1212-8. doi: 10.1093/gerona/gls178

Stein AC, Gaetano JN, Jacobs J, Kunnavakkam R, Bissonnette M, Pekow J. Northern Latitude but Not Season Is Associated with Increased Rates of Hospitalizations Related to Inflammatory Bowel Disease: Results of a Multi-Year Analysis of a National Cohort. PLoS One. 2016 Aug 31;11(8):e0161523. doi: 10.1371/journal.pone.0161523

Stiefel, K. M., and Ermentrout, G. B. (2016). Neurons as oscillators. J. Neurophysiol. 116, 2950–2960. doi: 10.1152/jn.00525.2015

Stoeva MK, Garcia-So J, Justice N, Myers J, Tyagi S, Nemchek M, McMurdie PJ, Kolterman O, Eid J. Butyrate-producing human gut symbiont, Clostridium butyricum, and its role in health and disease. Gut Microbes. 2021 Jan-Dec;13(1):1-28. doi: 10.1080/19490976.2021.1907272.

Straus MR, Bidon MK, Tang T, Jaimes JA, Whittaker GR, Daniel S. Inhibitors of L-Type Calcium Channels Show

Therapeutic Potential for Treating SARS-CoV-2 Infections by Preventing Virus Entry and Spread. ACS Infect Dis. 2021 Oct 8;7(10):2807-2815. doi: 10.1021/acsinfecdis.1c00023. Epub 2021 Sep 9. PMID: 34498840; PMCID: PMC8442615.

Su S, Xiao Z, Lin Z, Qiu Y, Jin Y, Wang Z. Plasma brain-derived neurotrophic factor levels in patients suffering from post-traumatic stress disorder. Psychiatry Res. 2015 Sep 30;229(1-2):365-9. doi: 10.1016/j.psychres.2015.06.038.

Su Y, Liu M, Liang K, Liu X, Song Y, Deng Y. Evaluating the Accelerated Blood Clearance Phenomenon of PEGylated Nanoemulsions in Rats by Intraperitoneal Administration. AAPS PharmSciTech. 2018 Oct;19(7):3210-3218. doi: 10.1208/s12249-018-1120-2

Subbanna M, Shivakumar V, Talukdar PM, Narayanaswamy JC, Venugopal D, Berk M, Varambally S, Venkatasubramanian G, Debnath M. Role of IL-6/RORC/IL-22 axis in driving Th17 pathway mediated immunopathogenesis of schizophrenia. Cytokine. 2018 Nov;111:112-118. doi: 10.1016/j.cyto.2018.08.016.

Suda, K., et al. (2024). Plasma membrane damage limits replicative lifespan in yeast and induces premature senescence in human fibroblasts. Nature Aging. doi.org/10.1038/s43587-024-00575-6.

Suda, M., Shimizu, I., Katsuumi, G. et al. Senolytic vaccination improves normal and pathological age-related phenotypes and increases lifespan in progeroid mice. Nat Aging (2021). https://doi.org/10.1038/s43587-021-00151-2

Suh, J., Lee, YS. Mitochondria as secretory organelles and therapeutic cargos. Exp Mol Med 56, 66–85 (2024). https://doi.org/10.1038/s12276-023-01141-722.

Sun L. Recent advances in the development of AHR antagonists in immuno-oncology. RSC Med Chem. 2021 Apr 6;12(6):902-914. doi: 10.1039/d1md00015b. PMID: 34223158; PMCID: PMC8221258.

Sung K, McCain J, King KR, Hong K, Aisagbonhi O, Adler ED, Urey MA. Biopsy-Proven Giant Cell Myocarditis Following the COVID-19 Vaccine. Circ Heart Fail. 2022 Apr;15(4):e009321. doi: 10.1161/CIRCHEARTFAILURE.121.009321.

Sung KY, Zhang B, Wang HE, Bai YM, Tsai SJ, Su TP, Chen TJ, Hou MC, Lu CL, Wang YP, Chen MH. Schizophrenia and risk of new-onset inflammatory bowel disease: a nationwide longitudinal study. Aliment Pharmacol Ther. 2022 May;55(9):1192-1201. doi: 10.1111/apt.16856.

Sung KY, Zhang B, Wang HE, Bai YM, Tsai SJ, Su TP, Chen TJ, Hou MC, Lu CL, Wang YP, Chen MH. Schizophrenia and risk of new-onset inflammatory bowel disease: a nationwide longitudinal study. Aliment Pharmacol Ther. 2022 May;55(9):1192-1201. doi: 10.1111/apt.16856.

Sung, K.; McCain, J.; et al. Biopsy-Proven Giant Cell Myocarditis Following the COVID-19 Vaccine. Circ Heart Fail 2022, 15 (4). https://doi.org/10.1161/CIRCHEARTFAILURE.121.009321.

Suzuki Y, Ishihara H. Difference in the lipid nanoparticle technology employed in three approved siRNA (Patisiran) and mRNA (COVID-19 vaccine) drugs. Drug Metab Pharmacokinet. 2021 Dec;41:100424. doi: 10.1016/j.dmpk.2021.100424.

Syed S, Moore KA, March E. A review of prevalence studies of Autism Spectrum Disorder by latitude and solar irradiance impact. Med Hypotheses. 2017 Nov;109:19-24. doi: 10.1016/j.mehy.2017.09.012.

Szeligowski T, Yun AL, Lennox BR, Burnet PWJ. The Gut Microbiome and Schizophrenia: The Current State of the Field and Clinical Applications. Front Psychiatry. 2020 Mar 12;11:156. doi: 10.3389/fpsyt.2020.00156.

Tabish SA. COVID-19 pandemic: Emerging perspectives and future trends. J Public Health Res. 2020 Jun 4;9(1):1786. doi: 10.4081/jphr.2020.1786.

Takami M, Fujimaki K, Nishimura MI, Iwashima M. Cutting Edge: AhR Is a Molecular Target of Calcitriol in Human T Cells. J Immunol. 2015 Sep 15;195(6):2520-3. doi: 10.4049/jimmunol.1500344. Epub 2015 Aug 14. PMID: 26276877; PMCID: PMC4561210.

Takata N, Mishima T, Hisatsune C, Nagai T, Ebisui E, Mikoshiba K, et al. Astrocyte calcium signaling transforms cholinergic modulation to cortical plasticity in vivo. J Neurosci. 2011 Dec 7;31(49):18155-65. doi: 10.1523/JNEUROSCI.5289-11.2011. Erratum in: J Neurosci. 2012 Aug 29;32(35):12303. PMID: 22159127; PMCID: PMC6634158.

Tam YY, Chen S, Cullis PR. Advances in Lipid Nanoparticles for siRNA Delivery. Pharmaceutics. 2013 Sep 18;5(3):498-507. doi: 10.3390/pharmaceutics5030498. PMID: 24300520; PMCID: PMC3836621.

Tang H, Mourad S, Zhai SD, Hart RJ. Dopamine agonists for preventing ovarian hyperstimulation syndrome. Cochrane Database Syst Rev. 2016 Nov 30;11(11):CD008605. doi: 10.1002/14651858.CD008605.pub3. Update in: Cochrane Database Syst Rev. 2021 Apr 14;4:CD008605.

Tang KY, Lickliter J, Huang ZH, Xian ZS, Chen HY, Huang C, Xiao C, Wang YP, Tan Y, Xu LF, Huang YL, Yan XQ. Safety, pharmacokinetics, and biomarkers of F-652, a recombinant human interleukin-22 dimer, in healthy subjects. Cell Mol Immunol. 2019 May;16(5):473-482. doi: 10.1038/s41423-018-0029-8.

Tang M, Hu X, Wang Y, Yao X, Zhang W, Yu C, et al. Ivermectin, a potential anticancer drug derived from an antiparasitic drug. Pharmacol Res. 2021 Jan;163:105207. doi: 10.1016/j.phrs.2020.105207. Epub 2020 Sep 21. PMID: 32971268; PMCID: PMC7505114.

Tarantino N, Leboyer M, Bouleau A, Hamdani N, Richard JR, Boukouaci W, Ching-Lien W, et al. Natural killer cells in first-episode psychosis: an innate immune signature? Mol Psychiatry. 2021 Sep;26(9):5297-5306. doi: 10.1038/s41380-020-01008-7.

Tarantino N, Leboyer M, Bouleau A, Hamdani N, Richard JR, Boukouaci W, Ching-Lien W, Godin O, Bengoufa D, Le

Corvoisier P, Barau C, Ledudal K, Debré P, Tamouza R, Vieillard V. Natural killer cells in first-episode psychosis: an innate immune signature? Mol Psychiatry. 2021 Sep;26(9):5297-5306. doi: 10.1038/s41380-020-01008-7.

Taubert J, Wardle SG, Ungerleider LG. What does a "face cell" want?'. Prog Neurobiol. 2020 Dec;195:101880. doi: 10.1016/j.pneurobio.2020.101880.

Taylor BV, Lucas RM, Dear K, Kilpatrick TJ, Pender MP, van der Mei IA, Chapman C, Coulthard A, Dwyer T, McMichael AJ, Valery PC, Williams D, Ponsonby AL. Latitudinal variation in incidence and type of first central nervous system demyelinating events. Mult Scler. 2010 Apr;16(4):398-405. doi: 10.1177/1352458509359724.

Teo, S.L.Y., Rennick, J.J., Yuen, D. et al. Unravelling cytosolic delivery of cell penetrating peptides with a quantitative endosomal escape assay. Nat Commun 12, 3721 (2021). https://doi.org/10.1038/s41467-021-23997-x

Terbeck S, Kahane G, McTavish S, McCutcheon R, Hewstone M, Savulescu J, Chesterman LP, Cowen PJ, Norbury R. β- Adrenoceptor blockade modulates fusiform gyrus activity to black versus white faces. Psychopharmacology (Berl). 2015 Aug;232(16):2951-8. doi: 10.1007/s00213-015-3929-7.

Theuerkauf SA, Michels A, Riechert V, Maier TJ, Flory E, Cichutek K, Buchholz CJ. Quantitative assays reveal cell fusion at minimal levels of SARS-CoV-2 spike protein and fusion from without. iScience. 2021 Mar 19;24(3):102170. doi: 10.1016/j.isci.2021.102170.

Thomas, Jaya Mary; Varkey, Joyamma; Augustine, Bibin Baby. Association between serum cholesterol, brain serotonin, and anxiety: A study in simvastatin administered experimental animals. International Journal of Nutrition, Pharmacology, Neurological Diseases 4(1):p 69-73, Jan–Mar 2014. | DOI: 10.4103/2231-0738.124617

Tischkau SA. Mechanisms of circadian clock interactions with aryl hydrocarbon receptor signalling. Eur J Neurosci. 2020 Jan;51(1):379-395. doi: 10.1111/ejn.14361.

Tonelli LH, Stiller J, Rujescu D, Giegling I, Schneider B, Maurer K,Schnabel A, Möller HJ, Chen HH, Postolache TT. Elevated cytokine expression in the orbitofrontal cortex of victims of suicide. ActaPsychiatr Scand. 2008 Mar;117(3):198-206. doi: 10.1111/j.1600-0447.2007.01128.x.

Tonelli LH, Stiller J, Rujescu D, Giegling I, Schneider B, Maurer K, Schnabel A, Möller HJ, Chen HH, Postolache TT. Elevated cytokine expression in the orbitofrontal cortex of victims of suicide. Acta Psychiatr Scand. 2008 Mar;117(3):198-206. doi: 10.1111/j.1600-0447.2007.01128.x.

Tost H, Meyer-Lindenberg A. I fear for you: a role for serotonin in moral behavior. Proc Natl Acad Sci U S A. 2010 Oct 5;107(40):17071-2. doi: 10.1073/pnas.1012545107.

Traina G. Mast Cells in Gut and Brain and Their Potential Role as an Emerging Therapeutic Target for Neural Diseases. Front Cell Neurosci. 2019 Jul 30;13:345. doi: 10.3389/fncel.2019.00345.

Tripathi, A., Bartosh, A., Whitehead, C. et al. Activation of cell-free mtDNA-TLR9 signaling mediates chronic stress-induced social behavior deficits. Mol Psychiatry 28, 3806–3815 (2023). https://doi.org/10.1038/s41380-023-02189-76.

Trumpff C, Marsland AL, Basualto-Alarcón C, Martin JL, Carroll JE, Sturm G, Vincent AE, Mosharov EV, Gu Z, Kaufman BA, Picard M. Acute psychological stress increases serum circulating cell-free mitochondrial DNA. Psychoneuroendocrinology. 2019 Aug;106:268-276. doi: 10.1016/j.psyneuen.2019.03.026.

Tsai RM, Miller Z, Koestler M, Rojas JC, Ljubenkov PA, Rosen HJ, et al. Reactions to Multiple Ascending Doses of the Microtubule Stabilizer TPI-287 in Patients With Alzheimer Disease, Progressive Supranuclear Palsy, and Corticobasal Syndrome: A Randomized Clinical Trial. JAMA Neurol. 2020 Feb 1;77(2):215-224. doi: 10.1001/jamaneurol.2019.3812. PMID: 31710340; PMCID: PMC6865783.

Tsantani M, Gray KLH, Cook R. New evidence of impaired expression recognition in developmental prosopagnosia. Cortex. 2022 Sep;154:15-26. doi: 10.1016/j.cortex.2022.05.008.

Uchiyama, K., Takagi, T., Mizushima, K. et al. Increased mucosal IL-12 expression is associated with relapse of ulcerative colitis. BMC Gastroenterol 21, 122 (2021). https://doi.org/10.1186/s12876-021-01709-5

Üçok, A.; Polat, A.; Çakır, S.; Genç, A. One year outcome in first episode schizophrenia: Predictors of relapse. Eur. Arch. Psychiatry Clin. Neurosci. 2005, 256, 37–43. [

ur Rehman Z, Hoekstra D, Zuhorn IS. Mechanism of polyplex- and lipoplex-mediated delivery of nucleic acids: real-time visualization of transient membrane destabilization without endosomal lysis. ACS Nano. 2013 May 28;7(5):3767-77. doi: 10.1021/nn3049494.

Urits I, Swanson D, Swett MC, Patel A, Berardino K, Amgalan A, Berger AA, Kassem H, Kaye AD, Viswanath O. A Review of Patisiran (ONPATTRO®) for the Treatment of Polyneuropathy in People with Hereditary Transthyretin Amyloidosis. Neurol Ther. 2020 Dec;9(2):301-315. doi: 10.1007/s40120-020-00208-1. Epub 2020 Aug 12. Erratum in: Neurol Ther. 2021 Jun;10(1):407. PMID: 32785879; PMCID: PMC7606409.

Vafadar A, Shabaninejad Z, Movahedpour A, et al. Quercetin and cancer: new insights into its therapeutic effects on ovarian cancer cells. Cell Biosci. 2020;10:32. Published 2020 Mar 10. doi:10.1186/s13578-020-00397-0

Van Gool WA , Weinstein HC , Scheltens P , et al . Effect of hydroxychloroquine on the progression of dementia in early Alzheimer's disease: an 18-month randomised, double-blind, placebo-controlled study. Lancet 2001;358:455–60.doi:10.1016/S0140-6736(01)05623-9

Vance TDR, Lee JE. Virus and eukaryote fusogen superfamilies. Curr Biol. 2020 Jul 6;30(13):R750-R754. doi:

10.1016/j.cub.2020.05.029. PMID: 32634411; PMCID: PMC7336913.

Vangoitsenhoven R, Cresci GAM. Role of Microbiome and Antibiotics in Autoimmune Diseases. Nutr Clin Pract. 2020 Jun;35(3):406-416. doi: 10.1002/ncp.10489. Epub 2020 Apr 22. PMID: 32319703.

Vargas DY, Raj A, Marras SA, Kramer FR, Tyagi S. Mechanism of mRNA transport in the nucleus. Proc Natl Acad Sci U S A. 2005 Nov 22;102(47):17008-13. doi: 10.1073/pnas.0505580102.

Varidaki A, Hong Y, Coffey ET. Repositioning Microtubule Stabilizing Drugs for Brain Disorders. Front Cell Neurosci. 2018 Aug 8;12:226. doi: 10.3389/fncel.2018.00226. PMID: 30135644; PMCID: PMC6092511.

Vauzour D. Dietary polyphenols as modulators of brain functions: biological actions and molecular mechanisms underpinning their beneficial effects. Oxid Med Cell Longev. 2012;2012:914273.

Vendemia JMC, Caine KE, Evans JR. Quantitative EEG Findings in Convicted Murderers (2005), Vol 9 No 3. DOI: https://doi.org/10.1300/J184v09n03_02

Venkatasubramanian G. Understanding schizophrenia as a disorder of consciousness: biological correlates and translational implications from quantum theory perspectives. Clin Psychopharmacol Neurosci. 2015 Apr 30;13(1):36-47. doi: 10.9758/cpn.2015.13.1.36.

Verma N, Mudge JD, Kasole M, Chen RC, Blanz SL, Trevathan JK, Lovett EG, Williams JC, Ludwig KA. Auricular Vagus Neuromodulation-A Systematic Review on Quality of Evidence and Clinical Effects. Front Neurosci. 2021 Apr 30;15:664740. doi: 10.3389/fnins.2021.664740. PMID: 33994937; PMCID: PMC8120162.

Viel T, Chinta S, Rane A, Chamoli M, Buck H, Andersen J. Microdose lithium reduces cellular senescence in human astrocytes - a potential pharmacotherapy for COVID-19? Aging (Albany, NY). 2020 Jun 13;12(11):10035-10040. doi: 10.18632/aging.103449. Epub 2020 Jun 13. PMID: 32534451; PMCID: PMC7346079

Vik-Mo AO, Fernø J, Skrede S, Steen VM. Psychotropic drugs up-regulate the expression of cholesterol transport proteins including ApoE in cultured human CNS- and liver cells. BMC Pharmacol. 2009 Aug 29;9:10. doi: 10.1186/1471-2210-9-10.

Villani A, Peri F. Microglia: Picky Brain Eaters. Dev Cell. 2019 Jan 7;48(1):3-4. doi: 10.1016/j.devcel.2018.12.013. PMID: 30620901.

Villemure E, Volgraf M, Jiang Y, Wu G, Ly CQ, Yuen PW, Lu A, Luo X, Liu M, Zhang S, Lupardus PJ, Wallweber HJ, Liederer BM, Deshmukh G, Plise E, Tay S, Wang TM, Hanson JE, Hackos DH, Scearce-Levie K, Schwarz JB, Sellers BD. GluN2A-Selective Pyridopyrimidinone Series of NMDAR Positive Allosteric Modulators with an Improved in Vivo Profile. ACS Med Chem Lett. 2016 Oct 31;8(1):84-89. doi: 10.1021/acsmedchemlett.6b00388.

Vivier E, Artis D, Colonna M, Diefenbach A, Di Santo JP, Eberl G, et al. Innate Lymphoid Cells: 10 Years On. Cell. 2018 Aug 23;174(5):1054-1066. doi: 10.1016/j.cell.2018.07.017.

Voronova O, Zhuravkov S, Korotkova E, Artamonov A, Plotnikov E. Antioxidant Properties of New Phenothiazine Derivatives. Antioxidants (Basel). 2022 Jul 14;11(7):1371. doi: 10.3390/antiox11071371.

Vucicevic L, Misirkic-Marjanovic M, Harhaji-Trajkovic L, Maric N, Trajkovic V. Mechanisms and therapeutic significance of autophagy modulation by antipsychotic drugs. Cell Stress. 2018 Oct 25;2(11):282-291. doi: 10.15698/cst2018.11.161. PMID: 31225453; PMCID: PMC6551804

Wallet, C.; De Rovere, M.; et al. Microglial Cells: The Main HIV-1 Reservoir in the Brain. Front Cell Infect Microbiol 2019, 9. https://doi.org/10.3389/fcimb.2019.00362.

Wang C, Zhang T, He L, Fu JY, Deng HX, Xue XL, Chen BT. Bacterial Translocation Associates With Aggression in Schizophrenia Inpatients. Front Syst Neurosci. 2021 Sep 29;15:704069. doi: 10.3389/fnsys.2021.704069.

Wang C, Zhang T, He L, Fu JY, Deng HX, Xue XL, Chen BT. Bacterial Translocation Associates With Aggression in Schizophrenia Inpatients. Front Syst Neurosci. 2021 Sep 29;15:704069. doi: 10.3389/fnsys.2021.704069.

Wang DF, Cao B, Xu MY, Liu YQ, Yan LL, Liu R, Wang JY, Lu QB. Meta-Analyses of Manganese Superoxide

Dismutase Activity, Gene Ala-9Val Polymorphism, and the Risk of Schizophrenia. Medicine (Baltimore). 2015 Sep;94(36):e1507. doi: 10.1097/MD.0000000000001507.

Wang LH, Rothberg KG, Anderson RG. Mis-assembly of clathrin lattices on endosomes reveals a regulatory switch for coated pit formation. J Cell Biol. 1993;123:1107–1117.

Wang Y, Ni J, Gao C, Xie L, Zhai L, Cui G, Yin X. Mitochondrial transplantation attenuates lipopolysaccharide- induced depression-like behaviors. Prog Neuropsychopharmacol Biol Psychiatry. 2019 Jul 13;93:240-249. doi: 10.1016/j.pnpbp.2019.04.010.

Wang Y, Ni J, Gao T, Gao C, Guo L, Yin X. Activation of astrocytic sigma-1 receptor exerts antidepressant-like effect via facilitating CD38-driven mitochondria transfer. Glia. 2020 Nov;68(11):2415-2426. doi: 10.1002/glia.23850.

Wang Y, Yu L, Zhou H, Zhou Z, Zhu H, Li Y, Zheng Z, Li X, Dong C. Serologic and molecular characteristics of hepatitis B virus infection in vaccinated schizophrenia patients in China. J Infect Dev Ctries. 2016 Apr 28;10(4):427-31. doi: 10.3855/jidc.7377. PMID: 27131009.

Warner, R. Recovery from Schizophrenia Psychiatry and Political Economy, 3rd ed.; Brunner-Routledge: Hove, UK; New York, NY, USA, 1997; p. 74

Watanabe M, Funahashi T, Suzuki T, Nomura S, Nakazawa T, Noguchi T, Tsukada Y. Antithymic antibodies in schizophrenic sera. Biol Psychiatry. 1982 Jun;17(6):699-710. PMID: 6125218.

Weber A, Prokazov Y, Zuschratter W, Hauser MJ. Desynchronisation of glycolytic oscillations in yeast cell populations. PLoS One. 2012;7(9):e43276. doi: 10.1371/journal.pone.0043276

Weber, N.S.; Gressitt, K.L.; Cowan, D.N.; Niebuhr, D.W.; Yolken, R.H.; Severance, E.G. Monocyte activation detected prior to a diagnosis of schizophrenia in the US Military New Onset Psychosis Project (MNOPP). Schizophr. Res. 2018, 197, 465–469

Wegrzyn M, Garlichs A, Heß RWK, Woermann FG, Labudda K. The hidden identity of faces: a case of lifelong prosopagnosia. BMC Psychol. 2019 Jan 22;7(1):4. doi: 10.1186/s40359-019-0278-z

Wei L, Yang X, Wang J, Wang Z, Wang Q, Ding Y, Yu A. H3K18 lactylation of senescent microglia potentiates brain aging and Alzheimer's disease through the NFκB signaling pathway. J Neuroinflammation. 2023 Sep 11;20(1):208. doi: 10.1186/s12974-023-02879-7

Wei, Jiao, and Ai-Min Hui. "The paradigm shift in treatment from Covid-19 to oncology with mRNA vaccines." Cancer Treatment Reviews (2022): 102405.

Weiland A, Wang Y, Wu W, Lan X, Han X, Li Q, Wang J. Ferroptosis and Its Role in Diverse Brain Diseases. Mol Neurobiol. 2019 Jul;56(7):4880-4893. doi: 10.1007/s12035-018-1403-3.

Weiss A, Touret F, Baronti C, et al. Niclosamide shows strong antiviral activity in a human airway model of SARS-

CoV-2 infection and a conserved potency against the Alpha (B.1.1.7), Beta (B.1.351) and Delta variant (B.1.617.2). PLoS One. 2021;16(12):e0260958. Published 2021 Dec 2. doi:10.1371/journal.pone.0260958

Wen X, Zhou X, Guo L. Berberine Inhibits Endothelial Cell Proliferation via Repressing ERK1/2 Pathway. Natural Product Communications. 2023;18(3). doi:10.1177/1934578X231152690

Westfall S, Dinh DM, Pasinetti GM. Investigation of Potential Brain Microbiome in Alzheimer's Disease: Implications of Study Bias. J Alzheimers Dis. 2020;75(2):559-570. doi: 10.3233/JAD-191328. PMID: 32310171.

Whiteley, C.M. (2021). Depression as a Disorder of Consciousness. The British Journal for the Philosophy of Science.

Whitlock JM, Chernomordik LV. Flagging fusion: Phosphatidylserine signaling in cell-cell fusion. J Biol Chem. 2021;296:100411. doi:10.1016/j.jbc.2021.100411

Wilson KE, Demyanovich H, Rubin LH, Wehring HJ, Kilday C, Kelly DL. Relationship of Interferon-γ to Cognitive Function in Midlife Women with Schizophrenia. Psychiatr Q. 2018 Dec;89(4):937-946. doi: 10.1007/s11126-018-9591-6

Wiwanitkit V. Psychosis and E. coli Infection: A Forgotten Issue. Indian J Psychol Med. 2012 Oct;34(4):407-8. doi: 10.4103/0253-7176.108241.

Wojnilowicz M, Glab A, Bertucci A, Caruso F, Cavalieri F. Super-resolution Imaging of Proton Sponge-Triggered Rupture of Endosomes and Cytosolic Release of Small Interfering RNA. ACS Nano. 2019 Jan 22;13(1):187-202. doi: 10.1021/acsnano.8b05151.

Wood PL, Unfried G, Whitehead W, Phillipps A, Wood JA. Dysfunctional plasmalogen dynamics in the plasma and platelets of patients with schizophrenia. Schizophr Res. 2015 Feb;161(2-3):506-10. doi: 10.1016/j.schres.2014.11.032. Epub 2014 Dec 12. PMID: 25497441.

Wu GWY, Wolkowitz OM, Reus VI, Kang JI, Elnar M, Sarwal R, Flory JD, Abu-Amara D, Hammamieh R, Gautam A, Doyle FJ 3rd, Yehuda R, Marmar CR, Jett M, Mellon SH; SBPBC. Serum brain-derived neurotrophic factor remains elevated after long long-term follow-up of combat veterans with chronic post-traumatic stress disorder. Psychoneuroendocrinology. 2021 Jul 22;134:105360. doi: 10.1016/j.psyneuen.2021.105360. Epub ahead of print. PMID: 34757255.

Wu Z, Li T. Nanoparticle-Mediated Cytoplasmic Delivery of Messenger RNA Vaccines: Challenges and Future Perspectives. Pharm Res. 2021 Mar;38(3):473-478. doi: 10.1007/s11095-021-03015-x

Xia QS, Wu F, Wu WB, Dong H, Huang ZY, Xu L, Lu FE, Gong J. Berberine reduces hepatic ceramide levels to improve insulin resistance in HFD-fed mice by inhibiting HIF-2α. Biomed Pharmacother. 2022 Jun;150:112955. doi: 10.1016/j.biopha.2022.112955.

Xiang J, Tian C, Niu Y, Yan T, Li D, Cao R, Guo H, Cui X, Cui H, Tan S, Wang B. Abnormal Entropy Modulation of the EEG Signal in Patients With Schizophrenia During the Auditory Paired-Stimulus Paradigm. Front Neuroinform. 2019 Feb 19;13:4. doi: 10.3389/fninf.2019.00004. PMID: 30837859; PMCID: PMC6390065.

Xie G, Raufman JP. Role of the Aryl Hydrocarbon Receptor in Colon Neoplasia. Cancers (Basel). 2015 Jul 31;7(3):1436-46. doi: 10.3390/cancers7030847. PMID: 26264025; PMCID: PMC4586780.

Xin M, Jin X, Cui X, Jin C, Piao L, Wan Y, Xu S, Zhang S, Yue X, Wang H, Nan Y, Cheng X. Dipeptidyl peptidase-4 inhibition prevents vascular aging in mice under chronic stress: Modulation of oxidative stress and inflammation. Chem Biol Interact. 2019 Dec 1;314:108842. doi: 10.1016/j.cbi.2019.108842.

Xiong Q, Tang F, Li Y, Xie F, Yuan L, Yao C, et al. Association of inflammatory bowel disease with suicidal ideation, suicide attempts, and suicide: A systematic review and meta-analysis. J Psychosom Res. 2022 Sep;160:110983. doi: 10.1016/j.jpsychores.2022.110983.

Xu J, Shi PY, Li H, Zhou J. Broad Spectrum Antiviral Agent Niclosamide and Its Therapeutic Potential. ACS Infect Dis. 2020 May 8;6(5):909-915. doi: 10.1021/acsinfecdis.0c00052. Epub 2020 Mar 10. PMID: 32125140; PMCID: PMC7098069.

Xue R, Zhang H, Pan J, Du Z, Zhou W, Zhang Z, Tian Z, Zhou R, Bai L. Peripheral Dopamine Controlled by Gut

Microbes Inhibits Invariant Natural Killer T Cell-Mediated Hepatitis. Front Immunol. 2018 Oct 17;9:2398. doi: 10.3389/fimmu.2018.02398.

Yadav M, Parle M, Jindal DK, Sharma N. Potential effect of spermidine on GABA, dopamine, acetylcholinesterase, oxidative stress and proinflammatory cytokines to diminish ketamine-induced psychotic symptoms in rats. Biomed Pharmacother. 2018 Feb;98:207-213. doi: 10.1016/j.biopha.2017.12.016.

Yamagishi M, Shirasaki Y, Funatsu T. Single-molecule tracking of mRNA in living cells. Methods Mol Biol. 2013;950:153-67. doi: 10.1007/978-1-62703-137-0_10. PMID: 23086875.

Yamamoto M, Gohda J, Kobayashi A, Tomita K, Hirayama Y, Naohiko Koshikawa, et al. Metalloproteinase-Dependent and TMPRSS2-Independent Cell Surface Entry Pathway of SARS-CoV-2 Requires the Furin Cleavage Site and the S2 Domain of Spike Protein. ASM Journal (2022). DOI: https://doi.org/10.1128/mbio.00519-22

Yamauchi Y, Greber UF. Principles of Virus Uncoating: Cues and the Snooker Ball. Traffic. 2016 Jun;17(6):569-92. doi: 10.1111/tra.12387.

Yan J, Liu W, Cai J, Wang Y, Li D, Hua H, Cao H. Advances in Phenazines over the Past Decade: Review of Their Pharmacological Activities, Mechanisms of Action, Biosynthetic Pathways and Synthetic Strategies. Mar Drugs. 2021 Oct 27;19(11):610. doi: 10.3390/md19110610. PMID: 34822481; PMCID: PMC8620606.

Yang J, Shen MH. Polyethylene glycol-mediated cell fusion. Methods Mol Biol. 2006;325:59-66. doi: 10.1385/1-59745-005-7:59. PMID: 16761719.

Yang X, Yang W, McVey DG, Zhao G, Hu J, Poston RN, Ren M, Willeit K, Coassin S, Willeit J, Webb TR, Samani NJ, Mayr M, Kiechl S, Ye S. FURIN Expression in Vascular Endothelial Cells Is Modulated by a Coronary Artery Disease-Associated Genetic Variant and Influences Monocyte Transendothelial Migration. J Am Heart Assoc. 2020 Feb 18;9(4):e014333. doi: 10.1161/JAHA.119.014333.

Yang Y, He M, Tian X, Guo Y, Liu F, Li Y, et al. Transgenic overexpression of furin increases epileptic susceptibility. Cell Death Dis. 2018;9(11):1058. doi: 10.1038/s41419-018-1076-x.

Yang, X.; Zhao, C.; Chen, X.; Jiang, L.; Su, X. Monocytes primed with GTS-21/α7 nAChR (nicotinic acetylcholine receptor) agonist develop anti-inflammatory memory. QJM Int. J. Med. 2017, 110, 437–445

Yanuck SF. Microglial Phagocytosis of Neurons: Diminishing Neuronal Loss in Traumatic, Infectious, Inflammatory, and Autoimmune CNS Disorders. Front Psychiatry. 2019 Oct 3;10:712. doi: 10.3389/fpsyt.2019.00712.

Yao BC, Meng LB, Hao ML, Zhang YM, Gong T, Guo ZG. Chronic stress: a critical risk factor for atherosclerosis. J Int Med Res. 2019 Apr;47(4):1429-1440. doi: 10.1177/0300060519826820.

Yenilmez C, Ozdemir Koroglu Z, Kurt H, Yanas M, Colak E, Degirmenci I, Gunes HV. A study of the possible association of plasminogen activator inhibitor type 1 4G/5G insertion/deletion polymorphism with susceptibility to schizophrenia and in its subtypes. J Clin Pharm Ther. 2017 Feb;42(1):103-107. doi: 10.1111/jcpt.12470.

Yeung, S.SH., Ho, YS. & Chang, R.CC. The role of meningeal populations of type II innate lymphoid cells in modulating neuroinflammation in neurodegenerative diseases. Exp Mol Med 53, 1251–1267 (2021). https://doi.org/10.1038/s12276-021-00660-5

Yin H, Pantazatos SP, Galfalvy H, Huang YY, Rosoklija GB, Dwork AJ, Burke A, Arango V, Oquendo MA, Mann JJ. A pilot integrative genomics study of GABA and glutamate neurotransmitter systems in suicide, suicidal behavior, and major depressive disorder. Am J Med Genet B Neuropsychiatr Genet. 2016 Apr;171B(3):414-426. doi: 10.1002/ajmg.b.32423.63.

Yoon, J.H.; Seo, Y.; Jo, Y.S.; Lee, S.; Cho, E.; Cazenave-Gassiot, A.; Shin, Y.S.; Moon, M.H.; An, H.J.; Wenk, M.R.; et al. Brainlipidomics: From functional landscape to clinical significance. Sci. Adv. 2022, 8, eadc9317. [CrossRef]

Yoshida S, Nakagami H, Hayashi H, Ikeda Y, Sun J, Tenma A, et al. The CD153 vaccine is a senotherapeutic option for preventing the accumulation of senescent T cells in mice. Nat Commun. 2020 May 18;11(1):2482. doi: 10.1038/s41467-020-16347-w. PMID: 32424156; PMCID: PMC7235045.

Yousefzadeh MJ et al. Tissue specificity of senescent cell accumulation during physiologic and accelerated aging of mice. Aging Cell 19, e13094 (2020). 10.1111/acel.13094

Youssef JG, Zahiruddin F, Youssef G, et al. G6PD deficiency and severity of COVID-19 pneumonia and acute respiratory distress syndrome: tip of the iceberg? Ann Hematol. 2021;100(3):667-673. doi:10.1007/s00277-021-04395-1

Yovel G, Sirota P, Mazeh D, Shakhar G, Rosenne E, Ben-Eliyahu S. Higher natural killer cell activity in schizophrenic patients: the impact of serum factors, medication, and smoking. Brain Behav Immun. 2000 Sep;14(3):153-69. doi: 10.1006/brbi.1999.0574. PMID: 10970677.

Yu CD, Xu QJ, Chang RB. Vagal sensory neurons and gut-brain signaling. Curr Opin Neurobiol. 2020 Jun;62:133-140. doi: 10.1016/j.conb.2020.03.006.

Yuan L, Zhang F, Shen M, Jia S, Xie J. Phytosterols Suppress Phagocytosis and Inhibit Inflammatory Mediators via ERK Pathway on LPS-Triggered Inflammatory Responses in RAW264.7 Macrophages and the Correlation with Their Structure. Foods. 2019 Nov 16;8(11):582. doi: 10.3390/foods8110582.

Zaiatz Bittencourt V, Jones F, Tosetto M, Doherty GA, Ryan EJ. Dysregulation of Metabolic Pathways in Circulating Natural Killer Cells Isolated from Inflammatory Bowel Disease Patients. J Crohns Colitis. 2021 Aug 2;15(8):1316-1325. doi: 10.1093/ecco-jcc/jjab014. PMID: 33460436;

Zaliunaite V, Steibliene V, Bode L, Podlipskyte A, Bunevicius R, Ludwig H. Primary psychosis and Borna disease virus infection in Lithuania: a case-control study. BMC Psychiatry. 2016;16(1):369. Published 2016 Nov 3. doi:10.1186/s12888-016-1087-z.

Zalsman G. Genetics of Suicidal Behavior in Children and Adolescents. In: Dwivedi Y, editor. The Neurobiological Basis of Suicide. Boca Raton (FL): CRC Press/Taylor & Francis; 2012.

Zhang B, Yao Y, Cornec AS, Oukoloff K, James MJ, Koivula P, et al. A brain-penetrant triazolopyrimidine enhances microtubule-stability, reduces axonal dysfunction and decreases tau pathology in a mouse tauopathy model. Mol Neurodegener. 2018 Nov 7;13(1):59. doi: 10.1186/s13024-018-0291-3. PMID: 30404654; PMCID: PMC6223064.

Zhang D, Tang Z, Huang H, Zhou G, Cui C, Weng Y, et al. Metabolic regulation of gene expression by histone lactylation. Nature. 2019;574(7779):575–80.

Zhang H, Han X, Alameh MG, Shepherd SJ, Padilla MS, Xue L, et al. Rational design of anti-inflammatory lipid nanoparticles for mRNA delivery. J Biomed Mater Res A. 2022 May;110(5):1101-1108. doi: 10.1002/jbm.a.37356.

Zhang L, Richards A, Barrasa MI, Hughes SH, Young RA, Jaenisch R. Reverse-transcribed SARS-CoV-2 RNA can integrate into the genome of cultured human cells and can be expressed in patient-derived tissues. Proc Natl Acad Sci U S

A. 2021 May 25;118(21):e2105968118. doi: 10.1073/pnas.2105968118.

Zhang L, Sander JW, Zhang L, Jiang XY, Wang W, Shuang K, et all. Suicidality is a common and serious feature of anti-N-methyl-D-aspartate receptor encephalitis. J Neurol. 2017Dec;264(12):2378-2386. doi: 10.1007/s00415-017-8626-5.

Zhang S, Xu X, Li Q, Chen J, Liu S, Zhao W, Cai H, Zhu J, Yu Y. Brain Network Topology and Structural-Functional Connectivity Coupling Mediate the Association Between Gut Microbiota and Cognition. Front Neurosci. 2022 Mar 29;16:814477. doi: 10.3389/fnins.2022.814477. PMID: 35422686; PMCID: PMC9002058.

Zhang X, Yao S, Zhu X, Wang X, Zhu X, Zhong M. Gray matter volume abnormalities in individuals with cognitive vulnerability to depression: a voxel-based morphometry study. J Affect Disord. 2012 Feb;136(3):443-52. doi: 10.1016/j.jad.2011.11.005.

Zhang Y, Gao X, Bai X, Yao S, Chang YZ, Gao G. The emerging role of furin in neurodegenerative and neuropsychiatric diseases. Transl Neurodegener. 2022 Aug 23;11(1):39. doi: 10.1186/s40035-022-00313-1.

Zhang Y, Yan R, Zhou Q. ACE2, B0AT1, and SARS-CoV-2 spike protein: Structural and functional implications. Curr Opin Struct Biol. 2022 Jun;74:102388. doi: 10.1016/j.sbi.2022.102388.

Zhang Y, Zhang Z, Luo L, Tong H, Chen F, Hou ST. 40 Hz Light Flicker Alters Human Brain Electroencephalography Microstates and Complexity Implicated in Brain Diseases. Front Neurosci. 2021 Dec 13;15:777183. doi: 10.3389/fnins.2021.777183.

Zhang, M.; Liang, J. Q.; et al. Expressional Activation and Functional Roles of Human Endogenous Retroviruses in Cancers. Rev Med Virol 2019, 29 (2). https://doi.org/10.1002/rmv.2025.

Zhang, X., Lang, Y., Sun, L. et al. Clinical characteristics and prognostic analysis of anti-gamma-aminobutyric acid-B (GABA-B)receptor encephalitis in Northeast China. BMC Neurol 20, 1(2020). https://doi.org/10.1186/s12883-019-1585-y

Zhang, X., Lang, Y., Sun, L. et al. Clinical characteristics and prognostic analysis of anti-gamma-aminobutyric acid-B (GABA-B) receptor encephalitis in Northeast China. BMC Neurol 20, 1 (2020). https://doi.org/10.1186/s12883-019-1585-y

Zhang, X., Norton, J., Carrière, I. et al. Preliminary evidence for a role of the adrenergic nervous system in generalized anxiety disorder. Sci Rep 7, 42676 (2017). https://doi.org/10.1038/srep42676

Zhao X, Li S, Gaur U, Zheng W. Artemisinin Improved Neuronal Functions in Alzheimer's Disease Animal Model 3xtg Mice and Neuronal Cells via Stimulating the ERK/CREB Signaling Pathway. Aging Dis. 2020 Jul

23;11(4):801-819. doi: 10.14336/AD.2019.0813. PMID: 32765947; PMCID: PMC7390534.

Zhao Y, Cong L, Lukiw WJ. Lipopolysaccharide (LPS) Accumulates in Neocortical Neurons of Alzheimer's Disease (AD) Brain and Impairs Transcription in Human Neuronal-Glial Primary Co-cultures. Front Aging Neurosci. 2017 Dec 12;9:407. doi: 10.3389/fnagi.2017.00407.

Zhao YC, Chi YJ, Yu YS, Liu JL, Su RW, Ma XH, Shan CH, Yang ZM. Polyamines are essential in embryo implantation: expression and function of polyamine-related genes in mouse uterus during peri-implantation period. Endocrinology. 2008 May;149(5):2325-32. doi: 10.1210/en.2007-1420.

Zhao, J., Zhu, H., Duan, K. et al. Dysbindin-1 regulates mitochondrial fission and gamma oscillations. Mol Psychiatry 26, 4633–4651 (2021). https://doi.org/10.1038/s41380-021-01038-9

Zhao, W.; Huang, Y.; et al. Dopamine Receptors Modulate Cytotoxicity of Natural Killer Cells via CAMP-PKA-CREB Signaling Pathway. PLoS One 2013, 8 (6), e65860. https://doi.org/10.1371/journal.pone.0065860.

Zhao, Y.; Cong, L.; Lukiw, W.J. Lipopolysaccharide (LPS) Accumulates in Neocortical Neurons of Alzheimer's Disease (AD) Brain and Impairs Transcription in Human Neuronal-Glial Primary Co-cultures. Front. Aging Neurosci. 2017, 9, 407.

Zhao, Y.; Cong, L.; Lukiw, W.J. Lipopolysaccharide (LPS) Accumulates in Neocortical Neurons of Alzheimer's Disease (AD) Brain and Impairs Transcription in Human Neuronal-Glial Primary Co-cultures. Front. Aging Neurosci. 2017, 9, 407.

Zheng L, Wen XL. Gut microbiota and inflammatory bowel disease: The current status and perspectives. World J Clin Cases. 2021 Jan 16;9(2):321-333. doi: 10.12998/wjcc.v9.i2.321. PMID: 33521100

Zhou Z, Zhen J, Karpowich NK, Law CJ, Reith ME, Wang DN. Antidepressant specificity of serotonin transporter suggested by three LeuT-SSRI structures. Nat Struct Mol Biol. 2009 Jun;16(6):652-7. doi: 10.1038/nsmb.1602.

Zhou, C., Ramaswamy, S., Johnson, D. et al. Novel Roles for Peroxynitrite in Angiotensin II and CaMKII Signaling. Sci Rep 6, 23416 (2016). https://doi.org/10.1038/srep23416

Zhu, F., Ju, Y., Wang, W. et al. Metagenome-wide association of gut microbiome features for schizophrenia. Nat Commun 11, 1612 (2020). https://doi.org/10.1038/s41467-020-15457-9

Zhu, F., Ju, Y., Wang, W. et al. Metagenome-wide association of gut microbiome features for schizophrenia. Nat Commun 11, 1612 (2020). https://doi.org/10.1038/s41467-020-15457-9

Zhu, H., Guan, A., Liu, J. et al. Noteworthy perspectives on microglia in neuropsychiatric disorders. J

Neuroinflammation 20, 223 (2023). https://doi.org/10.1186/s12974-023-02901-

Zhu, X.; Zhou, J.; Zhu, Y.; Yan, F.; Han, X.; Tan, Y.; Li, R. Neutrophil/lymphocyte, platelet/lymphocyte and monocyte/lymphocyte ratios in schizophrenia. Australas Psychiatry 2022, 30, 95–99. [Google Scholar] [CrossRef] [PubMed]

Ziegler, D.V., Czarnecka-Herok, J., Vernier, M. et al. Cholesterol biosynthetic pathway induces cellular senescence through ERRα. npj Aging 10, 5 (2024). https://doi.org/10.1038/s41514-023-00128-y

Zmijewski JW, Jope RS. Nuclear accumulation of glycogen synthase kinase-3 during replicative senescence of human fibroblasts. Aging Cell. 2004 Oct;3(5):309-17. doi: 10.1111/j.1474-9728.2004.00117.x. PMID: 15379854; PMCID: PMC1931580.

Żochowska A, Jakuszyk P, Nowicka MM, Nowicka A. Are covered faces eye-catching for us? The impact of masks on attentional processing of self and other faces during the COVID-19 pandemic. Cortex. 2022 Apr;149:173-187. doi: 10.1016/j.cortex.2022.01.015. Epub 2022 Feb 10. PMID: 35257944; PMCID: PMC8830153.

Zomorrodi, R., Loheswaran, G., Pushparaj, A. et al. Pulsed Near Infrared Transcranial and Intranasal Photobiomodulation Significantly Modulates Neural Oscillations: a pilot exploratory sA Pilot Exploratory Study. Sci Rep 9, 6309 (2019). https://doi.org/10.1038/s41598-019-42693-x

Zughaibi T.A., Suhail M., Tarique M., Tabrez S. Targeting PI3K/Akt/mTOR Pathway by Different Flavonoids: A Cancer Chemopreventive Approach. Int. J. Mol. Sci. 2021;22:12455. doi: 10.3390/ijms222212455. [PMC free article] [PubMed] [CrossRef] [Google Scholar]

www.ingramcontent.com/pod-product-compliance
Lightning Source LLC
Chambersburg PA
CBHW051130300726

48978CB00011B/222